Global Women's Health

Jürgen Wacker · Camilla Rothe ·
Maryam En-Nosse
Editors

Global Women's Health

Gynecology and Obstetrics Under Diverse Global Conditions

Springer

Editors
Jürgen Wacker
ehemaliger Chefarzt der Frauenklinik Bruchsal
Bruchsal, Germany

Maryam En-Nosse
Oberärztin Klinik für Gynäkologie und Geburtshilfe Universitätsklinikum Gießen und Marburg
Gießen, Germany

Camilla Rothe
Oberärztin Klinikum der LMU München
Medizinische Klinik IV Abteilung für Infektionen und Tropenmedizin
München, Germany

ISBN 978-3-662-69699-6 ISBN 978-3-662-69700-9 (eBook)
https://doi.org/10.1007/978-3-662-69700-9

Translation from the German language edition: "Globale Frauengesundheit" by Jürgen Wacker et al., © Der/die Herausgeber bzw. der/die Autor(en), exklusiv lizenziert an Springer-Verlag GmbH, DE, ein Teil von Springer Nature 2023. Published by Springer Berlin Heidelberg. All Rights Reserved.

This book is a translation of the original German edition "Globale Frauengesundheit" by Jürgen Wacker, published by Springer-Verlag GmbH, DE in 2023. The translation was done with the help of an artificial intelligence machine translation tool. A subsequent human revision was done primarily in terms of content, so that the book will read stylistically differently from a conventional translation. Springer Nature works continuously to further the development of tools for the production of books and on the related technologies to support the authors.

This Springer imprint is published by the registered company Springer-Verlag GmbH, DE, part of Springer Nature.
The registered company address is: Heidelberger Platz 3, 14197 Berlin, Germany

Foreword

The now available, very practical and at the same time scientific book, which was edited by Jürgen Wacker, Camilla Rothe and Maryam En-Nosse with the collaboration of Laeticia Nwaeburu, Eva Kantelhardt and Abdoulaye N'Diaye, is based on the well-known textbook "Obstetrics under simple conditions" also published by Jürgen Wacker, and on the Therapy Manual Gynecology and Obstetrics, which has now appeared in 3 editions, as well as on the manual "Obstetrics unplugged". These books, which have now become standard works, were also an integral part of the basis for the annual conference of the AG Women's Health in Development Cooperation (FIDE), which was successfully organized by Prof. Jürgen Wacker in Bruchsal two years ago, before the SARS-CoV2-related restrictions, where about 200 students, doctors and other related professions in Bruchsal discussed topics such as global women's health, population development, human nutrition and further development of agriculture, family planning, climate change, injuries from childbirth and rape, medical and ethical questions intensively.

The first edition of the book "Global Women's Health" deals with general topics such as population development, climate change, the influence of religions and traditions, Female Genital Mutilation (FGM), the right to self-determined family planning for women, etc., all of which threaten the health of women worldwide.

Using selected concrete examples such as preeclampsia, birth injuries, management of childbirth, breast cancer, etc., the book very competently and in clear language addresses the international guidelines and the different implementation in rich and poor countries. However, the authors of this book are always clearly driven by the insight that modern, Western medicine should not simply be imposed on colleagues in poorer countries of our world, such as Africa.

Colleague Jürgen Wacker, as a former development aid worker, has certainly gained experience through his decades of commitment, for example as the head of a hospital in Burkina Faso from 1986–1988, that we as German doctors have learned a lot through our work in poorer countries, for example in Africa, which we can then apply in Germany in obstetrics, but also in palliative medicine and the treatment of patients with cancer.

The prerequisite for this process of mutual learning from each other is the scientific processing of obstetrics under simple conditions, which Jürgen Wacker and his team have convincingly demonstrated, especially with regard to the topic of preeclampsia.

In this context, he quotes the motto: "Help and Learn Overseas" as well as the apt African proverb: "Wisdom is like the trunk of a baobab tree: One person alone cannot encompass it!"

Every day, about 800 women die from preventable causes related to pregnancy and childbirth, approximately 280,000 per year, with about 99% of these deaths occurring in LMICs. In addition, about 10 million women annually suffer life-threatening complications during pregnancy and childbirth, sometimes resulting in lifelong disabilities.

Maternal health is closely linked to a variety of issues such as family planning, migration, and economic growth, and the 2011 Nobel Peace Prize laureate and President of Liberia Ellen Johnson Sirleaf summed this up in the sentence "A Nation thrives when mothers survive—we must strive to keep them alive."

The Millennium Development Goal No. 5 focuses on reducing maternal mortality (MMR) by 75% between 1990 and 2015.

Maternal mortality is an indicator of a society's appreciation for its women, and inequalities based on gender, ethnicity, socioeconomic background, and regional origin can be analyzed for each country.

There was a significant improvement in maternal mortality from 550,000 deaths in 1990 to 280,000 in 2010 due to major international efforts since the Safe Motherhood Initiative in 1987.

The International Federation of Gynecology and Obstetrics, which was founded in Switzerland in 1954 and in which I was able to serve as an Officer and Honorary Treasurer for 6 years, has had a significant influence on this development, e.g. with the following resolutions during this time: Female Genital Mutilation (Montreal 1994), Violence Against Women (Copenhagen 1997), Women's Rights Related to Reproductive and Sexual Health (Washington DC 2000), Women's Sexual and Reproductive Rights—A Social Responsibility for Obstetricians-Gynecologists (Santiago 2003), FIGO Professional and Ethical Responsibilities concerning Sexual and Reproductive Rights (Santiago 2003).

Of the Non-Communicable Diseases, 80% of cardiovascular and diabetes-related deaths and approximately 90% of deaths from chronic obstructive pulmonary diseases occur in Low- and Middle-income countries (LMIC).

200 million women worldwide are affected by Female Genital Mutilation (FGM) with its negative consequences of severe pain, hemorrhage, tetanus, infections, sepsis, infertility, as well as psychological and sexual trauma.

The decline in maternal and infant mortality worldwide in recent years, despite all difficulties and setbacks, shows that the collective effort of individual governments, non-governmental organizations (NGOs), and local teams, promoted by the Sustainable Development Goals (SDGs), has made a visible change and can continue to achieve more.

The book now available from Jürgen Wacker, Camilla Rothe, and Maryam En-Nosse is therefore an important contribution to Maternal/Fetal Health, for which we are very grateful.

Prof. Dr. med. Dr. h.c. mult Wolfgang Holzgreve, MBA
Medical Director and Chairman of the Board of
University Hospital of Bonn

Preface

'Wisdom is like a baobab—no one can embrace it' (African proverb)

The Baobab (Adansonia digitata or Monkey Bread Tree) is one of the characteristic trees of the African savannah. It can live up to 2000 years, and the sprouting of its leaves at the end of the dry season heralds the approaching rainy season.

The Heidelberg psychiatrist and philosopher Karl Jaspers (23.02.1883 to 26.02.1969) once said:

'Nobody has the truth, we are all seeking it!'

The authors of the present book 'Global Women's Health' work in different disciplines and are, so to speak, sitting under a Baobab, the tree of knowledge, to collectively find answers to the questions of global women's health.

Some of the authors of this book have already worked on the textbooks 'Obstetrics under simple conditions', the manual 'Obstetrics unplugged', and the therapy manual 'Gynaecology and Obstetrics', and have collectively contributed to the success of these books. The idea to write a book about Global Women's Health was conceived in February 2020, during the 25th annual conference of the AG Women's Health in Development Cooperation (FIDE), which took place from February 6–9, 2020 in Bruchsal. This 25th FIDE conference, before the lockdown due to the Corona pandemic, brought together about 200 students, doctors, and members of other related professions at the Bruchsal Fürst-Stirum-Clinic and the Bruchsal Citizens' Centre. In numerous lectures and discussion forums, a wide range of topics related to international cooperation were addressed, which found their way into this book. The recipient of the Alternative Nobel Prize, the farmer Yacouba Sawadogo from Ouahigouya in Burkina Faso, impressively described his sustainable commitment to reforesting a forest in the middle of the eroded dry savannah of the Sahel. 'He adopted the regionally common cultivation method 'Zaï'—in which holes for the millet grains are beaten into the ground in weeks of hard work—to plant not only grain, but also many thousands of trees over decades of effort. Initially, he was still vilified as a madman and heretic because he dared to change the quasi-sacrosanct agricultural traditions'.

The findings of modern medicine can only be successfully applied to the preservation of the health of women and men in harmony with and in respect for nature.

What does Global Health mean to us?

Global health is the health of the population in a global context. Global women's health stands for modern gynecology and obstetrics of our time, which collaborates with other disciplines for the benefit of our patients and to maintain the health of women. The implementation of the ideas of Global women's health takes into account the current changes in climate, the consequences of the Corona pandemic, the increasingly difficult conditions of people in poor countries, and the globally observable shortage of food and raw materials.

Global means that we are in constant exchange with colleagues from other continents of our planet Earth, to mutually learn from each other, to better understand diseases and to be able to carry out treatments more successfully. 'Global' is not synonymous with 'totalitarian' and must not be confused with it! We do not intend to export German, European experiences to other regions of our Earth or even to impose them on other people! We have learned a lot for ourselves in the course of our commitment to humanitarian aid. The motto still applies: 'Helping and learning overseas!'

The authors of this book are convinced that mutual understanding and partnership-based mutual assistance are the most important foundations for a peaceful and fair coexistence—worldwide.

Albert Schweitzer summarized this realization in his book 'Reverence for Life' as follows:

'I am life that wants to live, in the midst of life that wants to live!'

What we all need is mutual understanding and mutual learning from each other.

All the authors of this book are inspired by this, and it can be read in all the chapters presented.

Due to current events, we have included the Ukrainian language in our glossary at the end of the book about the most important obstetric terms.

As doctors, scientists, and midwives, we cannot provide 'heavy weapons' to defend against a war of aggression, but instead of weapons, we can offer help and hope for suffering women and men!

Bruchsal, Germany — Jürgen Wacker
Munich, Germany — Camilla Rothe
Freiburg, Germany — Maryam En-Nosse
July 2022

Contents

Contributors

Margret Bauer Frauenklinik, Fürst-Stirum-Klinik Bruchsal, Bruchsal, Germany

Prof. Dr. med. Walter Bruchhausen Sektion Global Health, Institut für Hygiene und Public Health, Universitätsklinikum Bonn, Bonn, Germany

Dr. med. Rosemarie Burian Basel, Schweiz

Bhargavi Chekuri MD Department of Family Medicine, Columbia University, Aurora, USA

Madeleine Da Hebammenschule Saint-Edvige, Ouagadougou, Burkina Faso

Dr. med. Maryam En-Nosse Luisenhospital Aachen, Uniklinik Freiburg, Freiburg, Germany

Dr. Azadeh Farajpour Javazmi betterSoil e. V., Ulm, Germany

Anne Fritz Akademie für Gesundheitsberufe gGmbH, Heidelberg, Germany

Prof. Dr. med. Detlev Ganten Berlin Brandenburgische Akademie der Wissenschaften (BBAW), Berlin, Germany

PhD MD Claudia Hanson Department of Global Public Health, Karolinska Institutet, Stockholm, Sweden

Dr. med. Maria Eleni Hatzipanagiotou Departement of Gynecology and Obstetrics, University Medical Centre Regensburg, Regensburg, Germany

Dr. med. Laura Häusler Mannheim, Germany

Prof. Dr. Ulrich Hemel Weltethos-Institut, Universität Tübingen, Tübingen, Germany

Dr. med. Antje Henke Global & Planetary Health AG, Institut für Med. Epidemiologie, Biometrie u. Informatik, Proflizentrum Gesundheitswissenschaften, Medizinische Fakultät der Martin-Luther-Universität Halle-Wittenberg, Halle, Germany

Ramata Edvige Ilboudo Hebammenschule Saint-Edvige, Ouagadougou, Burkina Faso

Prof. Dr. med. Eva J. Kantelhardt Global & Planetary Health AG; Klinik und Poliklinik für Gynäkologie, Medizinische Fakultät der Martin-Luther-Universität Halle-Wittenberg, Universitätsklinikum Halle (Saale), Halle (Saale), Germany

Anne-Kathrin Klotzsch Hebamme, Bachelor of Science in International Midwifery Studies, Berlin, Germany

Anna Koch Graben-Neudorf, Germany

Diethard Kokoska Bruchsal, Germany

Grace Komuhangi Duisburg, Cham, Germany

Dr. med. Judith Lindert Klinik für Kinderchirurgie der Universität Rostock, Hamburg, Germany

Melanie Marwitz HebaVaria g.e.V., München, Germany

Prof. Dr. med. Michael Marx Heidelberger Institut für Global Health, Universitätsklinikum Heidelberg, Heidelberg, Germany

Dr. med. Abdoulaye N'Diaye Frauenklinik, Hopital Saint Camille, Ouagadougou, Burkina Faso;
Département de gynécologie, Hôpital Saint Camille de Ouagadougou, Centre de Santé Saint Camille, Ouagadougou, Burkina Faso

Dr. med. Laeticia Nwaeburu Klinikum Ingolstadt, Frauenklinik, Ingolstadt, Germany

Dr. med. Michel Odent London, Großbritannien

Dr. Tobias Orthen Forschungsinstitut für anwendungsorientierte Wissensverarbeitung, FAW/n Ulm, Ulm, Germany

Priv. Doz. Dr. med. Camilla Rothe Oberärztin Klinikum der LMU München Med. Klinik IV, Abt. f. Infektions- und Tropenmedizin, München, Germany

Dr. med. Britta Rutert Berlin Brandenburgische Akademie der Wissenschaften (BBAW), Berlin, Germany

MD Ali Saidi Muhimbili National Hospital, Muhimbili University of Health and Allied Health Science (MUHAS), Dar es Salaam, Tanzania

Dr. med. Zoubeida Saidane Frauenklinik der Fürst-Stirum-Klinik Bruchsal, Bruchsal, Germany

Prof. Dr. med. Nicole C. Schmidt Fakultät für Soziale Arbeit, Katholische Stiftungshochschule München (KSH), München, Germany;
Abteilung für Gynäkologie, Universitätsfrauenklinik Genf (HUG), Genf, Schweiz

Cecilia Sorensen PhD MD Mailman School of Public Health, Columbia University, New York, USA

Peggy Seehafer Hamburg, Germany

Natasha Sood MD, MPH, MEd Pennsylvania State University College of Medicine, Columbia University, Hershey, USA

Prof. Dr. Michael Stark c/o Regus (NESA), Unter den Linden, Berlin, Germany

Dr. med. Leonie Ströbele Klinik für Frauenheilkunde und Geburtshilfe, UKGM Standort Gießen, Gießen, Germany

Tobias Vorburg Fachbereich „Früherkennung besonderer Schutzbedarfe und psychischer Erkrankungen", Refugio München, München, Germany

Dr. med. Kees Waaldijk HC Gennep, Niederlande

Prof. Dr. med. Jürgen Wacker ehemaliger Chefarzt der Frauenklinik Bruchsal, Bruchsal, Germany

Dr. Yacouba Zanré Hôpital Schiphra, Ouagadougou, Burkina Faso

1 Introduction to the Topic: Global Justice in the Face of Recolonization in Africa, Climate Change, the Ukraine War, and the Corona Pandemic

Jürgen Wacker

Contents

The following illustration shows the framework and content of our book (Fig. 1.1).

We dedicate this book:
To all women of this world—of every origin, religion, skin color

1.1 Introduction to the Topic

As a former development aid worker of the German Development Service (DED) and head of the Bloc operatoire and the Maternité at the CHR in Dori (Burkina Faso), I regularly read and use the 'One World Calendar' of the Volker

J. Wacker (✉)
ehemaliger Chefarzt der Frauenklinik Bruchsal, Bruchsal, Germany
e-mail: wacker@menschenfuerfrauen.de

J. Wacker et al. (eds.), *Global Women's Health*,
https://doi.org/10.1007/978-3-662-69700-9_1

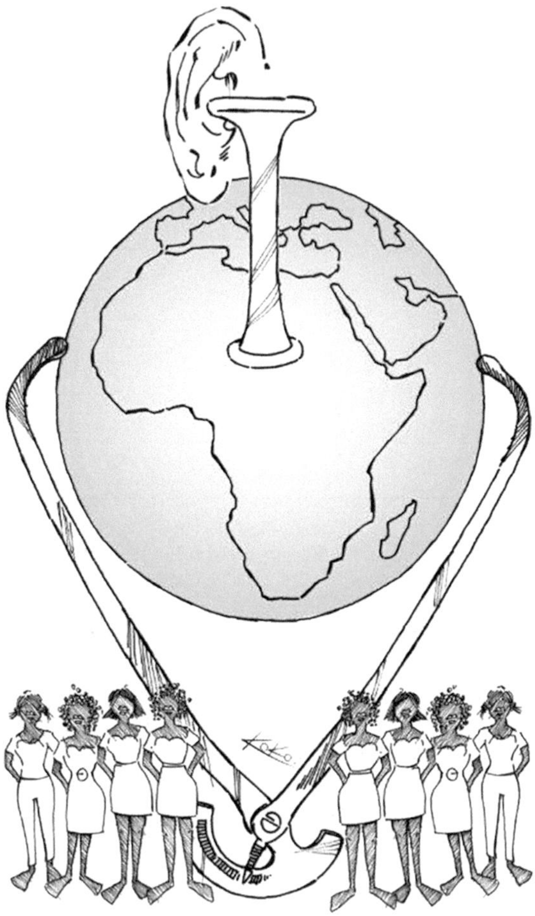

Fig. 1.1 Good listening and accurate measurement are the foundations of global thinking. (© Diethard Kokoska)

Harms publishing house. The 2022 edition features a remarkable article on the ‘Re-colonization of the Sahel’ by Dolly Katiutia Alima Afoumba. Ms. Afoumba holds a master’s degree in history, peace and conflict research. She is currently doing her doctorate at the Philipps University of Marburg in the department of Modern History. Ms. Afoumba writes:

> ‘The Sahel region is often referred to in the media as a powder keg (poudrière), an interesting play on words in two respects: On the one hand, it refers to the enormous amount of weapons and armed actors in the region, and on the other hand, it suggests that any tension in this risk area can quickly turn into a general conflict. However, the powder keg metaphor does not reveal who fills the powder keg and who lights its fuse. The following will explore the hypothesis that behind the hyper-militarization of the Sahel

> lies a campaign of re-colonization, driven by the increasing presence of foreign armies, expanded and consolidated by the subsequent settlement of multinational companies'. (Afoumba 2021)

In January 2022, I received news from former employees of the CHR Dori that in Gorgadji, a small town near Dori, about 30 km away, several terrorists had killed about 60 residents. They proudly reported that the terrorists were also killed by the defenders of Gorgadji.

On 15.01.2016, my surgical mentor, Dr. Ken Elliott, was kidnapped in Djibo (Sahel of Burkina Faso) along with his wife by Islamists. His wife, who suffered from diabetes mellitus, was released by the terrorists shortly afterwards. To this day, the fate of Ken Elliott remains unclear.

Our development servicebetween 1986 and 1988 began shortly after Mali declared war on Burkina Faso on 23.12.1985 because seven small Malian villages in the border area to Burkina Faso were included in a census by Burkinabe officials. The hostilities were stopped after less than two weeks due to a lack of fuel and ammunition on both sides. This so-called Christmas War was already over on 06.01.1986 when we landed in Ouagadougou. Although there was now a curfew from 6 p.m. to 6 a.m. and there were plenty of military checkpoints in the streets of the capital, no more shots were fired, and we were able to start our clinical work in the operating room and the Maternité in Dori.

I have been following the situation in the Sahel of Burkina Faso with great interest and increasing concern for 36 years. What has happened in the meantime, what has changed, that these peace-loving people in the Sahel must be afraid to visit the markets in Bani, Gorom-Gorom, Markoye, Oursi and Sebba to meet friends and relatives there?

We started our service in Burkina Faso with the conviction of doing something meaningful and peace-promoting for the coexistence and cohesion of the population of Burkina Faso, by working as doctors and midwives for the health of the people.

Dolly Afoumba writes about the fight against terrorism: 'As far as the armed deployment is concerned, the G 5 Sahel (Chad, Mali, Niger, Burkina Faso, Mauritania) has committed to forming an African army to combat terrorism. However, this initiative is not supported by the Western powers, according to Afoumba'.

We know that the Bundeswehrhas been stationed in Gao, in Mali, for years with hundreds of soldiers. These soldiers are part of one of the most casualty-heavy peace missions in the recent history of the United Nations. So far, 250 soldiers have been killed in their deployment. In June 2021, 12 German soldiers were seriously injured when a car bomb exploded in their camp. Meanwhile, Russian mercenaries are in Bamako, the capital of Mali, which is still plagued by ongoing coups, corruption, and terror.

In May 2022, the German Bundestag debated the deployment of the German Bundeswehr in Mali. Conflicts like the current ones in Mali and other West African states can always be traced back to the prevailing poverty of the population, their poor medical care, the corruption of the rulers, and the interference of foreign states, which mostly pursue their own interests in Africa's natural resources!

A "pull-out like in Afghanistan in the summer" is not a good example of German support and aid for the people in West Africa! We can, we must not leave the people there alone. We should help them to fight for their interests themselves and to determine their own fate, how they organize their states and elect their governments.

The phrase, 'Politics is medicine on a large scale!' comes from Rudolf Virchow. Virchow sees medicine as a social science, assigning the state the task of serving the health of the people (Fischer and Ganten 2021). In 1848, Virchow founded the Medical Reform and formulated his belief that education, prosperity, and freedom are the guarantees for the health of a nation. Already 64 years earlier, in the first volume of the 'System of a complete medical Policey', which appeared in Mannheim in 1784, the Bruchsal hospital doctor Johann Peter Frankadvocated: '...' "that the state must take responsibility for averting epidemics from large parts of the population by providing adequate living and working conditions, but also by careful (hygienic) handling of our most important food, drinking water (Wacker et al. 2021)."

Virchow and Frank described the situation of the poor population in Germany and some other European countries at their time. Meanwhile, the health situation of most people in Europe has significantly improved.

General globalization and the associated changes have made general health a field of politics. The dimensions in global health policy have shifted, they have become more political (Kickbusch 2013).

We must understand that globalization does not mean that the rich countries recolonize the poor countries, but that we can all only stay healthy and survive if we distribute the resources of our planet Earth more fairly and handle the nature surrounding us more carefully!

Global health is based on the 3 G's: Justice—Community—Common Sense

Our field of gynecology and obstetrics deals with the 3 G's (Wacker and Breitkopf 2008): Giving Birth—Thriving—Recovering

The editors of this book are convinced that these tasks of global women's health can only be accomplished in the future if we 'work interdisciplinary with other disciplines'.

The aim is to maintain the already high standard of curative medicine in the rich countries, but at the same time to build clinics in the poor countries to eliminate the current undersupply in clinical medicine there.

For all disciplines within medicine, it is important that in the future we strengthen not only the promotion of curative medicine but also the outpatient measures for the treatment of chronic diseases and the prevention of avoidable diseases.

1.2 From the Misery of the Poor and the Resource Depository of the Rich to Afrotopia

It is often lamented that poor countries, such as most states on the African continent, show no economic progress despite having received many financial contributions. It is known that many development funds disappear into dark, corruption-ridden black boxes controlled by governments. However, as the example of Burkina Faso (literally translated: Land of the Incorruptible) shows, even countries that have actively fought against prevailing corruption in the past (Thomas Sankara) can hardly, if at all, prosper economically.

Ulricke Herrmann addresses this problem in her article 'Forced into Free Trade': 'As history shows, it can be very sensible to deliberately opt for protectionism. This is especially true for developing countries that want to catch up with the technological gap to the market leaders'. Germany, France, and the USA are prime examples. They too were once developing countries—in the 19th century. At that time, Great Britain was the leading industrial country, while the other Europeans and the USA wanted to catch up with this lead. To protect their own industries against the superior British competition, the USA, for example, increased tariffs to values between 35 and 50% from 1820 until the Second World War. The increased tariffs were only abolished when their own industry belonged to the world market leaders (Herrmann 2019). According to Herrmann, today's developing countries have a much harder time overcoming the technological gap, as the minimum size for a new factory has steadily grown due to technological progress. We need new economic instruments to eliminate this disadvantage of poor countries.

The fact is the exploitationof the resources and nature of the African continent by foreign powers such as China, the USA, and some European countries.

The following caricature on the topic of 'Overfishing of the waters off Africa by foreign fishing fleets' from the One World Calendar of 2022 clearly illustrates this problem (Fig. 1.2).

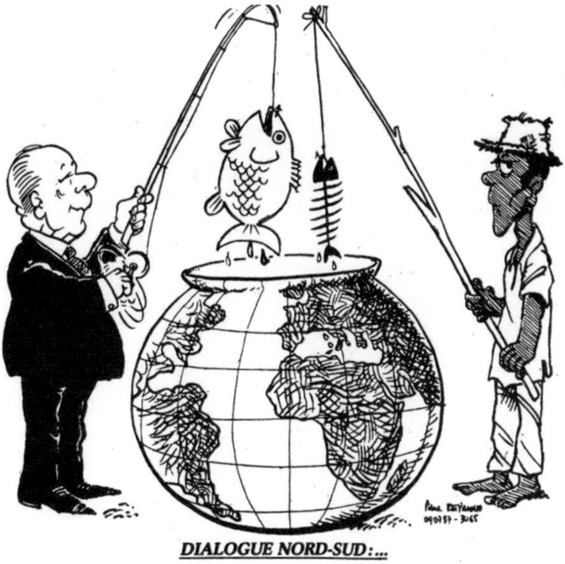

Fig. 1.2 Caricature "Two Fishermen". (With kind permission of Harms Verlag, Kiel)

This exploitation of Africa is unjust, and the conditions in the extraction sites and mines for the people living in the respective region of Africa are inhuman and unbearable! As part of fair cooperation within the framework of global collaboration, new, fairer ways must be found with the participation of the local population to avoid future conflicts.

In his book 'Afrotopia'—Rethinking Africa, the writer and professor of economics Felwine Sarr, born in Niodior, Senegal, writes: 'Considering the entire African continent is a difficult task, as one is confronted with stubborn clichés, stereotypes, and pseudo-certainties that lay like a veil of mist over reality. Since the 1960s and since the dawn of independence, Africa has been incessantly described by the Afro-pessimistic Vulgate as the continent that has made a false start and has been drifting ever since: a dying monster.' Sarr opposes these pessimistic statements with his optimism, his 'Afrotopia': 'Since the wind seems to have turned, a rhetoric of euphoria and optimism has blossomed in recent times. The future will henceforth be African. The continent is making progress in terms of economic growth and the prospects are good. According to economists, Africa will be the next target of international capital, as they can expect higher profits there than anywhere else. Thanks to the availability of natural resources and raw materials, the African continent will be the future El Dorado of world capitalism.'

Together with Felwine Sarr, I am not sure whether this development will help people in the big cities and rural regions of Africa to overcome their poverty.

The following illustration shows three satisfied fishermen, each catching fish off their coasts and not in foreign ponds (Fig. 1.3).

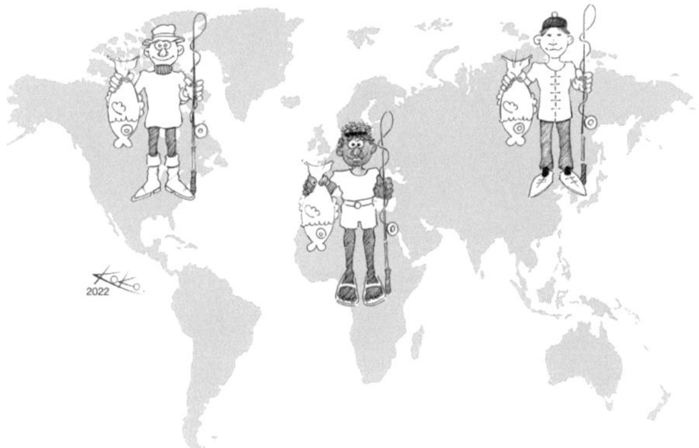

Fig. 1.3 Caricature "Three Satisfied Fishermen". (© Diethard Kokoska)

1.3 History of Development Policy—Decades in Development Cooperation

In order to assess the current state of development cooperation and to learn from old mistakes, let us quote from the overview article by Hubertus Büschel, who divides the time since the beginning of modern German development policy since 1966 into different decades (Büschel 2010):

- First development policy decade (1960–1970): It was assumed that injected capital promotes growth and prosperity ('Trickle-down effect'), i.e., the seepage of capital to the base of the population.
- Second decade (1970–1980): Time of revision. Time of securing basic needs. A basic needs strategy was developed, which recognized the satisfaction of basic needs of the people on the ground as the basis of economic growth.
- Third decade (1980–1990): Many developing countries were almost insolvent at the beginning of the 1980s. The oil crisis of the 1970s, the economic crisis at the beginning of the 1980s, and falling commodity prices led to a sharp increase in the foreign debt of developing countries.
- Fourth decade (1990–2000): Striving for sustainability; this decade was strongly influenced by the Conference on Environment and Development in Rio de Janeiro in 1992, during which Agenda 21 was established. Demand for sustainability and self-help.
- The time after 2000: Period of massive criticism of development cooperation. Several African authors criticize the previous development cooperation. They demand to stop any development aid immediately, because only then would Africans start to take responsibility and solve their economic problems. The Cameroonian Axelle Kabou points out the inevitable power imbalance between 'black elites' and white helpers on the one hand, and the recipients of development aid, the 'little people' on the ground, on the other hand (Kabou 2001).

1.4 Turning Point

Which period in international (development) cooperation is now ahead of us after the pandemic, climate crisis, and war-related turning point?

From now on, we should speak of global health, knowing that we in the North and South of our globe can learn from each other and help each other!

We need to develop ideas together for our common, global survival.

On the current occasion, let me briefly address the current problems that endanger the health of women, men, and children:

1.4.1 War of Aggression in Ukraine

Was this war foreseeable?

On 09.03.2022, in an interview on ARD, Joachim Gauck, the former President of Germany (2012–2017), made the following statement:

> "Yes! We should have recognized the seriousness of the situation as early as 2014 during the occupation of Crimea. Concurrently, possible war scenarios were publicly discussed in numerous talk shows on Russian television. Most European governments and American President Trump did not take these threats and the impending Russian war preparations seriously. In the West, we had become accustomed to ongoing peace and had succumbed to the illusion that this state of peaceful coexistence would last forever. Joachim Gauck knows from personal experience the effects of 'tank socialism' on citizens' freedom when people are spied on, lied to, and threatened in everyday life. We must support the people in Ukraine—ideologically, materially, and, if harsh sanctions against Putin's Russia do not help and the war continues to escalate, also militarily!"

Gauc explains that contrary to the understandable fear that quickly sets in, especially among Germans, a country can emerge strengthened from times of hardship. Helpers help other people, but always also themselves. The people in Ukraine are fighting for their rights, for their lives, but ultimately also for the preservation of our common European values and civil rights! We may have to restrict our current prosperity, freeze rather than sweat, but what does our 'freezing for freedom' mean to the people in Kyiv, Odessa, Mariupol, and the other cities compared to the unbridled killing in Ukraine!

In the issue of the Badische Neuesten Nachrichten (BNN) dated 27.04.2022, there are two headlines on the first page: on the left: Tanks for the Ukraine and on the right: Warning of World War!

We had become accustomed to peace in Europe, even though fighting and dying continue in Syria and Yemen. We had forgotten that we must also actively stand up for the preservation of peace. Passive pacifism cannot prevent wars.

As development aid workers, we saw ourselves as 'active fighters' for the preservation of peace, because we were convinced that if poverty and oppression eventually lead to conflicts and wars, our task is to eliminate these causes of wars and conflicts in a timely, i.e., preventive, manner!

The war of aggression on the Ukraine initiated by Russia has no comprehensible causes.

This war is solely caused by the imperial ambitions of its dictator. It cannot be accepted that women and girls are systematically made victims of sexual violence by the Russian government and that maternity clinics are destroyed by targeted Russian missile attacks!

1.4.2 Consequences of the Corona Pandemic

The author of Chap. 10 (Pandemic), Camilla Roth, goes into great detail about the collateral damage caused by the Corona Pandemic. Therefore, only a small excerpt from this Chap. 10 is found here:

The collateral damage caused by the COVID-19 pandemic is difficult to quantify. However, it is assumed to be considerable. Particularly in African countries, where the pandemic overall seems to have been much less severe than elsewhere, it is assumed that the sometimes drastic lockdown measures have caused greater economic, social, and medical damage than COVID-19 itself.

The pandemic has led to a deterioration in patient care in most countries around the world, due to lockdowns, fear of infection when in contact with medical facilities, blocked hospital beds, overloaded intensive care units, postponement of elective procedures, and staff shortages and reassignments. A German study showed a decrease in the number of inpatient oncology patients by 6% (Griewing et al. 2022). The number of births, on the other hand, increased by 11%. As a result of the local "Stay at home policy", a higher rate of stillbirths and ruptured ectopic pregnancies was reported from Israel. A higher rate of surgical deliveries and postpartum complications was reported from Austria.

The full medical, social, economic, and ecological implications of the pandemic will only be able to be conclusively assessed in a few years' time.

1.4.3 Climate Change

In light of the flood disaster and the devastation in the Ahrtal on 14.07.2021 and the resulting prolonged power outage, I wrote an article, also at the request of the editorial staff of the magazine Die Hebamme, titled "Sustainability in the Delivery Room" (Wacker 2021). In this article, I mentioned examples of obstetric methods and procedures that manage without or at least with less electricity consumption, Obstetrics unplugged (Wacker et al. 2020).

Cecilia Sorensen writes on the topic of climate change in Chap. 4:

The effects of climate change on health, including increased heat stress, poor air quality, extreme weather events, altered transmission of vector-borne diseases, poorer water quality, and reduced food security, affect men and women differently, depending on local cultural, socioeconomic, and physiological factors. Political—often changeable—measures that target these factors can both reduce negative health consequences and improve efforts to adapt to and mitigate climate change. It is urgently necessary to better understand how climate change affects sexual and gender minorities, and to explore more complex multidimensional and non-binary social interfaces that determine communities' responses to climate change.

1.5 Global Women's Health

Global health is the health of the population in a global context.

Global women's health stands for modern gynecology and obstetrics of our time, which collaborates with other disciplines for the benefit of our patients and to maintain the health of women. The implementation of the ideas of Global Women's Healthtakes into account the current changes in the climate, the consequences of the Corona pandemic, the increasingly difficult conditions of people in poor countries, and the globally observable shortage of food and raw materials.

Global means that we are in constant exchange with colleagues from other continents of our planet Earth to learn from each other, to better understand diseases and to be able to carry out treatments more successfully.

Medicine means more than the detection and treatment of diseases!

We are aware of the importance of the patient's family and social environment.

'Global' is not synonymous with 'totalitarian' and must not be confused with it!

We do not intend to export German, European experiences to other regions of our Earth or even to impose them on other people!

Out of reverence for life, Albert Schweitzer formulated:

> I am life that wants to live, in the midst of life that wants to live!

For me—us—this saying still applies today, only that in the view of Global Women's Health 'in the midst' means being surrounded by a globally running field of vision. The horizon of our medical responsibility has expanded!

In a conversation with the economist and author Dolly Katiutia Alima Afoumba, the saying was coined:

> In the North we need less of everything—in the South a little more of everything!

1.6 Addendum after Reviewing the Proof and Visits to Burkina Faso (November 22), Ethiopia (January 23), and Tanzania (February 23)

Burkina Faso in November 2022

On 15.10.22, the assassination of Thomas Sankara marked its 35th anniversary. On October 1, the second coup of the year 2022 took place in Ouagadougou, the capital of Burkina Faso. The new leader of Burkina Faso, Ibrahim Traoré, is 34 years old and already venerates himself as the 'New Thomas Sankara' (Roger 2022). In an interview with journalist Hubert Bado on 7.11.22, on the occasion of the topping-out ceremony of our maternity clinic in Ouagadougou, I was asked how I perceived the political changes introduced by Sankara when I worked as a doctor in the maternity and operating block of the regional hospital in Dori in the north of Burkina Faso from 1986 – 1988 (Bado 2022). Indeed, I still find it right that Sankara motivated his compatriots to become independent of international donors through their own efforts. He aimed for cooperation on an equal footing and rejected the role of the alms recipient. On the front page of the Burkinabe newspaper Sidwaya of November 8, 2022, above the title picture showing Capitaine Traoré with soldiers in the Sahel of Burkina Faso, it reads: **'Lutte contre le terrorisme: Le Capitain Ibrahim Traoré au front'**. One of the quotes from Thomas Sankara in the memorial in Ouagadougou reads: 'Si nous ne nous battons pas pour nous libérer, ils se battront pour nous garder esclaves à vie' (If we do not fight to free ourselves, they will fight to keep us slaves for life).

Addis Ababa in January 23
While we were conducting the topping-out ceremony for our new maternity clinic in Ouagadougou, I was invited to Addis Ababa to visit and evaluate a new cancer clinic (Cancer Competence Center). Indeed, we found in Addis an exemplary cooperation on an equal footing between Ethiopian and German doctors. In a joint session, the new guideline for the diagnosis and therapy of breast cancer was thoroughly and at a high level discussed together. I find the skyline of Addis with its many high-rise buildings of banks, insurance companies, and international administrative buildings impressive. It is noteworthy that these buildings are illuminated all night, and the high facades serve as a screen for many colorful advertising films until the early morning. In the Ethiopian Herald of 18.02.23, the Ethiopian Abbay Dam, which is nearing completion, was described as a good example of economic development ('It is a dam for development') for other African countries (Animut 2023). In conversations with Ethiopian colleagues, the economic importance of the newly founded **African Continental Free Trade Area (AfCFTA)** was pointed out. The main objectives of the agreement are **to increase intra-African trade, further promote industrialization, and build regional value chains. In the long term, the African community of states is aiming for a continental customs union and an African internal market with free movement of goods, services, and people.**

Arusha in Tanzania
During a visit to one of the Maasai villages in Northern Tanzania, we learned about the Maasai relocation program. The Maasai live in Tanzania and neighboring Kenya, with 110,000 in the Ngorongoro Conservation Area. Of these, 80,000 are to be relocated to Eastern Tanzania, as the Maasai and their animals have become too numerous, and the government and international conservation organizations fear that the unique ecosystem in the Ngorongoro Conservation Area could be destroyed (Böhm 2023). The Maasai are resisting and blocked the access to the Ngorongoro Conservation area in the spring of 2022. The question arises: Who determines where and how nature should be preserved? Who has to make way? Does 'untouched wilderness' mean nature without the people who have lived there for centuries?

Conclusion

The examples mentioned show that some African countries have realized that they can help themselves and increasingly need less interference from other foreign states like China, Europe, Russia, and the USA.

Colonialism was the day before yesterday!

Development aid was yesterday!

Partnership-based, economic, and global cooperation on an equal footing, without moralizing prescriptions and while respecting mutual interests, must begin as soon as possible!

References

Afoumba DKA (2021) Rekolonisierung des Sahel aus Wissenschaft und Frieden

Animut A (2023) Abbay Dam: Freeman advises Africans to emulate Ethiopia's Vision. The Ethiopian Herald 18.01.2023 ; No 111

Bado H (2022) Un homme au service de la femme burkinabè Sidwaya – Sociéte & Culture ; 11.11.22.

Böhm A (2023) Sie wollen hier nicht weg; Die ZEIT; N° 6; 2.02.2023

Büschel H (2010) Geschichte der Entwicklungspolitik; Version 1.0 in Docupedia – Zeitgeschichte, 11.02.2010

Fischer EP, Ganten D (2021) Die Idee des Humanen; Rudolf Virchow und Herrmann von Helmholtz. Das Erbe der Charité Hirzel, Stuttgart

Herrmann U (2019) Zum Freihandel gezwungen – Entwicklungsländer müssten jungen Branchen gegen die Konkurrenz der Industrieländer schützen können. In: Atlas der Globalisierung – Welt in Bewegung. Mahlke S (Hrsg). Le Monde diplomatique

Kabou A (2001) Weder arm noch ohnmächtig. Eine Streitschrift gegen schwarze Eliten und weiße Helfer. Basel, Kiel, Deutschland

Kickbusch I (2013) A game change in global health: the best is yet to come. Public Health Rev 35(1):1–20

Roger B (2022) Burkina Faso – La Mission (presque) impossible du Capitaine Traoré. Jeune Afrique N°3118 – Novembre 2022

Wacker J (2021) Nachhaltigkeit im Kreißsaal. Die Hebamme 34:55–61

Wacker J, Breitkopf B (2008) Gebären, Gedeihen und Genesen. Regionalkultur, Ubstadt-Weiher

Wacker J, Baldé MD, Bastert G (2020) Obstetrics unplugged. Regionalkultur, Ubstadt-Weiher

Wacker J, Ebert A, David M (2021) Johann Peter Frank (1745 –1821) zum 200. Todestag: Geburtshilfliche Aspekte im System einer vollständigen medicinischen Polizey. Geburtshilfe Frauenheilkd 81:506–510

Further Reading

Afoumba DKA (2022) Rekolonisierung des Sahel. Eine Welt Kalender. Harms, Arbeitsgemeinschaft für Frienden - und Konfliktforschung (AFK); Hochschule Rhein-Waal; Kleve; Deutschland, S 35–48

Carstens P (2022) Raus aus Mali? FAZ 10.01.2022

Fischer M (2022) Afrika als Spielball der globalen Rohstoffausbeutung. Eine Welt Kalender 2022:27–34

Harms V (2022) Eine Welt Kalender. Harms, Kiel, Deutschland

Sarr F (2019) Afrotopia. Matthes & Seitz, Berlin

Wacker J, Barth A, Harlfinger W, Kantelhardt E, Kunz K, Lange R (2017) Deutsche Gynäkologen in Afrika: Handfeste Taten statt hohler Worte. Frauenarzt 58:970–975

Global Population Development: Feeding People and the Advancement of Agriculture

2

Azadeh Farajpour Javazmi and Tobias Orthen

Contents

Introductory Questions

1. How many people currently live on our Earth and how are they distributed across the respective continents?
   A. A total of about 8 billion, of which 1 billion in Africa
   B. 6 billion, of which 3 billion in Africa
   C. 10 billion, of which 1 billion in Africa
2. What percentage of the world's population is responsible for about half of all greenhouse gas emissions?
   A. 30%
   B. 40%
   C. 10%

A. Farajpour Javazmi
betterSoil e. V., Ulm, Germany
e-mail: azadeh.farajpour@bettersoil.info

T. Orthen (✉)
Research Institute for Applied Knowledge Processing/n, FAW/n Ulm, Ulm, Germany
e-mail: orthen@fawn-ulm.de

J. Wacker et al. (eds.), *Global Women's Health*,
https://doi.org/10.1007/978-3-662-69700-9_2

3. Which is not one of the four principles for better soils with a lot of humus?
   A. Agroforestry
   B. Frequent ventilation
   C. Compost

2.1 The Full World

The Ulm Museum exhibits the "Lion Man", one of the oldest small works of art of mankind. The sculpture was found in the Lone valley near Ulm and was carved from mammoth ivory about 40,000 years ago. It shows a person about 30 cm tall with the head of a lion. The people back then lived from hunting, fishing, and gathering all kinds of fruits that nature provided. Essentially, it was about survival in a wild nature. Besides humans, the extinct cave bear, for example, was also interested in the caves that offered protection to humans.

As much as the lives of today's people may differ from those who created the Lion Man in the Neolithic Age, essential challenges still exist today. Then as now, the nutrition of mankind is a problem. Although technical and societal innovations, such as the invention of "land and cultural farming" about 10,000 years ago, have led to more and more people being able to be fed. But the generated surpluses do not equally benefit all people today: While a few billionaires have opened the door to space tourism in 2021, hundreds of millions of people are still struggling with the question of whether the next harvest will yield enough to feed their own family.

In contrast to the time of the "hunters and gatherers", humanity currently has the opportunity to shape living conditions on Earth in such a way that everyone gets their share: Some scientists call the current era the "Anthropocene". Because today, humans have as much impact on the Earth's ecosystem as only overarching physical forces could have had, which, for example, were responsible for the past ice ages. The problems of today are therefore essentially homemade and are also related to the increasing world population. Not surprisingly, the most important ones include the constantly advancing climate change and its adverse effects, but also the consistently high inequality. This is even increasing in parts of the world.

Looking at the development of human civilization over the last 2,000 years, one finds that the population has usually grown very slowly. For the year zero, the number of people is estimated at about 200 million. After that, it took 1,800 years for the population to grow to about one billion. At the time of the French Revolution, there were five times as many people as in the year zero, the industrialization had started in parts. However, the development in the last 200 years has been tremendous. Today, almost 8 billion people live on Earth. That's eight times as many people in a fraction of the time it took for the population to quintuple since the year zero. Currently, about the population of Germany is added each year (around 83 million people). The United Nations estimates that the world population will increase from currently 7.7 billion to just under 10 billion people in the next 30 years (UN 2019). This means that by 2050, the populations of India, Germany, the USA, Japan, and Canada combined will be added (see Fig. 2.1).

The exponential increase in the world's population has been accompanied by technical and societal innovations. In the current techno-economic system, more prosperity means higher pressure on the environment and particularly more climate change. This is because the system is based on the use of fossil energy.

The (still) growing world population needs to be fed! Looking at the development of agriculture over the last 10,000 years, it is very clear that climate and temperature fluctuations as well as regional weather conditions are among the most important factors influencing agriculture and its yield, yield security, but also the quality of the produce. Climate change and rising temperatures have led to an increase in extreme weather conditions, such as prolonged droughts, heavy rainfall and floods, erosion, landslides, salinization, and the loss of organic soil matter. While we in Europe have only recently experienced firsthand that climate change is real—witnessing extremely dry summers and heavy rainfall events— for many people in drier regions, living with such events has been a part of everyday life for decades.

In a full world with a growing population, these changes have a negative impact on agriculture, yield security, and nutrition. If the earth's temperature rises by an average of 3.7 to 4.8 °C, as stated in the 2014 report of the Intergovernmental Panel on Climate Change (IPCC), these negative effects on societies will drastically increase by the end of the century (IPCC 2014).

In order to limit the global increase in the average temperature of the earth to a maximum of 2 °C (preferably 1.5 °C), the countries of the world joined forces in 2015 and, after decades of struggle, concluded the Paris Climate Agreement. In

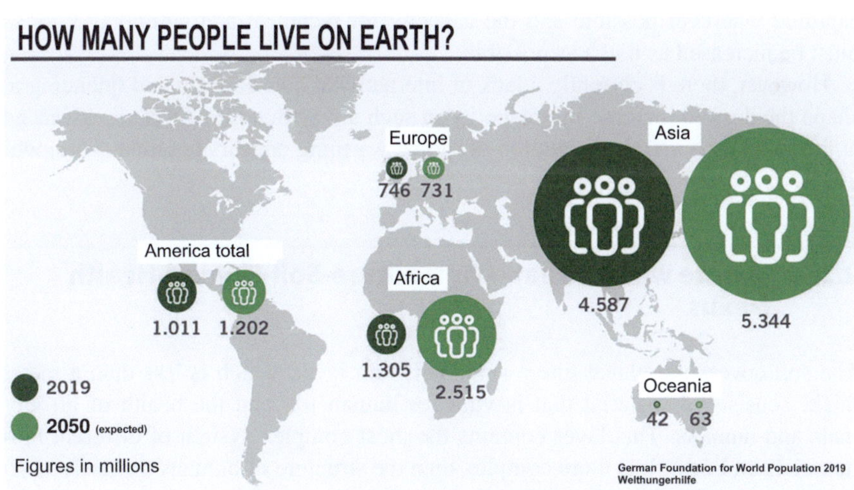

Fig. 2.1 Comparison between population growth in 2019 and 2050. *Source* World Hunger Aid 2022

the same year, the 17 Sustainable Development Goals (SDGs) were added to the international agenda. The SDGs define, in a way, under what conditions climate change should be limited—namely, not by limiting prosperity. Goal 8, for example, aims for an average economic growth for the poorest countries in the world of 7%.

This year (2022) marks the 50th anniversary of the United Nations Conference on the Human Environment, the so-called Stockholm Conference. The less wealthy countries demanded that social and economic development should have a priority over environmental protection measures, which the wealthier countries wanted to advance there. This paradigm has since become entrenched in international cooperation. The SDGs, also known as Agenda 2030, aim at advancing the three pillars of sustainability, namely that economy, ecology, and social concerns should be realized simultaneously. How the inherent contradictions between the individual pillars should be resolved was not discussed. Likewise, the growing world population is not an issue, although important closely related aspects are addressed: These include, for example, reproductive health, child mortality, and universal education.

If we want sustainable development and climate protection at the same time, it follows that people must become as wealthy as quickly as possible so that the number of children per family stabilizes at less than 2 and the population prospectively decreases again. The prosperity for people must be designed in such a way that nature is not further disrupted, but gradually restored. However currently, the increase in prosperity is associated with higher resource consumption. The basis for all this is provided by a tremendous increase in energy consumption. As widely known, the energy supply is currently predominantly of fossil origin, so CO_2-emissions are increasing. This mainly results in the need to successfully transition to a new energy system based on renewable energies. Along the way, CO_2 must be captured wherever possible and the capacity for technical and natural CO_2 sinks must be increased as much as possible.

However, there is currently a lack of international coordination and financing to shape the desired increase in prosperity in such a way that the SDGs are advanced at the same time and the limitation of global warming appears possible (Farajpour 2021).

2.2 We are what we eat—Agriculture-Soil-Human-Health Nexus

The soil covers the planet like a skin. This thin layer, which is less than a meter thick, consists of material that is vital for human life and the health of all animals and humans. This layer contains the most complex system of different biomaterials on Earth. It is more complex than the structure of humans themselves. At the Earth's surface, humans and soil meet. This means that humans influence the health of the soil and the soil influences the health of humans (Pepper 2013)! This happens directly and indirectly.

> *One teaspoon of soil contains more living organisms than there are people in the world. Without this "biological diversity" there would be no terrestrial life on earth.* (Capitals Coalition 2017)

Microorganisms, bacteria, and fungi are present in the soil by the trillions. They colonize plant roots and have no pathogenic effects on the plants. They protect the plant roots, improve and stimulate plant health and—what is especially important for us—they promote human health through their metabolic products. It has been shown that endophytes can produce new metabolic products such as antibiotics, antifungals, immunosuppressants, and cancer drugs (Strobel and Daisey 2003).

Soils influence human health particularly through food production and the quality of the cultivated food. The soil quality determines the nutritional value and production safety as well as the quality of the food (Zhu 2009). Health safety can be impaired, for example, when heavy metals and pathogens from contaminated soil are absorbed by plants and slowly enter the food chain. Naturally, soils contain many different elements that are necessary for the health and growth of plants as well as for human health. On one hand, the high concentration of these minerals negatively affects the health of all animals and humans. On the other hand, a deficiency of these minerals can be problematic. For example, fluoride-containing soil minerals, which are naturally present in groundwater, can contribute to the prevention of dental caries at moderate concentrations (0.7–1.2 mg/l). At a concentration of more than 4 mg/l water, they can be harmful and lead to harmful fluorosis (Burt and Tomar 2007). The same applies to mineral complexes with calcium, magnesium, and selenium. If the concentration of these mineral complexes is exceeded in the soil through agricultural activities, these can contaminate the groundwater and cause damage. Important minerals are also lost through soil loss and erosion.

Climate change exacerbates soil loss and erosion: A study by the University of Basel predicts that soil erosion by water and rain could increase by 30–66% by 2070, e.g., due to floods and heavy rainfall (Borrelli et al. 2020). Soil loss due to insufficient water is also a global challenge. In Europe, desertification could even progress faster than most people seem to be aware. Many European countries have already declared that they are severely affected by soil erosion and desertification. With advancing climate change and soil loss, food production, resilience of land areas, and water and food quality are decreasing. Since humans have the greatest impact on soils worldwide through agriculture (and more than 90% of our food comes from the soil), the type of agriculture plays a crucial role for human well-being.

2.3 Energy Consumption, Soils, and Emissions

The global energy consumption has almost doubled from more than 70,000 terawatt hours (TWh) in 1980 to more than 136,000 TWh in 2019. Still, more than 80% of the energy is fossil. In the building sector, a third of the energy is converted worldwide (Ahmad and Zhang 2020). Agriculture and human nutrition are also associated with high energy consumption. They cause about 23% of all human-made greenhouse gas emissions.

If agriculture only generated emissions, that would be one thing. However, important sinks for such emissions are also being destroyed. For agriculture, for example, large forest areas are converted into arable land, with the loss of biological diversity, pollution of aquatic ecosystems and groundwater, and the release of stored CO_2 into the atmosphere due to the type of soil management. According to the Food and Agriculture Organization of the United Nations in 2015, greenhouse gas emissions from agriculture, forestry, and fisheries have almost doubled in the last 50 years. Without greater efforts, the value could increase by another 30% by 2050 (FAO 2015).

Every year, 10 million hectares of arable land and good soils are lost. For illustration: This corresponds to the loss of 14 million football fields per year (Pimentel and Burgess 2013). Recent studies show, that these figures may even underestimate the problem. On a quarter of the world's soil, there is less humus and fewer nutrients than 25 years ago. Our soils are hungry, as hungry as the many poor people on the planet.

Depending on how land and soils are managed, they exacerbate problems or are part of the solution. If done correctly, soils can increase resilience to (temperature) changes in a world of weather extremes and climate change, remove and bind atmospheric greenhouse gas emissions, and improve human health. In general, they can contribute to sustainable development, the SDGs. If treated in a wrong way, the opposite happens: the negative impacts of climate change are exacerbated, the health of all people and animals is endangered, and poverty and hunger are intensified.

2.4 Balanced Inequality as a Driver for Sustainability

Climate change and the challenges of sustainable development are closely intertwined with economic inequality. Today, the richest 10% of the world's population earn about half of global income; they benefit most from the techno-economic system, including the global regulatory systems that are supposed to ensure its stability. Although the global economic performance has increased about tenfold since the Second World War. Particularly due to the rise of China, a global middle class has formed. Nevertheless, inequality has increased again in many states since the end of the 1980s. In some states, it is still rising. If one measures inequality across all people in the world, one finds that it is as high as in no nation-state. The situation is even more extreme when it comes to wealth than it is with income.

The distribution of financial resources must be taken into account because international climate protection and work on the SDGs naturally cost money. UNCTAD estimates that about 5–7 trillion US dollars per year are needed for their implementation for the period of the SDGs from 2015 to 2030 (UNCTAD 2014).

However, the prospect of raising this much money is far off. Not even the fund for supporting poorer states in adapting to climate change, which was decided within the framework of the Paris Agreement, is being sufficiently filled. The rich states should only pay 100 billion US dollars annually into this (UNFCCC 2011, 2019).

In the search for the necessary money, one should look at who causes the greenhouse gas emissions that in turn cause climate change. Historically, these are the rich states, which have, so to speak, generated high prosperity at the expense of the atmosphere. However, the states cannot handle the problem on their own. That's why the negotiations at the climate conferences are so tough. The private sector, on the other hand, today has about 5–7 times as much capital as the states (Chancel et al. 2017).

Emissions are almost one to one as unequally distributed as income. This implies that the richest 10% of the world's population cause about half of all emissions, while the poorest half of the world's population only cause about 10% of emissions (Chancel and Piketty 2015). But beware of jumping to conclusions: Actually, anyone who has a regular income and a steady job in a richer country belongs to the richest 10% worldwide.

These figures only refer to the source of emissions (polluter pays principle). For a fairer view, however, one should also take into account the individual capacity of the persons. Because within the richest 10% of the world's population are people who are not exactly rich in their respective home countries and, for example, have no wealth at all. This includes the lower half of the German income distribution. For social reasons, this group of people should not be burdened even more with levies or other measures for more climate protection.

A closer look at this question suggests that it would be most promising to hold the richest 30% of people in rich countries, the richest 10% in middle-income countries, and the richest 1% in poorer countries responsible (Orthen 2021). This would not only be fair, but also had the greatest impact in terms of financial resources and the existing influence that these people (the so-called top emitters) have. Moreover, the top emitters benefit most from progress in climate protection and sustainable development, because measures in this direction maintain the stability of the global economic system, from which the top emitters benefit most.

Empirically, it can be observed that rich states have a certain degree of inequality, not too much and not too little. Those who make an effort are rewarded, but broad prosperity is created through a functioning societal effort. Top earners can only benefit so much because everyone contributes and knows that they will not be left behind. Globally, we need to move towards such balanced inequality, anything else is unfair. At the same time, we need to ensure that this balanced inequality is not lost in the currently rich states. The fact that it is shaky can be seen in examples like Donald Trump or Brexit. If inequality gets out of balance, the stability of the global economic system is likely to fall apart as well. Stability is necessary to effectively address global challenges.

2.5 What needs to be done?

The agricultural sector is the backbone of the economy in many countries. It is also the key area of development cooperation. Sustainable practices must become economically viable for farmers. To this end, it is important that agriculture becomes a sink for greenhouse gas emissions, instead of continuing to cause emissions. Carbon must be stored in the soil and bound there permanently.

The so-called "organic matter (humus)" plays a central role for a better soil. The entirety of the organic soil substance is referred to as humus. So everything that has ever lived and died in the soil or still lives and is active there. Humus is responsible for soil fertility, consists of 58% carbon and 8% nitrogen (Dunst 2019). Globally, soils and humus are a huge carbon reservoir. Worldwide, between 1,500 and 2,400 gigatons of carbon are bound in the soil (Earth System Knowledge Platform n.d)—more than three times as much carbon as in the atmosphere and five times as much as in the world's plant mass (IPCC 2000). Humus can significantly improve soil properties. When a "clay-humus complex" forms, the carbon remains bound in the soil for centuries, ensuring soil fertility.

Through humus build-up, the 10 million hectares of good, fertile soils that are lost worldwide each year can be reclaimed. At the same time, humus management can produce food, reduce atmospheric greenhouse gas emissions, promote the health of all people and animals, bringing us closer to the SDGs.

As the climate crisis continues to intensify, interest in the topic of "soils for climate protection and sustainable development" has been increasing again in recent years. The authors' initiative "betterSoil—for a better world" has, for example, received a lot of support since 2020. Well-known personalities from politics, science, business, and practice support the discussion paper on the topic, which highlights the outstanding importance of soils.

Four scientific principles for better soils form the pillars for the practical work of the association betterSoil e.V.: (1.) the type of soil management, (2.) the application of compost, (3.) biochar and (4.) agroforestry systems. betterSoil e. V. is already active in several countries, including Kenya, Iran, Malawi, and Germany, and supports farmers in building up humus to improve their own living conditions, while at the same time protecting the climate (https://bettersoil.info). An important component is economic viability, so that working towards better soil is not a subsidized business, but can generate better incomes in the medium term.

As Fig. 2.2 shows, humus helps the soil in many ways and can promote human health as well. A soil well supplied with humus has a high water absorption capacity and can absorb up to 150 l of water per hour. This is because such soils are very porous with many holes and up to 600 earthworms per square meter live in them. In addition, a humus-rich soil can store up to 400 m^3 of water per hectare. These abilities help plants during long dry periods by absorbing moisture when it rains, facilitating the flow of water into the soil and preventing floods, while subsequently releasing water (Dunst 2019).

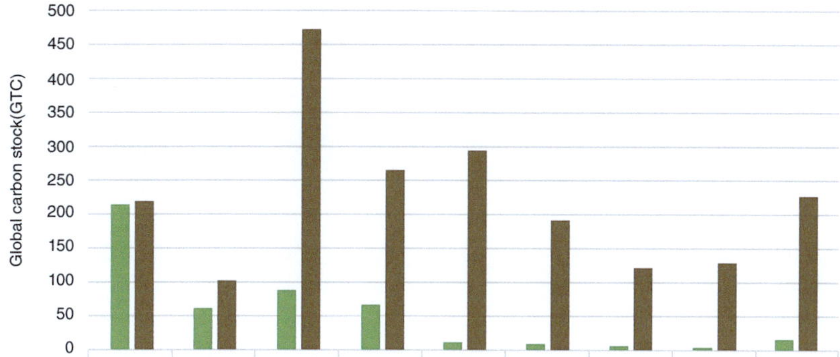

	Tropical forests	Forestsin temperate zones	Boreal forests	Tropical savannahs	Grassland in temperate zones	Deserts and semi-deserts	Tundra	Arable land	
Vegetation	212	59	88	66	9	8	6	3	15
Floor	216	100	471	264	295	191	121	128	225

Fig. 2.2 Global carbon stocks (Gt C) in vegetation and soil carbon pools up to a depth of 1 m. (IPCC 2000)

In times of global warming, these are exactly the properties that are essential for a more stable environment. Ecosystems with humus-rich soils are therefore more resilient. They prepare people for the extreme effects of a rapidly changing climate. "betterSoils" thus contribute to adaptation to climate change, but also to its mitigation, because they draw carbon from the atmosphere.

Such measures to promote soil quality and other nature-based projects, especially in combination with the promotion of the SDGs, should be financed by the top emitters. There are interesting points of contact with the voluntary carbon market, as promoted by the Development and Climate Alliance (https://allianz-entwicklung-klima.de). The alliance was founded by FAW/n in Ulm together with the Federal Ministry for Economic Cooperation and Development (BMZ) in fall 2019 and counts over 1,300 supporters at the time this article was written. Here, organizations, companies, cities, federal states, ministries, but also private individuals become climate-neutral or climate-positive by buying and retiring CO_2 certificates with high standards.

There are also interesting connections to the building sector, which is a major CO_2 emitter due to steel and cement. Healthy and strong soils are the prerequisite for the production of sustainable, renewable raw materials, primarily wood, which must be used more frequently in the building sector. We have already had good experiences replacing steel and cement in many places with resilient, durable, and fire-resistant wood constructions. The initiative "Bauhaus of the Earth" (https://bauhausdererde.org) by Hans Joachim Schellnhuber is intensively dedicated to this topic and has already made it to the European level with the establishment of a High-Level Roundtable "New European Bauhaus". Soils, wood, and buildings form an important triangle for the new "built environment" and for cleaning the atmosphere of greenhouse gas emissions.

Conclusion

To reduce the pressure of a growing world population on our planet, massive progress must be made in the area of the SDGs and international climate protection. The transformation of the energy system as well as the improvement of the quality of soils and the condition of natural carbon sinks in general, including the protection of (rain) forests and reforestation, play a special role for the basis of life and for feeding the world. To finance such measures, the top emitters should be held more accountable, so that the world society becomes more just through a balanced inequality.

Answers to the initial questions

1. A. Almost 8 billion in total, of which 1 billion in Africa
2. C. 10%
3. B. Frequent ventilation

References

Ahmad T, Zhang D (2020) A critical review of comparative global historical energy consumption and future demand: the story told so far. Energy Rep 6:1973–1991

Borrelli P et al (2020) Land use and climate change impacts on global soil erosion by water (2015-2070). Proc Natl Acad Sci 117(36):21994–22001

Burt BA, Tomar SL (2007) Changing the face of America: water fluoridation and oral health. In: Ward JW, Warren C (Hrsg) The history and practice of public health in twentieth century America. Oxford University Press, Oxford

Capitals Coalition (2017) One teaspoon of soil contains more living organisms than there are people in the world. https://capitalscoalition.org/one-teaspoon-of-soil-contains-more-living-organisms-than-there-are-people-in-the-world/. Accessed 31 Aug 2017

Chancel L et al. (2017) World inequality report 2018. World Inequality Lab. http://wir2018.wid.world. Accessed 17 Mar 2023

Chancel L, Piketty T (2015) Carbon and inequality: from Kyoto to Paris. Paris School of Economics,

Dunst G (2019) Humusaufbau: Chance für Landwirtschaft und Klima, 2. erw. Aufl. Sonnenerde Gerald Dunst Kulturerden GmbH, Riedlingsdorf

Earth System Knowledge Platform. (o. J.) Die Wissensplattform des Forschungsbereichs Erde und Umwelt der Helmholtz-Gemeinschaft. https://www.eskp.de/klimawandel/boeden-senken-oder-quellen-fuer-treibhausgase-935758/

FAO (2015) Soils help to combat and adapt to climate change by playing a key role in the carbon cycle. Food and Agriculture Organization. https://www.fao.org/documents/card/en/c/39058c2c-991b-4a24-a0bd-ccd0544e8320/

Farajpour A (2021) Humuswirtschaft und klimapositive Landwirtschaft – Brücke zwischen nachhaltiger Entwicklung und internationalem Klimaschutz. In: Gottwald F-T, Radermacher

F J, Plagge J (hrsg) Klimapositive Landwirtschaft; Mehr Wohlstand durch naturbasierte Lösungen, Nomos Verlagsgesellschaft
IPCC (2014) Climate change: mitigation of climate change. Contribution of working group III to the fifth assessment report of the intergovernmental panel on climate change. Edenhofer O et al. (hrsg). Cambridge University Press, Cambridge
IPCC (2000) Global carbon cycle Overview. International Panel on Climate Change. https://archive.ipcc.ch/ipccreports/sres/land_use/index.php?idp=3
Orthen TC (2021) Klimawandel, Ungleichheit und Top-Emitter – Wirkungszusammenhänge und die Rolle des wohlhabenden Privatsektors für Klimaschutz und eine nachhaltige Zukunft. Open Access Repositorium der Universität Ulm und Technischen Hochschule Ulm. Dissertation. https://doi.org/10.18725/OPARU-38785
Pimentel D, Burgess M (2013) Soil erosion threatens food production. Agriculture 3(3):443–463
UNCTAD (2014) World investment report 2014. Investing in the SDGs: an action plan. United Nations Conference on Trade and Development
UNFCCC (2011) Report of the conference of the parties on its sixteenth session. FCCC/CP/2010/7/Add.1. United Nations Framework Convention on Climate Change
UNFCCC (2019) Eighth report of the green climate fund to the conference of the parties to the United Nations framework convention on climate change. FCCC/CP/2019/3. United Nations Framework Convention on Climate Change
Strobel G, Daisey B (2003) Bioprospecting for microbial endophytes and their natural products. Microbiol Molec Biol Rev 67:491–502
UN (2019) Global issues population. United Nations. https://www.un.org/en/global-issues/population
Welthungerhilfe (2022) Bevölkerungswachstum. https://www.welthungerhilfe.de/informieren/themen/gesunde-ernaehrung-sichern/bevoelkerungswachstum-definition-entwicklung/
Zhu YG (2009) Soil science in the understanding of the security of food systems for health. Asia Pac. J. Clin. Nutr. 18:516–519
Pepper IL (2013) The Soil Health-Human Health Nexus Critical Reviews in Environmental Science and Technology 43(24) 2617-2652 10.1080/10643389.2012.694330

About the Self-Determined Family Planning of Women in Poor Countries and Female Migrants in Rich Countries

3

Laura Häusler, Jürgen Wacker, Zoubeida Saidane and Yacouba Zanré

Contents

L. Häusler
Mannheim, Germany
e-mail: Noreply@gmail.com

J. Wacker (✉)
ehemaliger Chefarzt der Frauenklinik Bruchsal, Bruchsal, Germany
e-mail: wacker@menschenfuerfrauen.de

Z. Saidane
Frauenklinik der Fürst-Stirum-Klinik Bruchsal, Bruchsal, Germany
e-mail: Zoubeida.Saidane@rkh-kliniken.de

Y. Zanré
Hôpital Shiphra, Ouagadougou, Burkina Faso

J. Wacker et al. (eds.), *Global Women's Health*,
https://doi.org/10.1007/978-3-662-69700-9_3

Introductory Questions

1. How many women worldwide have access to self-determined family planning (indication in %)?
   A. 20%
   B. 60%
   C. 80%
2. In which continent are the most unwanted pregnancies currently found?
   A. Asia
   B. Africa
   C. Latin America
3. What factors prevent the use of modern family planning methods among migrant women in Germany?
   A. Lack of language skills
   B. Religious regulations
   C. Lack of women's emancipation
   D. All answers are correct

3.1 The Importance of Family Planning Worldwide

Family planning saves lives. By preventing unwanted pregnancies and by extending the interval between birth and subsequent conception, modern family planning can reduce maternal and child mortality. In the past 20 years, the number of maternal deaths in developing countries has been reduced by 40% solely through the reduction of unplanned pregnancies and the reduction of high-risk pregnancies (Cleland et al. 2012; Mbizvo and Phillips 2014). The proportion of women using a modern contraceptive has doubled in the last 50 years and is currently almost 60%. However, according to the United Nations World Population Report, up to 217 million women worldwide still have an unmet need for modern contraception, and only every second woman can self-determine her physical integrity and sexual health. It is striking that women are more likely to influence the use of contraceptives than to be able to say "no" to sex. For a better understanding of this topic and to illustrate the limits of self-determined family planning, we have included the following cartoon as Fig. 3.1:

Self-determined family planning allows for an increasing emancipation of women in addition to health aspects (Okigbo et al. 2018). As of 2021, women worldwide only enjoy 75% of the legal rights that men are entitled to. The legal and economic disadvantage of women reduces their financial and societal independence and thus their ability to independently decide on issues such as sexuality, contraception, and health care. Adolescent girls are particularly at risk, especially if they are not married, as family planning is still reserved exclusively for married couples in many countries today. Sexual relationships outside of marriage are not recognized, leading to illegal and risky abortions. Furthermore, there is a significantly higher maternal mortality in the age group of pregnant women under 20

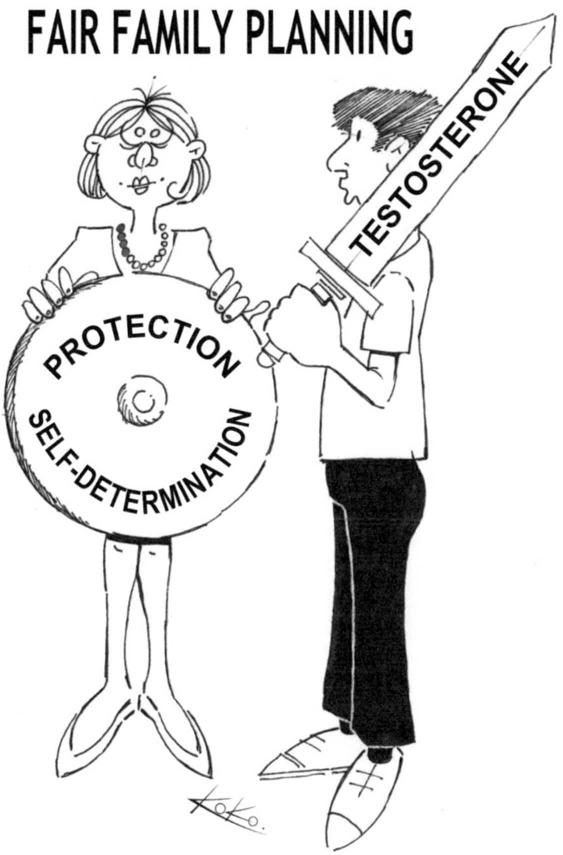

Fig. 3.1 Self-determined family planning. (© Diethard Kokoska)

years. Fortunately, the birth rate among adolescents is declining worldwide, but there are large regional differences. For example, 95% of births among adolescents come from poor countries. The Sub-Saharan region is particularly affected, with about 100 births per 1000 women in the age group of 15 to 19-year-olds each year. Table 3.1 shows the correlations between modern family planning and the occurrence of maternal complications during pregnancy and childbirth (Cleland et al. 2012).

In addition to regional factors, education level and wealth play a significant role. A lower contraceptive prevalence is evident among women who are poor, live in rural areas, or have a low level of education. These differences are particularly stark in African countries. Only through concentrated efforts to expand family planning services can they be overcome. Such government programs can be found in Bangladesh, Bhutan, Cambodia, and Thailand. This is evidenced, among other things, by the United Nations World Population Report, which shows

Table 3.1 Self-determined family planning—important facts at a glance. (Cleland et al. 2012)

The increasing use of modern contraceptives is responsible for 75% of the fertility decline in developing countries over the last 6 decades.	This means a significant reduction in maternal mortality through family planning. Exemplarily, this was reduced by 40% between 1990 and 2008.
In 2017, 217 million women worldwide had no access to modern family planning.	If all women in developing countries who want to prevent pregnancy had access to contraceptives, a further decrease in maternal deaths of up to 30% would be possible.
In 2003, there were approximately 42 million abortions, of which almost 50% took place under unsafe conditions. In 2017, 25.5 million abortions took place under unsafe conditions, 97% of them in developing countries.	This led to 47,000 deaths in 2003, corresponding to 13% of all maternal deaths that year, which could have been avoided by using modern contraceptives.
Maternal mortality is higher among adolescent mothers, particularly before the age of 15, among older pregnant women, in multiparity (> 4 children), and rapid pregnancy succession under 18 months.	The use of modern contraceptives can reduce high-risk pregnancies and lower maternal mortality: by 4.8 deaths per 100,000 births for each percentage point increase in the use of modern contraceptives.
The risk of prematurity and child maldevelopment as well as low birth weight significantly increases with a pregnancy interval of less than 18 months.	By increasing the pregnancy interval to 2 years, the risk of infant mortality (< 1 year) decreases by 10% and that for children between the ages of 1 and 4 by 21% in developing countries.
As of 2021, women worldwide only have 75% of the rights that men are entitled to. Due to more frequent school dropouts among adolescent pregnant women, their economic marginalization and financial dependence increase.	Self-determined family planning gives women the opportunity to at least partially control their bodies, and is thus a step towards gender equality.

a declining birth rate, especially in Asia and Latin America. In the African Sub-Saharan region, however, there was only a slight drop in the rate from 6.6 to 5.2 children per woman between 1960 and 2010. Despite progress in the field of family planning in many regions of the world, the global proportion of women who have access to modern contraception methods has stagnated at 80% since 2015. The effects of the Covid-19 pandemic, which has led to a reduced range of services from health facilities and a reduced demand from patients due to fear of infection, may have contributed to this stagnation. Thus, even today, up to 43% of all pregnancies in developing countries, especially in Africa, are unplanned, which corresponds to an estimated 89 million women who become pregnant unintentionally each year. This results in up to 48 million abortions per year, which are illegal in up to 50% of cases and take place under unsafe conditions.

In Europe too, contraceptive prevalence and the age at birth of the first child depend on economic factors and the level of education. This particularly affects migrant women from poorer countries (Helfferich 2013). The study "Family

Planning and Migration in Women's Life Course" by the Federal Centre for Health Education (BZgA) examined contraceptive behavior among migrant women from Turkey and the former CIS states. This showed not only a lower contraceptive prevalence compared to the German-born population, but also a higher rate of abortions, a younger age of women at the birth of the first child, and a lower marriage age. Sexuality is still linked to marriage in many cultures, and children are expected within marriage. Thus, in many cultures, contraception is only used after the first or second child. A retrospective study at the University Hospital Basel also showed a 2.5 times higher rate of interruptions among migrant women, mainly due to a lack of contraception. The main reasons for the lack of use of a contraceptive seemed to be linguistic and financial in nature (Kurth et al. 2010). In addition, there are issues related to residence status, which are also a priority in the advice given to migrant women by local authorities. There is a lack of low-threshold services to facilitate access to preventive measures of the health system, such as family planning (Keygnaert et al. 2014). In addition, cultural factors and misinformation hinder access to family planning services. Rasch et al. observed in a case-control study at seven Danish clinics that there was a great deal of ignorance about modern contraceptive methods, especially among migrant women. Many women were afraid of side effects or had already had bad experiences with contraceptives. Both were associated with an increased rate of abortions. Particularly among migrant women, there was often a negative attitude of the partner towards the use of contraceptives (Rasch et al. 2007). Many migrant women are also unaware of the existence of the "morning-after pill," as another study showed (Wolff et al. 2008).

In summary, the inadequate spread of self-determined family planning among migrant women in Western industrialized countries is multifactorial. The main factors are linguistic, financial, and cultural barriers, the lack of women's emancipation, and ignorance about modern contraception methods. Access to contraceptive counseling and self-determined family planning are among the sexual and reproductive rights of every human being, and the provision of appropriate programs is a state duty. The growing group of migrant women with different socio-cultural backgrounds must be given more focus. To reach this heterogeneous group of women and their partners, local awareness campaigns adapted to the respective cultural backgrounds are necessary.

3.2 What Methods are used Worldwide for Family Planning?

The most important step in preventing unwanted pregnancies is the use of a contraceptive. In 2012, nearly 20% of all women without contraception caused over 60% of all unwanted pregnancies (Darroch 2013). The switch to a contraceptive method with higher contraceptive effectiveness is also important. Long-acting reversible contraceptives can be considered safer due to a lower user error. This is particularly noticeable in comparison with condoms and oral contraceptives.

The "pill," for example, has an average effectiveness of 99.7% with perfect use, but with typical use, i.e., taking into account errors in use such as "forgetting the pill," 9% of women become unintentionally pregnant each year (Trussell 2011).

There are significant differences worldwide not only concerning contraceptive prevalence, but also the distribution of contraceptive methods. While in Western industrialized countries and some North African countries, the "pill" and the condom are the most common contraceptives, in South Asia, Latin America, and the Caribbean countries, female sterilization is the most popular method. In Central and West Asia, however, intrauterine devices, especially the copper coil, are most widespread. Long-acting hormonal methods such as depot progestogens are primarily used in the Sub-Saharan region and Southeast Asia (Darroch 2013). Overall, it is noticeable that in developing countries there is a smaller selection of different family planning methods and thus fewer alternatives are offered. This further reduces contraceptive prevalence and leads to more frequent discontinuation of the contraceptive method without switching to another contraceptive (Dagnew et al. 2021).

3.2.1 Natural Family Planning in Developing Countries

A widely used contraceptive method, especially in African developing countries, is natural family planning. Fears and superstitions are often associated with the topic of contraception. Thus, external family planning programs with per se highly secure methods such as the "pill" also fail due to cultural circumstances. In contrast, natural family planning enjoys high acceptance among the population of these countries. Depending on the study and method, failure of natural family planning was observed in up to 5% of cases with perfect application, but with typical application, an estimated quarter of women become unintentionally pregnant within a year (Trussell 2011). Despite the high failure rate, natural family planning can contribute to reducing the number of unwanted pregnancies solely due to its broad acceptance among the population of many developing countries. Another advantage is cost-effectiveness, which is given even with extensive initial care.

In addition to the Billings method, which is also widespread in Western countries, simplified concepts of natural family planning have been designed for women in developing countries. The Modified-Mucus-Method (MMM) is attributed to the Indian doctor Dorairaj and initially targeted illiterate women from the poorest strata of Indian society. The days with increased and spinnable cervical mucus and the two subsequent days are defined as the fertile period during which sexual intercourse should be avoided (Dorairaj 1991). The principle of the birth control chain, which is based on a simple calendar method, was developed in 1989 by the Viennese doctor and development aid worker Maria Hengstberger during a stay in Ethiopia. It consists of 30 teardrop-shaped beads in different colors: one red bead for the first day of menstruation, three red-yellow for the average duration of bleeding, eleven yellow beads for the infertile days and eight blue ones, which represent the fertile cycle phase, as well as 7 half-blue beads for the transition phases between the certainly fertile and infertile days. A small movable ring is attached to the chain, which is moved forward every day and thus shows the user in which cycle phase she is currently in. The main problem with this method is that it is only suitable for women with a very regular cycle and a cycle length of 26 to 32 days (Arévalo et al. 1999). The birth control chain developed by Ms. Hengstberger is shown in the following Fig. 3.2.

Another widely used method of natural family planning in developing countries is lactational amenorrhea. This method offers a high contraceptive safety of up to 98% when used correctly. Presumably due to the regular sucking stimulus on the mother's breast, egg maturation is inhibited. Consequently, amenorrhea occurs, i.e., the absence of menstruation. The contraceptive safety is only guaranteed as long as all three prerequisites of the lactational amenorrhea method are met: the persistent amenorrhea, the newborn's age under six months, and exclusive breastfeeding of the child day and night. The lactational amenorrhea method can be used to increase the interval between birth and subsequent pregnancy, and this time should be used to choose a subsequent contraceptive. In addition, this method promotes breastfeeding, an important aspect for the newborn's health, especially in developing countries where clean water for the preparation of baby food is not always available. This method is primarily limited by the increasing employment of women in many developing countries (Vekemans 1997).

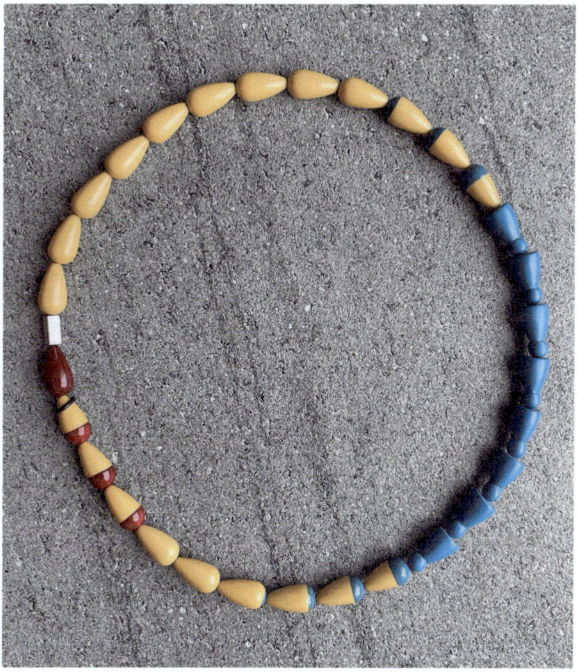

Fig. 3.2 Birth control chain, developed by Maria Hengstberger

3.2.2 Long Acting Reversible Contraceptives (LARC)

Long-acting reversible contraceptives can be divided into hormonal and non-hormonal contraceptives. Hormonal methods include progestogen implants such as the etonogestrel-containing Implanon® and intrauterine systems with levonorgestrel. The copper intrauterine device (IUD), the copper chain, and the copper ball belong to the group of hormone-free contraceptive methods. A major advantage of all long-acting reversible contraceptives is that there is no difference between perfect and typical use. This means that the contraceptive effectiveness of the method is independent of user compliance.

Intrauterine Devices (Copper or Hormonal Coil)
In 2015, 14% of all married or cohabiting women of reproductive age used an Intrauterine Device (IUD) for contraception. This makes IUDs the second most common contraceptive method in this group after female sterilization. However, the prevalence of IUD users varies greatly by region. Over 60% of women who use a coil for contraception live in China. In the least developed countries in the world, less than 1% of women use an IUD. The prevalence is particularly low in Africa, with the exception of some North African countries (Cleland et al. 2017). Possible reasons for the rare use of this contraceptive method in many developing countries could be the complex insertion process, a lack of expertise among health personnel, and the need for position control. In addition, government regulations and family planning programs are important. Regular training of health personnel and financial subsidization of IUDs, as well as a relaxation of the guidelines on who is authorized to insert them, would be necessary. In Egypt, for example, a country where 38% of women use a coil for contraception, the insertion and replacement of the IUD is not exclusively the responsibility of gynecologists, but can also be carried out by nursing staff, midwives, or general practitioners (Buhling et al. 2014). Furthermore, the approval of the copper coil is restricted in many countries. This affects nulliparous women, adolescents, as well as unmarried and promiscuous women, particularly due to concerns about an increased rate of ovarian inflammation among copper coil users, leading to subsequent sterility (Ali et al. 2019). However, the initial recommendation to use the copper coil only in women with at least one child has been revoked by the FDA, the WHO, and other international health authorities. The risk of infection appears to be slightly increased only in the first 30 days, which is presumably due to pre-existing infections (Bahamondes et al. 2020). Religious-cultural backgrounds can also play a role in the decision if bleeding disorders under IUDs are perceived as a hindrance to religious activities (Salem et al. 2006).

There is great potential to avoid risk pregnancies due to rapid pregnancy succession or multiparity by inserting a copper intrauterine device immediately after birth, also referred to as a post-partum IUD (PPIUD). To allow the maternal body to recover from pregnancy, the interval between birth and subsequent conception should be at least 18 months. A shorter pregnancy interval carries numerous risks such as the occurrence of cervical insufficiency with prematurity or uterine rupture in the case of a previous cesarean section. In addition, there is often a lack of development in children born very quickly in succession (Cleland et al. 2012). For this reason, a reliable method of contraception is initially required after delivery. The PPIUD is suitable for this: The copper coil TCu 380A, which has been approved by the FDA for 10 years, is used, but in several studies it has proven effectiveness for at least 12 years. Copper coils exert their contraceptive effect mainly through spermicidal effects and a sterile inflammation in the uterus (Bahamondes et al. 2020). The copper IUD is, apart from the condom, the only modern contraceptive approved by the WHO for immediate postpartum use for breastfeeding mothers. The insertion of a copper IUD within 48 hours of birth allows the initiation of a reliable method of contraception as part of inpatient or outpatient peripartum care. This saves the affected person an additional doctor's visit, which demonstrably increases compliance (Mohamed et al. 2003). The non-profit organization Jhpiego (John Hopkins Program for International Education in Gynecology and Obstetrics) and the United States Agency for International Development (USAID) have also recognized the potential of the PPIUD and have set up corresponding programs in several developing countries. The insertion is done high fundal using a special insertion technique to keep the risk of expulsion of the IUD as low as possible. The expulsion rates after six weeks were between 1.7 and 3.7% and were thus comparable to those when inserted at a later time (Pfitzer et al. 2015). However, it should be noted that the follow-up period in the described programs was only six weeks. Overall, slightly higher expulsion rates are probably to be expected than with later interval insertion. In general, the probability of expulsion is highest in the first three months after insertion. Celen et al. described an average expulsion rate of 12.3% over a follow-up period of 12 months, yet with very high user satisfaction (Celen et al. 2004). The infection rate, which averaged 1%, is not increased with the PPIUD. According to current knowledge, there is also no increased occurrence of uterine perforations (Kapp and Curtis 2009; Pfitzer et al. 2015). Limitations of the copper coil are mainly that it does not offer protection against sexually transmitted diseases. In addition, the copper coil often leads to bleeding disorders such as hyper- and dysmenorrhea (Ali et al. 2019).

The hormonal IUD is also recommended by some professional societies such as the American College of Obstetricians and Gynecologists (ACOG) for immediate postpartum insertion. Others recommend the insertion of the levonorgestrel IUD for breastfeeding mothers only from six weeks after delivery. The hormonal IUD can also be used for contraception in nulliparous women. The insertion is usually done during menstruation to rule out pregnancy, but in principle it is possible at any time of the cycle. Internationally available is the hormonal IUD with 52 mg of levonorgestrel. It has an effective duration of at least five to seven years. The hormonal IUD exerts its contraceptive effects through a thickening of the cervical mucus with obstruction of sperm ascension, it inhibits endometrial proliferation and partially ovulation. Due to its antiproliferative effect on the endometrium, the 52 mg LNG IUD can also be used therapeutically for bleeding disorders and endometriosis. In addition, the LNG IUD reduces the risk of endometrial and ovarian carcinomas (Bahamondes et al. 2020). Despite the positive side effects and the high contraceptive effectiveness, the hormonal IUD is rarely used in developing countries. This could be due to the higher costs and limited availability in the public health sector of many countries (Ali et al. 2019; Buhling et al. 2014; Pace et al. 2013).

Progestogen Implants

The progestogen implant Implanon® with 68 mg of etonogestrel is approved by the FDA for three years. The implant is inserted subcutaneously in the area of the inner upper arm. With a Pearl Index of 0.05, it is considered the safest contraceptive. Its contraceptive effect is primarily achieved by inhibiting ovulation, additional progestogen effects increase contraceptive safety. Despite its high contraceptive efficacy, progestogen implants play a rather subordinate role in family planning worldwide. Implanon® offers further advantages such as easy insertion with little effort, visibility and palpability with possible position control by the wearer, and approval for use during breastfeeding from 6 weeks postpartum. At the same time, several studies observed a high discontinuation rate among Implanon® users in developing countries. The main reasons cited for this were the occurrence of bleeding disorders, but also inadequate information about possible side effects and the benefits of Implanon®, as well as the lack of alternative contraceptive methods play a significant role (Aziz et al. 2018; Dagnew et al. 2021; Mrwebi et al. 2018). In addition, the cost factor of Implanon® is likely to be significant, even though there is state subsidization in some African countries like Ethiopia (Aziz et al. 2018).

3.2.3 Depot Progestogens

While depot progestogens play a rather subordinate role in Europe, they are used by 38% of users of a modern contraceptive in the Sub-Saharan region and by 47% in South Africa. The three-monthly intramuscular or subcutaneous application of depot medroxyprogesterone acetate (DMPA) is most commonly used (Fok and Blumenthal 2017; Smith et al. 2020). Depot progestogens exert their contraceptive effect by inhibiting follicle maturation and partly ovulation, as well as by thickening the cervical mucus with suppression of sperm ascension. Advantages are the high contraceptive safety, easy application, and the cost factor. On the other hand, it requires higher compliance than LARCs due to the shorter duration of action. In addition, several adverse events under depot progestogens should be mentioned. The effect on the bones with a possible decrease in bone density under DMPA should not be neglected, which is why long-term contraception over 2 years should only be carried out in the case of contraindications for other contraceptives. Due to the lack of long-term data to assess the effect on the bones in adolescents, depot progestogens are contraindicated in this group. Other side effects include a slightly increased risk of thrombosis, unfavorable effects on glucose-insulin metabolism, and a suspected increase in the risk of breast cancer. In the past, there were indications that the risk of HIV infection could increase under DMPA. In 2019, the randomized controlled ECHO study (Evidence for Contraceptive Options and HIV) was published. This compared the HIV infection risk in DMPA users with that of women who used copper or hormonal IUDs for contraception. A dramatic risk increase of more than 50% for DMPA users could be ruled out. Nevertheless, a slight increase in the risk of HIV infection under DMPA is not impossible. Considering the high HIV prevalence in many developing countries, even a slight risk increase could be significant. This aspect should be included in the patient's consultation if the HIV prevalence is appropriate. On the other hand, there are the health risks of an unplanned pregnancy if DMPA is discontinued without switching to another contraceptive method (Smith et al. 2020). Accordingly, after the publication of the ECHO study, the WHO decided to raise the recommendation for DMPA from level two back to level one (Polis and Curtis 2013).

3.2.4 Female Sterilization

Female sterilization is still the most common method of contraception among married or cohabiting women. However, with the introduction and spread of long-acting reversible contraceptives, it has lost its importance. The highest rate of female sterilizations is found in countries like India, as well as in Latin America and the Caribbean (Fang et al. 2021). In many parts of Africa, however, sterilization plays a subordinate role, partly due to the lack of infrastructure in the poorest developing countries with difficult access to a surgical center. In addition, there are high costs and a lack of expertise among health personnel due to the rare performance of the operation (Mbizvo and Phillips 2014).

3.2.5 The "Pill"

Oral contraceptives are mainly used for family planning in Western industrialized countries as well as in the North African countries of Morocco, Algeria, and Tunisia (Dimassi et al. 2017). A significant disadvantage of all oral contraceptives is that contraceptive safety depends on user compliance. Many women, especially in developing countries, are inadequately informed about oral contraceptives. Often these are freely available in pharmacies, without advice on correct intake or prior exclusion of contraindications (Mobark et al. 2019). This not only increases the risk of unwanted side effects, but also negatively affects reliable intake of the "pill" and thus reduces contraceptive effectiveness. Furthermore, misinformation and superstition prevail regarding hormonal contraceptives. A dramatic misconception is that these lead to permanent infertility. In many countries where a woman's value is largely dependent on the number of her healthy offspring, this has profound implications for the progress of family planning (Williamson et al. 2009).

3.2.6 The Condom

In addition to oral contraceptives, according to the BZgA in Germany, the condom is the second most common contraceptive. Among developing countries, it is mainly prevalent in Central Africa (Darroch 2013). The condom is associated more with protection against sexually transmitted diseases in many regions of the world and is less often used to prevent unwanted pregnancies. Accordingly, it often stands for promiscuity. This leads to many women not demanding their partner to use a condom (Williamson et al. 2009). Furthermore, a significant portion of men reject the condom anyway, as it is perceived as uncomfortable and inhibiting pleasure. This is also reflected in the Pearl Index, which is two in the case of perfect use, but 12 in typical use. Nevertheless, the condom is essential for sexual and reproductive health, as it is an easily accessible and cost-effective contraceptive that provides protection against sexually transmitted diseases.

3.2.7 Emergency Contraception

The “morning-after pill" is part of the WHO list of essential medicines. Unfortunately, it is only limitedly available in many poor countries and is often not listed in state health programs. In addition, in poorer countries, Levonorgestrel-based emergency contraceptives are primarily offered, as Ulipristal acetate is more expensive. However, the latter has a higher effectiveness especially with a larger distance to unprotected sexual intercourse and in overweight women. The safest emergency contraception is the copper IUD, which is approved up to 7 days after unprotected intercourse (Glasier 2013; Westley et al. 2013)

3.3 What Options are there to Facilitate Access to Family Planning?

In conclusion, it can be stated that the unmet need for family planning is declining both globally and in Germany. Nevertheless, there is a lack of modern contraceptives, primarily among women with low socioeconomic status and education. Not only the high health risks of pregnancy and childbirth, especially in developing countries with high maternal mortality, are important, but also the financial and societal dependence on the partner that women enter into through pregnancy.

There is also a need for improvement in the area of modern family planning in Germany, especially among migrant women and marginalized groups. These lack low-threshold access to the health system. Although there are generally accessible counseling centers in this country, since counselors is not a protected term, they have very different qualifications. At the same time, the counseling centers are inadequately networked with gynecologists. In gynecological practices, on the other hand, there is often a lack of time for the complex contraceptive counseling of vulnerable groups. Better cooperation between counseling centers and gynecologists is needed here. It would also be conceivable to have a regular rotation of doctors into the relevant counseling centers to support and train the local staff. In times of increasing migration, there is a need for an interpreter service in the health care system that is always available online or by phone to overcome the often existing language barrier. It would also make sense to train health personnel in dealing with people from other cultural circles in order to create a better understanding of cultural circumstances and thus simplify access to the corresponding patients. The cost factor should not be forgotten. In addition to professional and individualized contraceptive counseling, it is necessary to assume the cost of contraceptives for vulnerable groups.

Without contraceptive counseling, choosing a suitable contraceptive is difficult. Self-determined family planning and thus also contraceptive counseling are human rights. These must be consistently implemented in order to protect the health and well-being of millions of women and girls and to promote their equality.

Answers to the initial questions

1. C. 80%
2. B. Africa
3. D. All answers are correct

References

Ali M, Folz R, Farron M (2019) Expanding choice and access in contraception: an assessment of intrauterine contraception policies in low and middle-income countries. BMC Public Health 19(1):1707. https://doi.org/10.1186/s12889-019-8080-7

Arévalo M, Sinai I, Jennings V (1999) A fixed formula to define the fertile window of the menstrual cycle as the basis of a simple method of natural family planning. Contraception 60(6):357–360. https://doi.org/10.1016/s0010-7824(99)00106-7

Aziz MM, El-Gazzar AF, Elgibaly O (2018) Factors associated with first-year discontinuation of Implanon in Upper Egypt: clients' and providers' perspectives. BMJ Sex Reprod Health. https://doi.org/10.1136/bmjsrh-2017-101860

Bahamondes L, Fernandes A, Monteiro I, Bahamondes MV (2020) Long-acting reversible contraceptive (LARCs) methods. Best Pract Res Clin Obstet Gynaecol 66:28–40. https://doi.org/10.1016/j.bpobgyn.2019.12.002

Buhling KJ, Zite NB, Lotke P, Black K (2014) Worldwide use of intrauterine contraception: a review. Contraception 89(3):162–173. https://doi.org/10.1016/j.contraception.2013.11.011

Celen S, Möröy P, Sucak A, Aktulay A, Danişman N (2004) Clinical outcomes of early postplacental insertion of intrauterine contraceptive devices. Contraception 69(4):279–282. https://doi.org/10.1016/j.contraception.2003.12.004

Cleland J, Conde-Agudelo A, Peterson H, Ross J, Tsui A (2012) Contraception and health. Lancet 380(9837):149–156. https://doi.org/10.1016/s0140-6736(12)60609-6

Cleland J, Ali M, Benova L, Daniele M (2017) The promotion of intrauterine contraception in low- and middle-income countries: a narrative review. Contraception 95(6):519–528. https://doi.org/10.1016/j.contraception.2017.03.009

Dagnew GW, Gelaw YM, Asresie MB, Anteneh ZA (2021) Level and timing of implanon discontinuation and associated factors among women who used implanon in andabet district,

public health facilities, North-West ethiopia. Biomed Res Int 2021:6647660. https://doi.org/10.1155/2021/6647660
Darroch JE (2013) Trends in contraceptive use. Contraception 87(3):259–263. https://doi.org/10.1016/j.contraception.2012.08.029
Dimassi K, Douik F, Douzi MA, Saidi O, Ben Romdhane H (2017) Social determinants of contraceptive use in Tunisia. Rev Epidemiol Sante Publique 65(1):53–59. https://doi.org/10.1016/j.respe.2016.06.330
Dorairaj K (1991) The modified mucus method in India. Am J Obstet Gynecol 165(6 Pt 2):2066–2067. https://doi.org/10.1016/s0002-9378(11)90584-5
Fang NZ, Advaney SP, Castaño PM, Davis A, Westhoff CL (2021) Female permanent contraception trends and updates. Am J Obstet Gynecol. https://doi.org/10.1016/j.ajog.2021.12.261
Fok WK, Blumenthal PD (2017) HIV and contraception. Curr Opin Obstet Gynecol 29(6):419–426. https://doi.org/10.1097/gco.0000000000000405
Glasier A (2013) Emergency contraception: clinical outcomes. Contraception 87(3):309–313. https://doi.org/10.1016/j.contraception.2012.08.027
Helfferich C (2013) Reproductive health of women. Family planning and „reproductive rights" in Germany. Bundesgesundheitsbl Gesundheitsforsch Gesundheitsschutz 56(2):192–198. https://doi.org/10.1007/s00103-012-1603-3
Kapp N, Curtis KM (2009) Intrauterine device insertion during the postpartum period: a systematic review. Contraception 80(4):327–336. https://doi.org/10.1016/j.contraception.2009.03.024
Keygnaert I, Guieu A, Ooms G, Vettenburg N, Temmerman M, Roelens K (2014) Sexual and reproductive health of migrants: does the EU care? Health Policy 114(2-3):215–225. https://doi.org/10.1016/j.healthpol.2013.10.007
Kurth E, Jaeger FN, Zemp E, Tschudin S, Bischoff A (2010) Reproductive health care for asylum-seeking women – a challenge for health professionals. BMC Public Health 10:659. https://doi.org/10.1186/1471-2458-10-659
Mbizvo MT, Phillips SJ (2014) Family planning: choices and challenges for developing countries. Best Pract Res Clin Obstet Gynaecol 28(6):931–943. https://doi.org/10.1016/j.bpobgyn.2014.04.014
Mobark DM, Al-Tabakha MM, Hasan S (2019) Assessing hormonal contraceptive dispensing and counseling provided by community pharmacists in the United Arab Emirates: a simulated patient study. Pharm Pract (Granada) 17(2):1465. https://doi.org/10.18549/PharmPract.2019.2.1465
Mohamed SA, Kamel MA, Shaaban OM, Salem HT (2003) Acceptability for the use of postpartum intrauterine contraceptive devices: Assiut experience. Med Princ Pract 12(3):170–175. https://doi.org/10.1159/000070754
Mrwebi KP, Goon DT, Owolabi EO, Adeniyi OV, Seekoe E, Ajayi AI (2018) Reasons for discontinuation of implanon among users in Buffalo City metropolitan municipality, South Africa: a cross-sectional study. Afr J Reprod Health 22(1):113–119. https://doi.org/10.29063/ajrh2018/v22i1.11
Okigbo CC, Speizer IS, Domino ME, Curtis SL, Halpern CT, Fotso JC (2018) Gender norms and modern contraceptive use in urban Nigeria: a multilevel longitudinal study. BMC Womens Health 18(1):178. https://doi.org/10.1186/s12905-018-0664-3
Pace LE, Dusetzina SB, Fendrick AM, Keating NL, Dalton VK (2013) The impact of out-of-pocket costs on the use of intrauterine contraception among women with employer-sponsored insurance. Med Care 51(11):959–963. https://doi.org/10.1097/MLR.0b013e3182a97b5d
Pfitzer A, Mackenzie D, Blanchard H, Hyjazi Y, Kumar S, Lisanework Kassa S, Marinduque B, Mateo MG, Mukarugwiro B, Ngabo F, Zaeem S, Zafar Z, Smith JM (2015) A facility birth can be the time to start family planning: postpartum intrauterine device experiences from six countries. Int J Gynaecol Obstet 130(Suppl 2):S54–S61. https://doi.org/10.1016/j.ijgo.2015.03.008
Polis CB, Curtis KM (2013) Use of hormonal contraceptives and HIV acquisition in women: a systematic review of the epidemiological evidence. Lancet Infect Dis 13(9):797–808. https://doi.org/10.1016/s1473-3099(13)70155-5

Rasch V, Knudsen LB, Gammeltoft T, Christensen JT, Erenbjerg M, Christensen JJ, Sorensen JB (2007) Contraceptive attitudes and contraceptive failure among women requesting induced abortion in Denmark. Hum Reprod 22(5):1320–1326. https://doi.org/10.1093/humrep/dem012

Salem RM, Setty V, Williamson RT, Schwandt H (2006) When contraceptives change monthly bleeding. Popul Rep J 54(1):3–19

Smith JA, Beacroft L, Abdullah F, Buthelezi B, Makua M, Morroni C, Ramjee G, Velasquez C, Hallett TB (2020) Responding to the ECHO trial results: modelling the potential impact of changing contraceptive method mix on HIV and reproductive health in South Africa. J Int AIDS Soc 23(10):e25620. https://doi.org/10.1002/jia2.25620

Trussell J (2011) Contraceptive failure in the United States. Contraception 83(5):397–404. https://doi.org/10.1016/j.contraception.2011.01.021

Vekemans M (1997) Postpartum contraception: the lactational amenorrhea method. Eur J Contracept Reprod Health Care 2(2):105–111. https://doi.org/10.3109/13625189709167463

Westley E, Kapp N, Palermo T, Bleck J (2013) A review of global access to emergency contraception. Int J Gynaecol Obstet 123(1):4–6. https://doi.org/10.1016/j.ijgo.2013.04.019

Williamson LM, Parkes A, Wight D, Petticrew M, Hart GJ (2009) Limits to modern contraceptive use among young women in developing countries: a systematic review of qualitative research. Reprod Health 6:3. https://doi.org/10.1186/1742-4755-6-3

Wolff H, Epiney M, Lourenco AP, Costanza MC, Delieutraz-Marchand J, Andreoli N, Dubuisson JB, Gaspoz JM, Irion O (2008) Undocumented migrants lack access to pregnancy care and prevention. BMC Public Health 8:93. https://doi.org/10.1186/1471-2458-8-93

Global Climate Change and Women's Health

4

Bhargavi Chekuri, Natasha Sood, Cecilia Sorensen and Maryam En-Nosse

Contents

B. Chekuri
Department of Family Medicine, University of Colorado School of Medicine, Aurora, Colorado, USA
e-mail: Bhargavi.chekuri@cuanschutz.edu

N. Sood
Pennsylvania State University College of Medicine, Columbia University, Hershey, USA
e-mail: nsood@pennstatehealth.psu.edu

C. Sorensen
Mailman School of Public Health, Columbia University, New York, USA
e-mail: cjs2282@cumc.columbia.edu

M. En-Nosse (✉)
Oberärztin Klinik für Gynäkologie und Geburtshilfe, Universitätsklinikum Gießen und Marburg, Gießen, Germany
e-mail: maryam.en-nosse@uk-gm.de

J. Wacker et al. (eds.), *Global Women's Health*,
https://doi.org/10.1007/978-3-662-69700-9_4

Introductory Questions

1. For which groups does climate change worsen the current global health outcomes?
   A. Non-pregnant women
   B. Sexual and gender minorities
   C. Pregnant women
   D. Men
   E. All of the above groups
2. Which of the following factors is the most important in driving gender-specific health differences that are exacerbated by climate change?
   A. Pregnancy status
   B. Geographical location
   C. Gender inequality
   D. Exposure to heat
   E. Stress from climate-related disasters
3. Which of the following climate action strategies help to reduce gender-based health differences?
   A. Collection of gender-disaggregated data
   B. Promotion of gender equality
   C. Gender-specific policy
   D. Gender mainstreaming
   E. All of the above

4.1 Introduction

climate change exacerbates current global health inequalities, and gender-specific impacts are increasingly recognized as needing more understanding and attention. This chapter deals with gender-specific differences in the health impacts of climate change, as well as with indications of adaptation and mitigation measures that can promote and protect the health of women and sexual and gender minorities (SGM). These groups are disproportionately affected by the health risks of climate change due to a combination of direct and indirect exposures, reflecting differences in health needs as well as differences in behaviors, social and cultural constructs. For example, women have unique reproductive health needs and are also more likely to live in poverty, making them vulnerable to climate-related health risks such as floods, extreme weather events, heat-related diseases, droughts, and changing infectious diseases. This is particularly true for low and middle income countries (LMIC), where gender disparities are the widest (WHO 2014). There are large, unacceptable research gaps regarding the impacts of climate change on SGM, who may be particularly at risk due to additional issues such as discrimination worldwide (Goldsmith et al. 2021; Van Daalen et al. 2020). Although climate change, poverty, and gender inequality are complex global problems that can compound each other, leveraging the unique abilities and social roles of women and SGM offers significant opportunities for adapting to climate change and climate protection (UNFCCC 2015). Integrating gender-diverse perspectives into climate protection measures and programs helps to eliminate existing disparities and also offers more cost-effective, sustainable climate protection plans that promote increased political and social cooperation (Burns et al. 2017; Cook et al. 2019; UNFCCC 2015).

4.1.1 Definitions

Biological Sex refers to the biological characteristics that define people as female or male.

Gender refers to the socially constructed characteristics, norms, roles, and behaviors attributed to women, men, girls, boys, and non-binary people. Since gender is a social construct, ideas about it vary across societies and over time (WHO n.d.).

Sexual and gender minorities (SGM), broadly refers to population groups whose sexual orientation and/or gender identity as well as reproductive development lies outside cultural, societal, or physiological norms (NIH n.d.; O'Malley and Holzinger 2018; Rushton et al. 2019).

Gender equality refers to the equal rights, responsibilities, and opportunities of all genders (U N Women n.d.; UNDP 2015).

Gender responsiveness refers to outcomes and efforts to promote equal participation as well as an equitable and fair distribution of benefits, reflecting an understanding of gender roles and inequalities (UNDP 2015).

Gender mainstreaming is defined by the United Nations as "the process of assessing the implications for women and men of any planned action, including legislation, policies or programmes, in all areas and at all levels. It is a strategy for making women's as well as men's concerns and experiences an integral dimension of the design, implementation, monitoring and evaluation of policies and programmes in all political, economic and societal spheres so that women and men benefit equally and inequality is not perpetuated. The ultimate goal is to achieve gender equality." (U N Women n.d.; UNDP 2015).

4.2 Impacts of Climate Change on the Health of Women

4.2.1 General

Global climate change affects health through multiple exposure pathways, including degraded air quality, altered patterns of vector-borne diseases(VBD), extreme weather events, wildfires, and droughts. These exposure pathways exacerbate existing physiological, cultural, and socioeconomic vulnerabilities and disproportionately affect the health of women around the world. While both men and women are susceptible to the health impacts of climate change, women's distinct health needs, such as nutritional needs during pregnancy, places them at increased risk of suffering from climate-related events. In addition, women are more affected by poverty, which further increases their risk for climate-related exposures. In 2015, 736 million people worldwide lived in extreme poverty, with the largest gender gap in *LMIC* and among women of reproductive age (World Bank 2018). It is expected that climate change will push an additional 32 to 132 million people into extreme poverty by 2030 (Jafino et al. 2020). A lack of data on the nuances of climate impacts on women leads to a lack of awareness of their specific needs and responses under these circumstances (Sorensen et al. 2018). Measuring the disease burden from climate-sensitive events is crucial to provide more resources for climate protection and adaptation services for women (Chersich et al. 2020). To protect women's health in our changing climate, it is crucial that local, national, and even global decision-makers and healthcare workers advocate for gender-responsive solutions (U N Women n.d.).

4.2.2 Extreme Temperatures

Human-induced climate change is caused by the burning of fossil fuels, which has led to an unprecedented increase in the CO_2 concentration in the atmosphere, now exceeding 410 parts per million(ppm) (IPCC 2021a). The increase in CO_2 concentration has led to a warming of the Earth's surface by 1.1°C compared to pre-industrial times and an increase in the frequency and intensity of extreme heat events (IPCC 2021b). Extreme heat events lead to a variety of health harms, many of which disproportionately affect women, ultimately leading to an increase in their morbidity and mortality in the context of these events (Van Steen et al. 2019)

During heatwaves, women have a higher risk of death, primarily due to indirect effects related to unequal resource distribution. With the exception of reproductive outcomes, global variability in health of women exposed to extreme heat suggests that health inequalities are more associated with differences in underlying social and cultural norms and gender equality than with physiological differences between the sexes (Global Gender and Climate Alliance 2016; "Mapped" 2020). Some ways in which social and cultural norms can impact gendered health outcomes of individuals exposed to extreme heat have been described. For example, if women are isolated due to social and cultural norms during extreme heat events, they may have a higher mortality rate than men (Sorensen et al. 2018).

The effects of high temperatures during pregnancy are particularly harmful, as heat exposure can lead to numerous acute and subacute negative consequences, such as preterm birth (Kuehn and Cormick 2017), congenital malformations, pregnancy-induced hypertension and preeclampsia, low birth weight, and peripartum bleeding (Chersich et al. 2020; Cil and Cameron 2017). There may also be a lag between heat exposure in pregnancy and adverse outcomes that can range from months to years and decades (Chersich et al. 2020).

Heat can increase the risk of heat-related morbidity and mortality in pregnant women through the following mechanisms:

- Physiological and anatomical changes related to pregnancy limit the ability to thermoregulate and increase susceptibility to dehydration, maternal heat illnesses, and premature labor (Bekkar et al. 2020; Chersich et al. 2020; Roos et al. 2021)
- Hormonal changes increase the production of vasoactive substances that influence blood pressure, increase blood viscosity, and impair endothelial cell function. This alters blood flow in the placenta and can increase propensity for hypertensive crises and stillbirths (Ha et al. 2017a).
- Additional exposure to excessive heat can reduce blood flow in the uterus, further impairing the exchange between placenta and fetus and fetal growth (Ha et al. 2017c).
- As pregnancy progresses, internal heat production rises with fetal and placental metabolism; at the same time, increased body mass requires additional external cooling measures (Chersich et al. 2020)
- Hyperthermia is teratogenic and disrupts the normal sequence of gene activity during organogenesis (Van Zutphen et al. 2012). This can lead to early fetal death and neural tube defects (Auger et al. 2017).

Elevated temperatures can also lead to premature rupture of membranes (Ha et al. 2018), decreased amniotic fluid volume (Bekkar et al. 2020) or placental abruption (He et al. 2018). Studies have shown that the odds of preterm birth during heatwaves is increased by 1.16 fold (95% confidence interval 1.10 to 1.23) (Chersich et al. 2020). Higher ambient temperatures have also been associated with increased rates of Group B Streptococcus colonization and cardiovascular events in pregnant women (Dadvand et al. 2011; Ha et al. 2017b). Pregnant women with risk factors such as young age, gestational hypertension, and gestational diabetes are at increased risk for heat-related illnesses (Basu et al. 2017). As a result of these health risks, pregnant women are more frequently admitted to the emergency room during heatwaves (Davis and Novicoff 2018).

Extreme heat exposure in the last weeks of pregnancy appears to have the greatest significance for preterm births and stillbirths (Chersich et al. 2020). Some evidence suggests that pregnant women in LMIC are exposed to extreme heat throughout pregnancy, due to poor access to cooling centers and other heat reduction measures. In high-income countries (HIC), susceptibility to heat may be most pronounced in the last weeks of pregnancy. (Chersich et al. 2020).

The association between heat and adverse pregnancy outcomes is particularly pronounced in LMIC where there are already high rates of preterm births (Chawanpaiboon et al. 2019).

Lower socioeconomic status increases the relative risk of a heat-related preterm birth worldwide, and in HIC, racial and ethnic disparities have a similar, amplifying effect (Basu et al. 2017; Chersich et al. 2020). This may be stem from historical disparities in occupational settings, housing, and other manifestations of marginalization due to systemic racism (Cushing et al. 2022).

External factors such as limited access to shade, especially in urban areas (Cushing et al. 2022), cooling, and barriers to healthcare access, exacerbatewomen's susceptibility to heat-related illness. Furthermore, women in LMIC, who often continue to do the majority of household chores during pregnancy (e.g., wood and water procurement, farming), may be exposed to extreme heat for extended periods (Chersich et al. 2020). Exposure to extreme heat during agricultural or other outdoor work may occur even before pregnancy is confirmed. Late in pregnancy, women may work beyond their heat tolerance limits to avoid wage losses (Flocks et al. 2013).

Extreme heat has significant impacts on the health of women and can be particularly harmful during pregnancy. Associations between socioeconomic status, structural racism, and heat-related illnesses during pregnancy are strongest.

4.2.3 Climate-related Disasters and Forced Migration

Climate-related disasters, including hurricanes, wildfires, droughts, and floods, have increased fivefold since 1970 (Zhongming and Wei 2021). From 2017 to 2019, the number of people affected by natural disasters rose from 129 million to 134 million, and a quarter of those affected were women of reproductive age (UNOCHA 2017). Preparedness plans that specifically address the needs of women in disaster and emergency situations are underdeveloped, yet women are disproportionately affected in both resource-poor and resource-rich environments (Sorensen et al. 2018).

Globally, women suffer disproportionately from disasters, and female survivors have a lower life expectancy than males (Erman et al. 2021). Gender disparities in disasters are directly related to gender inequality and socioeconomic status (Neumayer and Plümper 2007). In LMIC, more women die from extreme disasters than in HIC (WHO 2002), due to limited mobility and access to information about disaster preparedness and public emergency shelters (Erman et al. 2021). These factors are further exacerbated by health status, literacy level, communication barriers in language or dialect, economic status, and caregiving responsibilities, which compromise their ability to evacuate during a disaster (Global Gender and Climate Alliance 2016; Moosa and Tuana 2014).

After a disaster, nutritional deficiencies in women can lead to worse outcomes and increased vulnerability (Raham 2013). Pregnant women who give birth in post-disaster settings are at greater risk of complications such as preeclampsia and low birth weight (Tong et al. 2011). Damaged facilities result in compromised prenatal and peripartum care (Harville et al. 2009). Cultural and social norms, as well as beliefs related to menstruation are associated with health problems such as genitourinary infections due to lack of sanitary facilities (WHO 2002).

More than half, i.e., 21 million, of the internally displaced persons at the end of 2018 were women and girls, and the majority were from LMIC (Cazabat 2020; UNHCR 2021). Forced migration and repeated short distance relocations are especially significant for women's health, as they disrupt social support systems and family networks (WHO 2002). This is further exacerbated by low socioeconomic status. Moreover, women may not be able to migrate to areas with better economic living conditions, and those who do migrate are faced with caregiving burdens during transit or in unfamiliar new environments (Lemery et al. 2021). Women are also typically excluded from post-disaster workforces and suffer from stagnated economic recoveries (Sorensen et al. 2018). This is physiologically and psychologically stressful, leading to poor health outcomes, which are further exacerbated by the lack of health services, housing, and sanitary facilities during migration (Sorensen et al. 2018).

After climate-related disasters, girls, women and SGM are at higher risk of sexual violence, sexual exploitation, physical and sexual abuse, human trafficking, as well as a higher risk of domestic violence and intimate partner violence (IFRC 2007; Velasco and Dupar 2021). Women and girls may be forced into transactional sex in exchange for basic needs, food, shelter, and security (WHO 2002). As a result, women are at increased risk of contracting HIV, especially in resource-limited areas, and may be unable to access usual medications, resulting in serious HIV complications (Joshi et al. 2020). Women may also have limited access to contraception (Ellington et al. 2013) andsafe family planning services when clinics are impaired (Joshi et al. 2020; Leyser-Whalen et al. 2020). Lastly, women are more likely to experience mental health issues such as depression, anxiety, and post-traumatic stress disorder after climate-related disasters, especially women with low social support (McGuire et al. 2018).

4.2.4 Food Insecurity

Food security is achieved when a person has physical and economic access to sufficient, safe, and nutritious food that meets the requirements of a healthy life (FAO 2019). Though LMIC carry the global burden of malnutrition and food insecurity, it is important for the health and well-being of people in both HIC and LMIC (FAO 2011).

Although women are significant contributors to local and global food security—producing half of the world's food—they are among the most food insecure (Visser and Wangu 2021). The COVID-19 pandemic has dramatically increased acute food insecurity in 2020 - 2021 (Visser and Wangu 2021). Currently, 60% of the chronically hungry people in the world are women and girls (Visser and

Wangu 2021) and they are at risk in all aspects of food security: availability, access, use, and stability (OXFAM 2019). Whilewomen play a crucial role in food production and household food security (through unpaid work on family farms,in domestic care, and through paid housework), less than 13% of agricultural land is owned by women, due to sociopolitical, discriminatory policies and practices regarding land ownership (UN 2020; UNDP 2016). This results in women being excluded from agricultural contracts, land ownership, access to technology, and financial incentives (FAO 2011). Further, entrenched gender norms limit women's opportunities in agriculture, as well as in decision-making regarding resources, household income and expenditure, and access to financial credit (Visser and Wangu 2021).

Global climate change threatens to exacerbate existing inequities in food and nutrition security, as it fuels rising temperatures and shifting precipitation patterns, impairing crop, livestock, and fishery yields (Lemery et al. 2021). Worldwide, women suffer from higher rates of anemia and malnutrition and are especially sensitive to climate-driven food insecurity due to increased nutrient needs during menstruation, pregnancy, and breastfeeding. Food insecurity has been associated with lower intake of micronutrients in women (Ivers and Cullen 2011). Food insecurity can be exacerbated by cultural practices that prioritize feeding men and children over women, worsening in anemia in women (FAO 2019). Anemia is associated with cognitive and physical impairments, chronic fatigue, depressed mood, adverse cardiovascular outcomes, and increased maternal morbidity and mortality (Benson et al. 2021). Poor pregnancy outcomes related to food insecurity can be attributed to increased nutrient needs, difficulties in food preparation, and the need for pregnant women to retire from work, leading to financial strain (Laraia et al. 2006).

Women make up more than 40% of the agricultural workforce worldwide in LMIC, making food scarcity both a health and an economic issue. As climatic conditions negatively impact agricultural yields, women's access to food and economic prosperity is further diminished (FAO 2011). Women in LMIC and rural areas also face gender-specific mobility restrictions (Diiro et al. 2018), increasing their reliance on men for food procurement. Women exposed to persistent food insecurity are more likely to experience domestic violence and be forced to participate in transactional sex (Miller et al. 2011; Weiser et al. 2007). Limited access to education about nutrition further exacerbates food insecurity in women (Visser and Wangu 2021).

Women are particularly vulnerable to food insecurity due to gender-specific cultural norms, especially in LMIC. Addressing these barriers is crucial for understanding the health challenges that food insecurity poses for women and provides a basis for creating resilient food systems.

4.2.5 Uncertain Water Supply and Wastewater Disposal

In LMIC, women and girls bear the primary responsibility for managing household water supply and sanitation, *Water Sanitation Hygiene* (WASH) (UN 2021b). Freshwater resources are strained globally, with areas of increasing scarcity near areas of large population density. Up to 1.7 billion people currently lack access to an adequate freshwater supply (UN 2021a), resulting in a large global burden of disease from unsafe water, poor sanitation, and limited hygiene (WRI 2019). As the number of people living in water-stressed areas increases, its scarcity leads to myriad of effects.

It is estimated that a family of five needs 100 liters of water per day, weighing 100 kg (WHO 2014). Women are largely responsible for the procurement and use of water in the household, with mean travel times for fetching water as high as 54 minutes (Holvoet et al. 2016). In some regions, fetching water can consume up to 85% of a woman's daily energy intake (Duncan 2006). As water availability changes, women may be forced to fetch water from geographically and biologically more dangerous sources. Women face increased risk of abuse or attack in water transportation or sanitation needs as women often empty sanitation buckets at night increasing the threat of violence of sexual assault (UN 2021b; Winter et al. 2019).

The term water security consists of four domains: availability, access, use, and stability of access over time (Young et al. 2021). Water insecurity occurs when barriers arise in any of these areas. Women are particularly susceptible to the lack of a safe and sufficient water supply, as they bear the time-consuming responsibility of searching for and transporting water, leaving them less time for other activities such as livelihood procurement, education, and other tasks (UN 2021b; Shiva and Jalees 2005). This simultaneously increases their exposure to environmental stressors such as heat-related diseases or dehydration, which is particularly harmful during pregnancy (Kuehn and McCormick 2017). As primary water purveyors, women are at increased risk of musculoskeletal trauma (Geere et al. 2018). Further, limited material and financial access to resources for menstrual hygiene hygeine management and pregnancy needs may force women and girls to refrain from practicing hygiene for fear of violence, assault, or stigmatization (Winter et al. 2019). Globally, poor WASH practices increase the risk of waterborne diseases (e.g., cholera, bacterial infections) (Mahamud et al. 2012). Dependence on biologically contaminated water can lead to both the transmission of diseases and the direct toxin ingestion (Duncan 2006), which is exacerbated by water scarcity. Cultural restrictions that prioritize the needs of men and children put women at even greatest risk from the sequelae of water shortages (Lemery et al. 2021).

Globally, economic access to water can be restricted by poverty, caste, restrictions on women being unaccompanied outside the home, , or other socio-political processes (Young et al. 2021). In North America water insecurity is predominantly experienced by Black, Indigenous and people of color (BIPOC) (Meehan et al. 2020; Young et al. 2021).

Women are disproportionately burdened by poor access to WASH, which is reflected in a disproportionately high health burden for women. More needs to be done to understand the intersectionality between water and gender, as eliminating the WASH inequalities is a crucial factor in achieving gender and health justice in the 21st century.

4.2.6 Infectious Diseases and Vector-Borne Diseases

Infectious diseases and VBD present a heavy burden to LMIC, though HIC are still at risk. Rising global temperatures and altered precipitation patterns are changing the geographical distribution of vectors that transmit human diseases. VBD can be transmitted to humans by arthropods such as mosquitoes, ticks, and fleas. The prevalence of VBD such as malaria, Lyme disease, Dengue virus, and Zika virus is increasing and spreading to new geographical areas.

Women are disproportionately susceptible to VBD for a variety of physiologic and cultural reasons. As women are primarily responsible for water collection, they often spend more time near standing water sources and other areas that can place them in close contact with mosquito breeding sites (Gunn et al. 2018). Pregnant women are particularly susceptible to mosquito-borne diseases as they produce more CO_2 during pregnancy (CO_2 is a chemo-attractant for mosquitoes) and peripheral blood flow is increased in pregnancy, making them more prone to mosquito bites (Lindsay et al. 2000; Mbonye et al. 2006).

Once infected, pregnant women are at greaterrisk of complications and severe illness from a variety of diseases such as malaria, Zika, and Dengue fever. Pregnant women have a higher risk of severe malaria than infected non-pregnant women (O'Kelly and Lambert 2020), and the development of Dengue hemorrhagic fever is 3.4 times higher in pregnancy (Machado et al. 2013). Dengue virus infections during pregnancy are also associated with an increased risk of intrauterine growth disorders, eclampsia, cesarean delivery, and postpartum hemorrhage.

Hormonally induced changes in the immune system lead to a higher intensity of parasitemia when infected with malaria in pregnancy (Lindsay et al. 2000; Mbonye et al. 2006). Zika virus, which has devastating fetal effects including microcephaly, central nervous system malformations, and impaired cognitive development (Petersen et al. 2016), has recently increased in prevalence. Maternal infection during pregnancy can lead to acute rash, fever, and myalgia and rarely to neurological complications such as Guillain-Barré syndrome. (Pomar et al. 2019). Limited or completely absent access to prenatal and obstetric care further worsens pregnancy and birth outcomes in this setting.

The impacts of extreme heat, air pollution, extreme weather conditions (e.g., disasters, forced migration), and vector-borne diseases on women are summarized in Fig. 4.1.

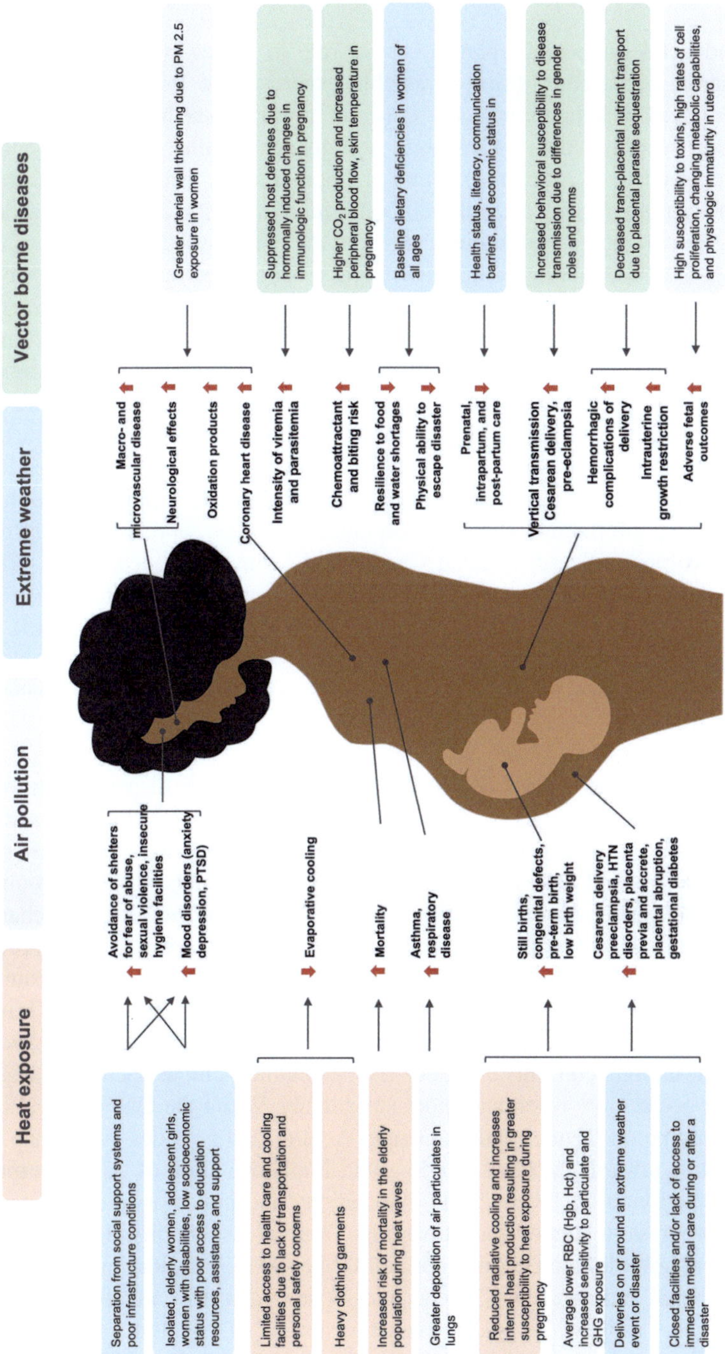

Fig. 4.1 Impacts of climate change on women's health by exposure pathways. (Created by: Natasha Sood, MPH, Emily Sbriolo, MD, Celilica Soerensen, MD)

4.3 The Role of Gender in Climate Policy and Planning

Women and gender-minorities play a crucial role in mitigating and adapting to climate change becausethey bring invaluable expertise and leadership necessary to make progress with interconnected issues of poverty, health disparities, water security, food security, energy transitions, and gender equality. Including gender-minority perspectives in all climate action policies, through gender mainstreaming is critical for improving health and well-being in communities around the world. Improving the current state of knowledge about the gender-specific impacts of climate change and conducting comprehensive assessments of the strengths, weaknesses, opportunities, and threats to women and other minorities is a fundamental step to make progress. When women are included in the development of climate solutions and empowered to take leadership positions, gender equality improves and the effectiveness of climate-related projects and measures increases (Cook et al. 2019). Some studies have shown, for example, that countries with more women in leadership positions have a smaller national carbon footprint or more protected land areas (Global Gender and Climate Alliance 2016). Likewise, companies are more likely to disclose information about carbon emissions when more women are represented on corporate boards (Global Gender and Climate Alliance 2016). When women are not involved in these processes, climate action plans are often less effective and existing gender gaps worsen (Buckingham et al. 2005; UNFCCC 2015).

4.4 Summary

Global climate change exacerbates current gendered health disparities through a variety of exposure pathways. These diferences are primarily due to existing social, economic, cultural, and political gendered inequalities. Pregnancy and other reproductive and sexual health needs add additional burdens for women and sexual and gender minorities. The evidence base about how climate change impacts women, as well as how women's exper-tise can be leveraged to improve health outcomes and climate action must be strengthened. Gender mainstreaming is the policy decided by the United Nations Framework Convention on Climate Change (UNFCCC) and other international bodies to improve gender-gaps in health. When nations commit to gender mainstreaming, climate action has been shown to be occur more often and more sustainably. While the UNFCCC's Lima Work Programme on Gender and its Gender Action Plan provides a roadmap for nations to shift towards capacity building and implementation of gender-responsive climate action at all levels, it lacks specificity and indicators and targets for measuring progress in gender mainstreaming. There is also an urgent need to better understand how climate change impacts SGM as well as explore more complex multidimensional and non-binary social intersections that drive communities' climate responses. Lastly, while gender mainstreaming is an essential way to achieve gender equality, progress is stymied if nations continue to make slow progress in limiting global warming to 1.5 degrees.

Answers to the Initial Questions

1. E. All of the above. Global climate change worsens health outcomes for men, women and sexual and gender minorities. Climate change also exacerbates existing gender health disparities.
2. C. Gender equality. Gender inequality is the reason for the existing gender-specific global health differences, which are further exacerbated by the climate change.
3. E. All of the above.

References

Auger N, Fraser WD, Arbour L, Bilodeau-Bertrand M, Kosatsky T (2017) Elevated ambient temperatures and risk of neural tube defects. Occup Environ Med 74(5):315–320. https://doi.org/10.1136/oemed-2016-103956

Basu R, Chen H, Li DK, Avalos LA (2017) The impact of maternal factors on the association between temperature and preterm delivery. Environ Res 154:109–114. https://doi.org/10.1016/j.envres.2016.12.017

Bekkar B, Pacheco S, Basu R, DeNicola N (2020) Association of air pollution and heat exposure with preterm birth, low birth weight, and stillbirth in the US: a systematic review. JAMA Netw Open 3(6):e208243. https://doi.org/10.1001/jamanetworkopen.2020.8243

Benson CS, Shah A, Stanworth SJ, Frise CJ, Spiby H, Lax SJ, Murray J, Klein AA (2021) The effect of iron deficiency and anaemia on women's health. Anaesthesia 76:84–95. https://doi.org/10.1111/anae.15405

Buckingham S, Reeves D, Batchelor A (2005) Wasting women: the environmental justice of including women in municipal waste management. Local Environ 10(4):427–444. https://doi.org/10.1080/13549830500160974

Burns B, Sharma A, Hall L, Zhou V, Garma, S (2017) Pocket guide to gender equality under the UNFCCC. European Capacity Building Initiative

Cazabat C (2020) Hidden in plain sight. I. Displacement. https://www.internal-displacement.org/sites/default/files/publications/documents/202003-twice-invisible-internally-displaced-women.pdf

Chawanpaiboon S, Vogel JP, Moller AB, Lumbiganon P, Petzold M, Hogan D, Landoulsi S, Jampathong N, Kongwattanakul K, Laopaiboon M, Lewis C, Rattanakanokchai S, Teng DN, Thinkhamrop J, Watananirun K, Zhang J, Zhou W, Gülmezoglu AM (2019) Global, regional, and national estimates of levels of preterm birth in 2014: a systematic review and modelling analysis. Lancet Glob Health 7(1):e37–e46. https://doi.org/10.1016/S2214-109X(18)30451-0

Chersich MF, Pham MD, Areal A, Haghighi MM, Manyuchi A, Swift CP, Wernecke B, Robinson M, Hetem R, Boeckmann M, Hajat S, Climate C, Heat-Health Study, G (2020) Associations between high temperatures in pregnancy and risk of preterm birth, low birth weight, and stillbirths: systematic review and meta-analysis. BMJ (Clinical research ed.) 371:m3811. https://doi.org/10.1136/bmj.m3811

Cil G, Cameron TA (2017) Potential climate change health risks from increases in heat waves: abnormal birth outcomes and adverse maternal health conditions. Risk Anal 37(11):2066–2079. https://doi.org/10.1111/risa.12767

Cook NJ, Grillos T, Andersson KP (2019) Gender quotas increase the equality and effectiveness of climate policy interventions. Nat Clim Chang 9(4):330–334. https://doi.org/10.1038/s41558-019-0438-4

Cushing L, Morello-Frosch R, Hubbard A (2022) Extreme heat and its association with social disparities in the risk of spontaneous preterm birth. Paediatr Perinat Epidemiol 36(1):13–22. https://doi.org/10.1111/ppe.12834

Dadvand P, Basagana X, Figueras F, Sunyer J, Nieuwenhuijsen MJ (2011) Climate and group B streptococci colonisation during pregnancy: present implications and future concerns. BJOG 118(11):1396–1400. https://doi.org/10.1111/j.1471-0528.2011.03044.x

Davis RE, Novicoff WM (2018) The impact of heat waves on emergency department admissions in Charlottesville, Virginia, U.S.A. Int J Environ Res Public Health 15(7). https://doi.org/10.3390/ijerph15071436

Diiro GM, Seymour G, Kassie M, Muricho G, Muriithi BW (2018) Women's empowerment in agriculture and agricultural productivity: evidence from rural maize farmer households in western Kenya. PLoS One 13(5):e0197995. https://doi.org/10.1371/journal.pone.0197995

Duncan K (2006) Global climate change, air pollution, and women's health. WIT Transactions on Ecology and the Environment Bandnummer: Vol. 99, Seitenzahlen: S. 633–643

Ellington SR, Kourtis AP, Curtis KM, Tepper N, Gorman S, Jamieson DJ, Zotti M, Barfield W (2013) Contraceptive availability during an emergency response in the United States. J Women Health (2002) 22(3):189–193. https://doi.org/10.1089/jwh.2012.4178

Erman A, De Vries Robbé SA, Fabian Thies S, Kabir K, Maruo M (2021) Gender dimensions of disaster risk and resilience: existing evidence. World Bank, Washington, DC

FAO (2011) The state of food and agriculture 2010–2011, women in agriculture: closing the gender gap for development. F. a. A. Association, Rome

FAO (2019) The state of food security and nutrition in the world. The state of food. Food and Agriculture Organization. http://www.fao.org/state-of-food-security-nutrition/en/

Flocks J, Thien Mac V, Runkle J, Tovar-Aguilar JA, Economos J, McCauley LA (2013) Female farmworkers' perceptions of heat-related illness and pregnancy health. J Agromedicine 18(4):350–358. https://doi.org/10.1080/1059924X.2013.826607

Geere JA, Bartram J, Bates L, Danquah L, Evans B, Fisher MB, Groce N, Majuru B, Mokoena MM, Mukhola MS, Nguyen-Viet H, Duc PP, Williams AR, Schmidt WP, Hunter PR (2018) Carrying water may be a major contributor to disability from musculoskeletal disorders in low income countries: a cross-sectional survey in South Africa, Ghana and Vietnam. J Glob Health 8(1):010406. https://doi.org/10.7189/jogh.08.010406

Global Gender and Climate Alliance (2016) Gender and climate change: a closer look at existing evidence. Global Gender and Climate Alliance, New York. https://wedo.org/wp-content/uploads/2016/11/GGCA-RP-FINAL.pdf

Goldsmith L, Raditz V, Méndez M (2021) Queer and present danger: understanding the disparate impacts of disasters on LGBTQ + Communities. Disasters. https://doi.org/10.1111/disa.12509

Gunn JKL, Ernst KC, Center KE, Bischoff K, Nunez AV, Huynh M, Okello A, Hayden MH (2018) Current strategies and successes in engaging women in vector control: a systematic review. BMJ Glob Health 3(1):e000366. https://doi.org/10.1136/bmjgh-2017-000366

Ha S, Liu D, Zhu Y, Soo Kim S, Sherman S, Grantz KL, Mendola P (2017a) Ambient temperature and stillbirth: a multi-center retrospective cohort study. Environ Health Perspect 125(6):067011. https://doi.org/10.1289/EHP945

Ha S, Nguyen K, Liu D, Männistö T, Nobles C, Sherman S, Mendola P (2017b) Ambient temperature and risk of cardiovascular events at labor and delivery: a case-crossover study. Environ Res 159:622–628. https://doi.org/10.1016/j.envres.2017.09.010

Ha S, Zhu Y, Liu D, Sherman S, Mendola P (2017c) Ambient temperature and air quality in relation to small for gestational age and term low birthweight. Environ Res 155:394–400. https://doi.org/10.1016/j.envres.2017.02.021

Ha S, Liu D, Zhu Y, Sherman S, Mendola P (2018) Acute associations between outdoor temperature and premature rupture of membranes. Epidemiology 29(2):175–182. https://doi.org/10.1097/EDE.0000000000000779

Harville EW, Xiong X, Buekens P (2009) Hurricane Katrina and perinatal health. Birth 36(4):325–331. https://doi.org/10.1111/j.1523 536X.2009.00360.x

He S, Kosatsky T, Smargiassi A, Bilodeau-Bertrand M, Auger N (2018) Heat and pregnancy-related emergencies: risk of placental abruption during hot weather. Environ Int 111:295–300. https://doi.org/10.1016/j.envint.2017.11.004

Holvoet N, Dewachter S, Molenaers N (2016) Look who's talking. Explaining water-related information sharing and demand for action among Ugandan villagers. Environ Manage 58(5):780–796. https://doi.org/10.1007/s00267-016-0760-9

IFRC (2007). World disasters report 2007: focus on discrimination. I. F. o. t. R. Cross. https://www.ifrc.org/document/world-disasters-report-2007-focus-discrimination

IPCC (2021a) IPCC sixth assessment technical report AR6 climate change 2021: the physical science basis. I. P. o. C. Change

IPCC (2021b) IPCC special report

Ivers LC, Cullen KA (2011) Food insecurity: special considerations for women. Am J Clin Nutr 94(6):1740S–1744S. https://doi.org/10.3945/ajcn.111.012617

Jafino BA, Walsh B, Rozenberg J, Hallegatte S (2020) Revised estimates of the impact of climate change on extreme poverty by 2030. W. B. Group,

Joshi R, Andersen PT, Thapa S, Aro AR (2020) Sex trafficking, prostitution, and increased HIV risk among women during and after the 2015 Nepal earthquake. SAGE Open Med 8:2050312120938287. https://doi.org/10.1177/2050312120938287

Kuehn L, McCormick S (2017) Heat exposure and maternal health in the face of climate change. Int J Environ Res Public Health 14(8). https://doi.org/10.3390/ijerph14080853

Laraia BA, Siega-Riz AM, Gundersen C, Dole N (2006) Psychosocial factors and socioeconomic indicators are associated with household food insecurity among pregnant women. J Nutr 136(1):177–182. https://doi.org/10.1093/jn/136.1.177

Lemery J, Knowlton K, Sorensen C (2021) Global climate change and human health: from science to practice. John Wiley & Sons,

Leyser-Whalen O, Chaleshtori SZ, Monteblanco A (2020) Another disaster: access to abortion after Hurricane Harvey. Health Care Women Int 41(10):1111–1127. https://doi.org/10.1080/07399332.2020.1833883

Lindsay S, Ansell J, Selman C, Cox V, Hamilton K, Walraven G (2000) Effect of pregnancy on exposure to malaria mosquitoes. Lancet 355(9219):1972. https://doi.org/10.1016/S0140-6736(00)02334-5

Machado CR, Machado ES, Rohloff RD, Azevedo M, Campos DP, de Oliveira RB, Brasil P (2013) Is pregnancy associated with severe dengue? A review of data from the Rio de Janeiro surveillance information system. PLoS Negl Trop Dis 7(5):e2217. https://doi.org/10.1371/journal.pntd.0002217

Mahamud AS, Ahmed JA, Nyoka R, Auko E, Kahi V, Ndirangu J, Nguhi M, Burton JW, Muhindo BZ, Breiman RF, Eidex RB (2012) Epidemic cholera in Kakuma Refugee Camp, Kenya, 2009: the importance of sanitation and soap. J Infect Dev Ctries 6(3):234–241. https://doi.org/10.3855/jidc.1966

Mapped: How Climate Change Disproportionately Affects Women's Health (2020) Carbon brief. https://www.carbonbrief.org/mapped-how-climate-change-disproportionately-affects-womens-health

Mbonye AK, Neema S, Magnussen P (2006) Preventing malaria in pregnancy: a study of perceptions and policy implications in Mukono district, Uganda. Health Policy Plan 21(1):17–26. https://doi.org/10.1093/heapol/czj002

McGuire AP, Gauthier JM, Anderson LM, Hollingsworth DW, Tracy M, Galea S, Coffey SF (2018) Social support moderates effects of natural disaster exposure on depression and post-traumatic stress disorder symptoms: effects for displaced and nondisplaced residents. Journal of Traumatic Stress 31(2):223–233. https://doi.org/10.1002/jts.22270

Meehan K, Jurjevich JR, Chun NMJW, Sherrill J (2020) Geographies of insecure water access and the housing-water nexus in US cities. Proc Natl Acad Sci U S A 117(46):28700–28707. https://doi.org/10.1073/pnas.2007361117

Miller CL, Bangsberg DR, Tuller DM, Senkungu J, Kawuma A, Frongillo EA, Weiser SD (2011) Food insecurity and sexual risk in an HIV endemic community in Uganda. AIDS Behav 15(7):1512–1519. https://doi.org/10.1007/s10461-010-9693-0
Moosa CS, Tuana N (2014) Mapping a research agenda concerning gender and climate change: a review of the literature. J Fem Philos. https://doi.org/10.1111/hypa.12085
Neumayer E, Plümper T (2007) The gendered nature of natural disasters: the impact of catastrophic events on the gender gap in life expectancy, 1981–2002. Ann Assoc Am Geogr 97(3):551–566. https://doi.org/10.1111/j.1467-8306.2007.00563.x
O'Malley J, Holzinger A (2018) Sexual and gender minorities and the sustainable development goals. United Nations Development Programme,
O'Kelly B, Lambert JS (2020) Vector-borne diseases in pregnancy. Ther Adv Infect Dis 7:2049936120941725. https://doi.org/10.1177/2049936120941725
OXFAM (2019) Gender inequalities and food insecurity: ten years after the food price crisis, why are women farmers still food-insecure?
Petersen LR, Jamieson DJ, Powers AM, Honein MA (2016) Zika Virus. N Engl J Med 374(16):1552–1563. https://doi.org/10.1056/NEJMra1602113
Pomar L, Musso D, Malinger G, Vouga M, Panchaud A, Baud D (2019) Zika virus during pregnancy: from maternal exposure to congenital Zika virus syndrome. Prenat Diagn 39(6):420–430. https://doi.org/10.1002/pd.5446
Raham S (2013) Climate change, disaster and gender vulnerability: a study on two divisions of Bangladesh. Am J Hum Ecol 2:72–82
Roos N, Kovats S, Hajat S, Filippi V, Chersich M, Luchters S, Scorgie F, Nakstad B, Stephansson O, Consortium C (2021) Maternal and newborn health risks of climate change: a call for awareness and global action. Acta Obstet Gynecol Scand 100(4):566–570. https://doi.org/10.1111/aogs.14124
Rushton A, Gray L, Canty J, Blanchard K (2019) Beyond binary: (re)defining „gender" for 21st century disaster risk reduction research, policy, and practice. Int J Environ Res Public Health 16(20):3984. https://doi.org/10.3390/ijerph16203984
Shiva V, Jalees K (2005) Water & women: a report by research foundation for science, technology, and ecology for National Commission for Women. Navdanya/RFSTE
Sorensen C, Murray V, Lemery J, Balbus J (2018) Climate change and women's health: Impacts and policy directions. PLoS Med 15(7):e1002603. https://doi.org/10.1371/journal.pmed.1002603
Tong VT, Zotti ME, Hsia J (2011) Impact of the Red River catastrophic flood on women giving birth in North Dakota, 1994-2000. Matern Child Health J 15(3):281–288. https://doi.org/10.1007/s10995-010-0576-9
UN (2020) Realizing womenis rights to land and other productive resources, 2. Aufl. United Nations. Office of the High Commissioner for Human Rights, New York and Geneva
UN (2021a) Goal 6: Ensure access to water and sanitation for all. United Nations Sustainable Development Goals. https://www.un.org/sustainabledevelopment/water-and-sanitation/
UN (2021b) Water and gender. United Nations. https://www.unwater.org/water-facts/gender/
UN OCHA (2017) Global humanitarian overview
UNDP (2015) Gender responsive national communications toolkit
UNDP (2016) Gender and climate change. Gender, climate change and food security. United Nations Development Programme
UNFCCC (2015) Implementation of gender-responsive climate action in the context of sustainable development: report of the expert group meeting. https://unfccc.int/files/gender_and_climate_change/application/pdf/egmreport.pdf
UNHCR (2021) Women. United Nations High Commissioner for Refugees. https://www.unhcr.org/en-us/women.html
Van Daalen K, Jung L, Dhatt R, Phelan AL (2020) Climate change and gender-based health disparities. Lancet Planet Health 4(2):e44–e45. https://doi.org/10.1016/s2542-5196(20)30001-2

Van Steen Y, Ntarladima AM, Grobbee R, Karssenberg D, Vaartjes I (2019) Sex differences in mortality after heat waves: are elderly women at higher risk? Int Arch Occup Environ Health 92(1):37–48. https://doi.org/10.1007/s00420-018-1360-1

Van Zutphen AR, Lin S, Fletcher BA, Hwang S-A (2012) A population-based case-control study of extreme summer temperature and birth defects. Environ Health Perspect 120(10):1443–1449. https://doi.org/10.1289/ehp.1104671

Velasco P, Dupar M (2021) Advancing gender equality and climate action: a practical guide to setting targets and monitoring progress. In: Climate and Development Knowledge Network (CDKN)

Visser J, Wangu J (2021) Women's dual centrality in food security solutions: the need for a stronger gender lens in food systems' transformation. Current Res Environ Sustain 3:100094. https://doi.org/10.1016/j.crsust.2021.100094

Weiser SD, Leiter K, Bangsberg DR, Butler LM, Percy-de Korte F, Hlanze Z, Phaladze N, Iacopino V, Heisler M (2007) Food insufficiency is associated with high-risk sexual behavior among women in Botswana and Swaziland. PLoS Med 4(10):1589–1597; ; discussion 1598. https://doi.org/10.1371/journal.pmed.0040260

WHO (2002) Gender and health in disasters. World Health Organization. https://apps.who.int/iris/handle/10665/68886

WHO (2014) Gender, climate change, and health. W. H. Organization. https://www.who.int/globalchange/GenderClimateChangeHealthfinal.pdf

Winter S, Dreibelbis R, Barchi F (2019) Women's sanitation practices in informal settlements: a multi-level analysis of factors influencing utilisation in Nairobi, Kenya. Glob Public Health 14(5):663–674. https://doi.org/10.1080/17441692.2018.1534256

World Bank (2018) Poverty and shared prosperity 2018: piecing together the poverty puzzle. World Bank,

WRI (2019) Updated global water risk atlas reveals top water-stressed countries and states. World Resources Institute. wri.org/news/release-updated-global-water-risk-atlas-reveals-top-water-stressed-countries-and-states. Zugegriffen am 25.03.2023

Young SL, Frongillo EA, Jamaluddine Z, Melgar-Quiñonez H, Pérez-Escamilla R, Ringler C, Rosinger AY (2021) Perspective: the importance of water security for ensuring food security, good nutrition, and well-being. Adv Nutr 12(4):1058–1073. https://doi.org/10.1093/advances/nmab003

Zhongming Z, Wei L (2021) Atlas of mortality and economic losses from weather, climate and water extremes (1970–2019)

Further reading

U N Women. (o. J.) OSAGI gender mainstreaming – concepts and definitions. https://www.un.org/womenwatch/osagi/conceptsandefinitions.htm

A Holistic View of Women's Health in a Rapidly Changing World

5

Detlev Ganten and Britta Rutert

Contents

5.1 Introduction—Women's Health in a Rapidly Changing World

The world is currently changing faster than ever. The COVID-19 pandemic, the war in Ukraine, wildfires in California or Brandenburg, floods and heavy rain in all parts of the world—hardly a day goes by without new threatening headlines in the media and their real effects on the entire world, individual states and communities. Health and lives of families and individuals, women, men and children are always directly affected. In almost all countries, women with their children bear the greatest danger and heaviest burden for body, life and health. Climate change, increasing environmental destruction in many ways and inhumane living conditions in cities and in the countryside, as well as recurring epidemics show that a

D. Ganten (✉) · B. Rutert
Berlin Brandenburgische Akademie der Wissenschaften (BBAW), Berlin, Germany
e-mail: detlev.ganten@virchow.foundation.de

B. Rutert
e-mail: Noreply@gmail.com

J. Wacker et al. (eds.), *Global Women's Health*,
https://doi.org/10.1007/978-3-662-69700-9_5

rethink must take place in order to secure the future of this planet and to enable humane living conditions.

The effects of the increasing local and global crises affect all spheres of life, from economy and politics to transport and mobility, to the health and education system. If health can no longer be offered as a reliable component of societal life, the various areas of societal functions can no longer act stably and the functionality of society and the individual is fundamentally endangered. Human health is only possible on a healthy planet, therefore it is necessary, in order to ensure the survival of subsequent generations, to anchor the topic of health holistically, holistically, more strongly in the consciousness and action of global politics. The health of women is always particularly at risk and particularly important in the care for children and the family. In particular, women of the global South are, as this book shows, often particularly vulnerable.

In this chapter, we deal with global health and especially with the role of women in a rapidly and ever faster changing world. Reference is made to the World Health Summit(WHS) in Berlin, which has committed itself in a special way to the implementation of the United Nations' (UN) Sustainable Development Goals (SDGs) in the sense of a holistic view of health. In order to better and more systematically deal with the complexity of the broad topic of global health, a "health formula" was developed and recently published (Ganten and Rutert "Restart! For the Future of our Health System" (2021), Niehaus and Ganten "The Health Formula" (2014)). This formula does not magically create health, but it helps to capture the complexity of this large area in a new systematics, to better understand and to approach specific points in order to contribute to an improvement of the situation, without losing sight of the holistic complexity. The Sustainability Goalsof the UN in connection with the health formula can thus help to view women's health from a holistic perspective, in which environment, biology and behavior play just as big a role as socio-economic inequalities. They can thus serve as a specific approach for interventions and for practical improvements.

5.2 Global Health and the World Health Summit

The World Health Summit(WHS) has been held annually in Berlin since 2009 and brings together up to 6000 delegates from around the world. The aim is to discuss developments and challenges in global health. The WHS is committed to a holistic view of health. This means that global health is seen here in an interdisciplinary interplay of science, politics, the private sector, and civil society, improvements are discussed, and the results are made accessible to all people.

The World Health Summit is organized by the Charité in Berlin and is integrated into the international, worldwide academic network of the "M8 Alliance" of over 30 academic health centers, universities, and all 130 academies of sciences and medicine worldwide. With the WHS Regional Meetings around the world, various symposia of experts, and the M8 Alliance Statements, the WHS influences key developments in global health in politics, science, business, and civil society.

In recent decades, various holistic approaches have been developed in research and practice, all of which explicitly deal with the complexity, the continuum, and the interrelationships between biological, socioeconomic, and ecological systems in the field of health: "One Health" primarily addresses the mutual dependencies of human health, plant health, and animal health; "Planetary Health" emphasizes the connections between human health and an intact environment, especially the consequences of climate change; "Global Health" furthermore focuses on health equity and comprehensive health strategies across the entire planet. Koplan et al. (2009) define global health as "... an area for study, research, and practice that places a priority on improving health and achieving health equity for all people worldwide". With this definition, global health differs from other terms such as international health or public health by focusing on equal access to healthcare for all (Beaglehole and Bonita 2010).

Approaches such as *Universal Health Coverage*, universal access to healthcare (WHO 2021), or the *health-in-all-policy-approach*, the attempt to integrate health comprehensively into all major political strategies (HiaP approach 2014), are supported by the World Health Summit. Healthcare should be equally accessible to all people and therefore must be included in all areas of life. These approaches are also central steps in the attempt to achieve the United Nations' sustainability goals. The sustainability goals (Sustainable Development Goals, SDGs) defined by the United Nations in 2015 have made global health one of the central themes. The total of 17 goals cover a wide range of topics. Areas of action include, for example, increased efforts for peace and rule of law (SDG 16), education for all (SDG 4), the protection of our climate and resources (SDG 13), or gender equality (SDG 5). "Healthy life and well-being for all" (SDG 3) is linked to all other goals. Disease, for example, is both a cause and a consequence of poverty, and health is an important basis for economic development. Because of this close link, progress towards individual goals can only be achieved through holistic approaches that take into account the interactions.

5.3 Health is more than medicine: a formula that redefines health

Health is a complex construct. And yet, as the literature and theater critic Ludwig Börne expressed in the 19th century: "There are a thousand diseases, but only one health" (Börne 1862, p. 195). But what exactly is this health (van der Eijk et al. 2021)?

The World Health Organization (WHO) defined health as a "state of complete physical, mental and social well-being and the absence of disease" (WHO 2006). This definition includes an optimal state, which is rarely ever achieved and which leaves out the cultural aspects of understanding health as well as (environmental) conditions. Therefore, this chapter offers another definition of health that includes determinants missing in the WHO definition. Ganten and Niehaus (2014) discussed an alternative, evolutionary definition of health in the book "The Health

Formula: Understanding and Preventing the Major Civilizational Diseases" (2014). This health formula is an attempt to summarize a complex issue like health in a formula that condenses the complexity to the essentials. Health is more than medicine and biology (Ganten and Rutert 2021). A person can only live healthily where the conditions allow it. The greatest possible health will only be achievable for the individual and for a society when living conditions, behavior, and environment are optimally aligned with human biological possibilities and needs.

Biology, environment, and behavior are each highly complex and variable in themselves. But health depends on each individual parameter and the complex interplay of biology, environment, and behavior. Put into a simple formula, health is defined as a function of our inherited biology, the environment in which we live, and our behavior: Health = Function (f) (Biology (B) × Environment (E) × Behavior (B)) or even simpler: H = f (B × E × B). Biology includes all living things, from the genome to cell function, organs, and the entire body function. The environment includes land, water, atmosphere, climate, but also the socio-economic and other living worlds. Behavior in relation to health is essentially characterized among other things by education, nutrition, and movement (Ganten and Rutert 2021, p. 260). From a conceptual point of view, biology, environment, and behavior and their interactions are crucial parameters because the evolution of life as a whole is determined by them. This health formula is thus both comprehensive and offers a holistic, evolutionary view of life and health.

5.4 Women's Health in the Context of Global Health

What does a holistic approach to medicine and health mean in practice for a vulnerable group such as women in countries of the global South, who, as childbearers and physically weaker individuals, are particularly affected by the impacts of crises such as epidemics, climate change, and wars, and whose lifestyles and behaviors are strongly determined by socio-cultural influences, dietary rules, or environmental influences? It will be difficult to convey that women should eat better or exercise more, i.e., optimize their behavior for health, if they are in a socio-cultural space that does not allow movement beyond housework and farm work. If women are in an environment affected by drought or floods, or simply under household conditions that hardly allow for healthy living (e.g., due to sooty wood fires indoors, a common factor for respiratory infections and lung diseases), this moral claim can hardly be demanded. Rather, the external conditions should be considered as parameters for improving health conditions. Especially in times of crisis, special attention should be paid to these conditions. Because only in a healthy environment can healthy life take place.

Women not only occupy a special position in global health due to restrictive environments, but also due to changing environmental conditions. Especially as childbearers and mothers, they are vulnerably exposed to environmental conditions in times of crisis, droughts, floods, or fires. For example, the paths to vital resources such as food, wood, or water become longer due to dried up sources or dried up forests. Due to these conditions explicitly caused by climate change, they are among other things at a higher risk of physical abuse (Sorensen et al. 2018). Although the research data in this area still needs to be expanded, the fact that women are exposed to climate change in a different way than men is scientifically proven. It is primarily the physically weaker position and childbirth that make women more vulnerable. Despite significant improvement in the last 20 years, about 800 women still die every day from the consequences of childbirth complications worldwide. The COVID-19 pandemic has unfortunately led to setbacks because midwives could not or were not allowed to work, transport was not available, or entire clinics were closed (UNICEF 2021). Socio-economic inequality also exacerbates vulnerability. Women work in large parts of the world as unpaid forces in the care of children or (older) family members and are thus excluded from paid work or even from positions at management level. They can less often live independently of men and are dependent on them. Situations of dependence are often created and perpetuated in a brutal way. Changing this is an important step to achieve SDG 5 "Gender Equality" (Datt et al. 2017). This is also one of the central goals of the organization "Women in Global Health" (WGH), which among other things advocates for women to have an equal say in leadership roles in health as men do.

Education is essential to overcome gender inequality. Education means, for example, understanding the connections between environmental protection and health protection or the right to health. Women and young girls are more often excluded from educational institutions such as schools than young men. Helpful here would be internet-based learning and training programs (Ganten and Rutert 2021, p. 271), which could be accessible to everyone via mobile phones. The internet is sometimes more accessible for girls and women in countries of the global South than school. This is where the Sustainable Development Goal 4 "Education for All" comes into play. But education does not only mean factual knowledge, but also "creation, creativity, shaping. Education goes through the person. It enables a person to reflect on themselves and the world around them through explanation and interpretation, to position themselves with greater independence and freedom in every respect" (Ganten and Rutert 2021, p. 272). This level of education is difficult to achieve if it is not desired. Therefore, SDG 4 as a formal political goal is so significant, because such politically and internationally authorized guidelines increase the chance of achieving these goals step by step.

It becomes clear that the Sustainable Development Goals of the United Nations are all intertwined. The third SDG "Health and Well-being for All" can hardly be thought of without including the other goals. Health is only really achievable in an intact environment with the appropriate education, which in turn can influence behaviors. Especially in times of constant global change, it is all the more important to work with optimism on the implementation of the sustainability goals, especially where the most vulnerable groups, women and children, suffer most from the consequences of a changing world. The responsibility for changing living conditions cannot be imposed on women. Instead, in line with the previously described health formula, the (environmental) conditions must be consistently improved. Planetary Health with an emphasis on the importance of climate is thus directly linked to Global Health. Ultimately, climate protection and nature conservation also mean health protection. Health can therefore only be thought of and achieved with a holistic perspective.

5.5 Summary

Much research has already been conducted, said, and written about women's health. Therefore, this article focused on the holistic view of the health formula and thus on improving external conditions and especially on women's education. Education enables women to reflect and position themselves in their environment and to become more aware of their health. Even though this is a long process fraught with many challenges, it is essential, especially in the face of the many changes brought about by climate change and pandemics, to continually work towards making SDG 3 "Health and Well-being for All" achievable. The health of women and mothers has already been significantly improved globally, but there is still much to do. The implementation of the SDGs must therefore be driven forward much more strongly by 2030. The World Health Summit also continues to feel obliged to postulate the holistic approach to health and the sustainability goals as an international forum and to work significantly on their implementation under the umbrella of global and planetary health. This does not mean, of course, that partial aspects of the sustainability goals or special efforts to address very specific problems would be less important. Every progress towards the big goal is important and needs support. Every disease that can be treated or prevented means a better and happier life. The great challenge of the future, however, is dealing with complexity. This also includes global health. Holistic concepts can more effectively address social, socio-economic, and environmental problems and tasks in their interdependence. Improving global health is such a humanitarian, noble task. For the individual as well as for society as a whole, there is nothing more important than health. Women play a big role in this, as they, being a vulnerable group, require special protection. Therefore, the holistic view of health should be emphasized even more in political strategies and guidelines.

References

Beaglehole R, Bonita R (2010) What is global health? Glob Health Action 2010:3. https://doi.org/10.3402/gha.v3i0.5142

Börne L (1862) Gesammelte Schriften von Ludwig Börne. Neue vollständige Auflage. Bd 7. Hoffman & Campe, Hamburg

Dhatt R, Theobald S, Buzuzi S, Ros B, Vong S, Muraya K, Molyneux S, Hawkins K, González-Beiras C, Rosin K, Lichtenstein D, Wilkins K, Thompson K, Davis K, Jackson C (2017) The role of women's leadership and gender equity in leadership and health system strengthening. Global Health Epidemiol Genomics 2:e8. page 1 of 9. https://doi.org/10.1017/gheg.2016.22

van der Eijk P, Ganten D, Marek R (2021) Was ist Gesundheit? Interdisziplinäre Perspektiven aus Medizin, Geschichte und Kultur. De Gruyter Humanprojekt 18, Warsaw/Berlin

Ganten D, Niehaus J (2014) Die Gesundheitsformel: Die großen Zivilisationskrankheiten verstehen und verhindern. Albrecht Knaus, München

Ganten D, Rutert B (2021) Gesundheit ist mehr als Medizin. Die Gesundheitsfomel. In: Klapper B, Cichon I (Hrsg) Neustart! Für die Zukunft unseres Gesundheitswesens. Medizinische Verlagsgesellschaft, Berlin

Health in all policies (HiAP) framework for country action (2014) Health Promot Int 29(Suppl. 1):19–28. https://doi.org/10.1093/heapro/dau035

Koplan JP, Bond TC, Merson MH, Reddy KS, Rodriguez MH, Sewankambo NK et al (2009) Towards a common definition of global health. Lancet 373:1993–1995

Sorensen C, Murray V, Lemery J, Balbus J (2018) Climate change and women's health: impacts and policy directions. PLoS Med 15(7):e1002603. https://doi.org/10.1371/journal.pmed.1002603

Unicef (2021) Maternal and newborn health and COVID-19. https://data.unicef.org/topic/maternal-health/covid-19/

World Health Organization (2006) Definition of health. https://www.who.int/governance/eb/who_constitution_en.pdf

World Health Organization (2021) Factsheet: universal health coverage. https://www.who.int/news-room/fact-sheets/detail/universal-health-coverage-(uhc)

The Influence of Religions on Women's Health

6

Ulrich Hemel

Contents

Introductory Questions

1. The five world religions include: Christianity, Islam, Hinduism, Buddhism, and Judaism. Which two of the mentioned world religions have more than one billion followers each?
   A. Buddhism and Judaism
   B. Hinduism and Buddhism
   C. Christianity and Islam
   D. Islam and Hinduism
2. Which two world religions call their followers to proselytize those of other faiths?
   A. Hinduism and Judaism
   B. Buddhism and Hinduism
   C. Islam and Judaism
   D. Christianity and Islam

U. Hemel (✉)
Weltethos-Institut, Universität Tübingen, Tübingen, Germany
e-mail: Hemel@weltethos-institut.org

J. Wacker et al. (eds.), *Global Women's Health*,
https://doi.org/10.1007/978-3-662-69700-9_6

3. In hospitals strongly oriented towards natural sciences, there is often a lack of space and time for the practice of religion and spirituality for the sick people! Examples of practiced religious rituals for seriously ill patients are:
   A. Visit from the hospital chaplain
   B. Receiving the last rites
   C. Valet or farewell blessing
   D. Ritual washings

Religions have a massive influence on the physical and mental health of people, and thus also of women, but are often overlooked in medicine and especially in development policy. The widely known 17 Sustainable Development Goals of the United Nations (17 SDGs) do mention gender equality (SDG 5) and quality education (SDG 4). However, possible impacts due to membership and practice of religions are not mentioned—even though over 80% of people are religiously influenced, especially by the so-called world religions.

Religions are therefore still underestimated in their effect as essential actors of civil society, or rather perceived as inhibiting factors of modern medical practice. However, they can also act as their allies.

6.1 Religions as Actors of Civil Society and Coexistence in Religious Diversity

The reason for this chapter is a consideration of the role change of religions. They mutated from the adversary of the state as in medieval Europe to the responsible actor of the global civil society. This term deserves a clear distinction. In the terminology of the Institute for Social Strategy, founded in 2009 by Ulrich Hemel (www.institut-fuer-sozialstrategie.org), any person or institution that is not supported by the state or shaped by organized crime is considered an actor of civil society (Hemel 2019a).

This definition goes beyond a previously widespread description of civil society, which primarily sees it represented by non-governmental organizations (NGOs) and activist groups. The advantage of such a broad, but clearly delineated definition is that sports, music, art, business enterprises, and religions can also be understood as actors of civil society.

Religious diversity, religious competition, global migration flows, and global communication demand peaceful coexistence. Different religions with very different ideas about life and death, health and illness, nutrition and gender roles must be tolerated (Höpflinger et al. 2021). In this context, a discussion is currently emerging about the possible introduction of a 18th Sustainable Development Goal of the United Nations (SDG 18), specifically on the topic of "good religious and world-view practices" (Hemel 2022). Good religious and world-view practices can be indicated by the following keywords:

1. Freedom of religion
2. Freedom of worship
3. Freedom of conversion
4. Religious tolerance as freedom for and as freedom from religion
5. Rejection of human rights-hostile religious practice

Religions follow their own, specifically religious logic. They deal with fundamentally truth-capable, but undecidable questions such as life after death, the position of humans in the world, but also the "good life" and moral duties according to the ideas of a religious community. Religions therefore have a massive impact on education, training and action, but also on health and health-relevant behavior, including by and of women.

The peculiarity of the demand for good religious and world-view practices (SDG 18) consists, on the one hand, in the fact that this goal does not abolish the possible truth and validity claim of a religion. Rather, it combines this in favor of the good coexistence of all with a "right to error and provisionality" understood from the inherent logic of the respective religion. After all, it is either true that, for example, Jesus Christ is the Son of God and Savior of the world or that Mohammed is the final prophet of God. We cannot decide these questions, but we can live well together if we do not subject them to the pressure of political enforcement.

The view of religions as actors of civil society does not always correspond to the self-understanding in certain interpretations of religious world and life design. This is especially comprehensive in fundamentalist currents, leaving no room for alternatives. In such cases, there is regularly religious coercion and religiously motivated violence, also against women. An example would be the stoning of women known from the Old Testament and from Islam, especially in the case of adultery (Bar 2021).

The civilizing effect of democratic living conditions with their demand for a democracy-capable religion is the background of the formulation of principles of "good religious and world-view practices". Because it includes freedoms to be granted and tolerated, such as in the case of voluntary religious change (conversion), but also for agnostic or atheistic people who want to live without religion.

The demand for a departure from human rights-hostile practice is fundamentally shared by all religions, as the so-called World Ethos values show (Hemel 2019a; Ziebertz 2010). These were adopted in 1993 and 2018 by the Parliament of the World's Religions with the participation of numerous religious communities including all world religions (Kuschel 2019). However, whether the circumcision of boys (circumcision) can be considered as bodily harm or as valuable and human rights-compliant religious practice remains controversial.

World religions are defined here as particularly powerful and widespread religions. These therefore include not only Christianity and Islam, which together influence about half of the world population, but also Hinduism and Buddhism with a total of also over one billion followers. Judaism, which is numerically smaller (with around 15 million religious members worldwide), also belongs to the world religions, because it is basically the root of Christianity and Islam. The patriarch Abraham is recognized in these three world religions, so they are often also referred to as "Abrahamic world religions".

The Parliament of the World's Religions also includes numerous other older and newer religious communities , from the Bahai to the Sikhs, from shamanistic natural religions to Caodaism in Vietnam. In addition, within large religions there are numerous denominations, currents and separate communities up to sects. They all have a massive influence on nutrition, on the female body, on the education and self-image of girls and thus on women's health.

In sociocultural practice, different influences regularly mix. When it comes to religious ideas, this is referred to as "syncretism" as a form of mixing traditional ideas with the practices of a world religion. However, much more essential for the question of women's health is a mixture of religious, political, and traditional societal ideas about the relationship between men and women. Both in Christianity and in Islam, for example, there is a lively discussion about how far patriarchal ideas from the time of Jesus and Mohammed are part of authentic religious faith or rather time-bound elements that can no longer have a normative claim today. It is the task of theological research to interpret its own religious tradition to the best of its knowledge and conscience for its value and validity in the context of the time of its origin and its ability to connect to the respective time.

The same applies to time-bound scientific or, in a narrower sense, natural philosophical ideas that seem downright offensive today. If the man's semen is considered the transmitter of human life, then masturbation or "onanism" (according to the biblical figure of Onan) comes close to mass murder: it becomes the "culpable waste of creative life force" (Levinson 1984). In Judaism, coitus interruptus was critically viewed for similar reasons (Levinson 1984). Conversely, if the woman's body is merely considered a vessel for the unfolding of life donated by the man, because the connections of genetics were not known before Gregor Mendel, then patriarchal ideas of the superiority of the man over the woman are close at hand. It often takes decades to centuries for religions to overcome such shadows of the past in their practice.

However, the inherent logic of religions surprisingly depends little on overcoming time-typical constraints. Therefore, religious change is repeatedly associated with partly drastic changes in religious beliefs, without this being recognized or acknowledged at first glance. A well-known example, of course also relevant to health, is the death penalty. For example, it was long accepted in the Catechism of the Catholic Church for extreme cases, but has since been removed from it and religiously outlawed as a punitive measure.

6.2 World Religions, Health and Disease

Religions offer their members a complex symbolic world interpretation and a series of specific religious practices that are intended to give the individual person orientation, meaning, and support. Their holistic claim to interpretation is reflected in the unfolding and transmission of a rich symbolic universe, a life-shaping "narrative" or narration, and a frequently enough behavior-controlling everyday relevance. This includes, among other things, self- and world-images, body- and gender-related role images, but also views on the "correct" social order, on decency and morality, power and powerlessness, nutrition and sexuality.

Typical is the linking of an external event with a specific interpretation.

Over time, however, it often becomes apparent that other and alternative interpretations are possible, so that different explanatory models can be assigned to an event.

The event "disease" can then, for example, be interpreted as a "test of God" or as a "punishment", as was the case, for example, with the emergence of AIDS. Because AIDS originally emerged strongly in the homosexual scene, which is rejected by many religious people as unnatural, some religious interpretations were voiced that considered AIDS as a punishment for homosexual practices. However, this highly controversial thought could not be maintained when it became clear that even children could become infected in the womb.

To this day, questions of proper nutrition, sexual orientation, the self-image of boys and girls, and the social order of power and powerlessness in a society shape the relationship between religion, health, and disease. A special role is played by **the respective understanding of what is considered nature and what is considered natural**.

Homosexuality in men and women was considered a disease that required treatment. It was not removed from the manual of psychiatric disorders (DSM) used in the USA until 1973 and from the classification of diseases (ICD) published by the WHO until 1992 (Wolf 2004). Currently, such an issue is evident, for example, in the relationship of religious communities to persons of a non-binary sexual orientation. LGBQTI* people were (and are) not taken seriously in their concerns, but instead discriminated against because of their supposedly sinful lifestyle (Gräve et al. 2021). However, resistance is now growing against this, which is also theologically justified. Then it is argued, for example, that the primary concern is to honor the person as desired by God. What sexual orientation he or she has is then of secondary importance.

Another link is the connection of health and disease with the real or supposed will of God, often associated with patriarchal orders. In many religions, a **do-experience correlation** is addressed, in which good deeds lead to a good life, and bad actions lead to a bad life. The Book of Job, known to Jews, Christians, and Muslims, takes up this correlation, which cannot be maintained in real life, and argues in a differentiated way: If even a righteous man like Job is hit by strokes of fate, these should not be unreflectively interpreted as "punishment from God". The astonished question of why not every smoker dies earlier than others or why someone dies too early despite the best fitness can still be observed today.

The consideration of the male and female body also plays a role to this day. Who has which rights over their own body and when? The example of menstruation shows how a biological event (BE) was linked with religious interpretations (RI) on the subject of purity and gender roles. Already in Old Testament Judaism, women were obliged to maintain full-body hygiene, to bathe and take a ritual immersion bath after menstruation, and men were obliged to satisfy the woman for her physical and emotional well-being (Levinson 1984). The obvious connection between women's health and the transmission of human life also led to lively controversies around contraception and abortion in numerous religious contexts (Jütte 2003; Maguire 2003).

Regulations on sexuality, like norms around nutrition or dealing with property and possessions, serve not only to maintain a certain social order, but also a spiritual purpose. In modern language, we could speak of the **training of self-control**. Whether it is generally about fasting or specifically about the separation of dairy and meat dishes as in Judaism, the avoidance of pork and alcohol in Islam, or other dietary rules around holy days and holy times—it is fundamentally clear that the eating habits supported by a community have physiological consequences that, like the prevalence of beauty and body ideals, affect individual and collective human health.

Within a religious worldview, it is repeatedly a matter of questioning the events of physical and social reality with regard to the will and action of God. The privilege of healing was assigned to the shaman in a number of prehistoric cultures. Religious rituals were and are also practiced in medical contexts (Brauer 2020).

Physical and mental health were considered connected long before all psychosomatics in religious worldviews. It is also worth taking a look at the boundaries between world religions and officially unrecognized religion-related practices such as magic, spiritual healing, and prayer healing. That effects occur within the framework of such practices is undisputed. The interpretation of the causes, which range from the placebo and nocebo effect to psychologically effective causal chains of cursing and blessing, is controversial.

The difference between world religions and magical practices lies in the fact that world religions do not construct a direct connection between a certain religious action and its desired success, such as healing from a disease, but in their own religious logic refer to the inscrutable decree of divine will.

Finally, the influence of world religions on the emergence of a modern health care system should not be underestimated. Hospitals first emerged along the pilgrimage routes, precisely because pilgrims could not be cared for in home care. Furthermore, specific religious motives became effective in the health care system, such as the service to the sick as a service to the neighbor, which in Christianity became a "another Christ" as a medium of encountering God. Such ideas were given social form through the founding of religious communities for the purpose of nursing and care for the poor.

6.3 World Religions and Women's Health

Religions are particularly focused on crucial life situations in their social practice. Through initiation rites, rituals, and sacraments, they mark transitions and help to cope with life crises. The focus is always on the classification of life events into an overarching context. The "framing", i.e., the assignment of a given situation to a certain class of events (Goffman 1974), thus becomes the door to coping with concrete life tasks, which can also be called "coping" (Eckenrode 1991; Hemel 2019b; Hemel 2020). The main effect is the experienced self-efficacy of a person or a community, which can be experienced, for example, when praying for a sick person.

The particular logic of each religion requires a basic level of religious competence in the sense of basic knowledge of a religion, whether it is a Christian, Islamic, or Hindu background. In everyday clinical practice, this is often referred to as "intercultural competence" or interculturally sensitive ethics consultation (Grützmann 2015). In fact, at least three topics overlap here: the specific religious background (e.g., that of an Alevi Turkish woman in a German women's clinic), the linguistic and sociocultural background (such as the role of an Alevi woman in Turkish origin society), and the interaction background in one's own country (for example, with a Protestant Lutheran gynecologist).

Consequently, a **triad of sensitization** is required in response to three essential facets:

- depending on religious religion or denomination (example: an Alevi woman),
- depending on linguistic-cultural origin (example: Turkish culture) and
- depending on the religious and cultural context of interaction (example: German Protestant gynecologist).

Let's take the certainly drastic example of female genital mutilation (FGM). It is particularly prevalent in western and northeastern Africa, but also in parts of Asia, and is also practiced illegally in Germany (estimated between 3000 to 10,000 cases) and Europe. Women's, children's and human rights organizations unanimously condemn the corresponding practice. It leads to the death of many young women and girls, to physical and emotional suffering.

Now, genital mutilation is not practiced in all Islamic countries. It is the result of the interaction of local, patriarchal traditions with certain religious-Islamic interpretations. In the meantime, there is a fatwa, a binding Islamic legal opinion, that condemns FGM. The inclusion of religion makes the fight against a human rights-hostile religiously motivated practice more effective and promising.

Since women give birth to children, the religious interpretation of family planning practices, conception and contraception, birth, artificial insemination, but also abortion and surrogacy is a universal field of religious influences on women's health. In many religions, such as Judaism and Islam, a pragmatic attitude prevails. The decision about the chosen practice is predominantly up to the woman.

In the context of Christianity, however, the not so much biblical, but late antique hostility towards the body had a long-lasting effect. Combined with a normatively narrowed concept of nature and naturalness, it led to a very restrictive view of sexuality and to the decades-long rejection of many forms of contraception, especially in the Catholic Church, from the pill to the condom (Aschmann

2021; comprehensive: Maguire 2003). In the meantime, it is also officially recognized by the church that sexuality should not only be narrowed down to the procreation of life among married partners, but should also be an expression of love and affection in a couple. This sounds self-evident, but it has direct effects on sexual practice and women's health, because family planning becomes fundamentally legitimate even in the context of Catholic doctrine and morals.

Particularly controversial, but of great importance for women's health, is legal access to abortion. On this field, scientific, religious and political considerations mix. For example, the Jewish term "Nefesch" refers to an independent person. However, the fetus in the womb is not considered a person until its birth, but as part of the mother. This results in a comparatively liberal attitude towards abortion. In Hinduism and Buddhism, on the other hand, the question arises whether an abortion could be harmful to the unborn life in the cycle of rebirth (Lecso 1987; Poggendorf-Kakar 2017).

Especially in Catholic Christianity, however, every form of human life is perceived as a soul-filled person from the beginning, so that an abortion, even at a very early stage of development, is generally considered as killing innocent life and is largely rejected.

In Islam, unborn life is considered "property of the Creator" (Surah 10, 68). However, the embryo only becomes human with the formation of limbs and the "breathing in of the soul", which is assumed from day 40 or from day 120 of a pregnancy, depending on the school of law (Tworuschka 1984). Without a valid reason, abortion is also forbidden in Islam. However, the rules vary greatly. For example, Tunisia and Morocco have a broad medical indication with a deadline solution and greater understanding for emergencies involving the life and health of the mother (Tworuschka 1984).

World religions have a direct impact on physical and mental women's health. A telling example is the **valuation of virginity**, associated with notions of "purity" or "decency" and "honor". After the wedding night, for example, a cloth stained with hymen blood must be publicly shown as proof of virginity. Corresponding practices have been reported from both Sicily and Arab countries, both in Christian and Islamic environments.

As in the case of female genital mutilation, world religions play an ambivalent role here, because on the one hand they legitimized certain misogynistic sociocultural practices over a long period of time, but over time they also knew how to distance themselves from them. For example, many religious and legal scholars of Islam spoke out in favor of banning female genital mutilation at a conference at the University of Cairo in 2006 (Mauer 2009). In other words: religious and theological arguments have contributed both to the oppression and to the liberation of women from patriarchal conditions that burden women's health. This ability to change, especially of world religions, clearly distinguishes them from magical or traditional, sociocultural-ethnic practices without religious backgrounds.

An example of this relationship is provided by the Christian resurrection narrative. Jesus first appeared to the women, even though they had no right to testify in court at the time (Heiler 1977). Today, this is considered a strong argument in favor of equal rights for men and women, for example in the Catholic Church in the discussion about admission to the priesthood (Leimgruber 2021).

For this reason, it is worthwhile to include world religions in topics related to women's health, also with regard to mental aspects of women's health. Because to this day, women are strong actors in the field of education, including religious education in the family. Current reports show how stressful the traditional condemnation of a homosexual orientation can still be in the experience of children, adolescents, and adults (Gräve et al. 2021). While religions do reflect societal developments, they can also promote or inhibit them. This applies to dealing with one's own body and sexuality, as well as to questions of nutrition or the evaluation of health and illness, the attribution of value and self-worth, or indeed of condemnation and disregard.

6.4 The Role of Religions in Combating Epidemics and Diseases

The diaconal side of religions in the narrower sense is particularly expressed through their activities in the field of nursing and elderly care and in the fight against epidemics. While this is true for all religions, it is particularly pronounced in Christianity due to the demand for harmony between self-love and love for others. The founding of public hospitals, the activities of charitable religious communities, as well as hospices and offers for specific target groups such as sick homeless people, prostitutes (e.g., the Solwodi initiative) or women who have committed crimes (Halbhuber-Gassner and Pravda 2013) speak volumes. The Maltese, Johanniter, Green Crescent, and Red Cross are examples of corresponding, often specifically religiously motivated organizations.

Physical and mental health go hand in hand. Religions, for example, offer a way of dealing with one's own stressful life situations through the provision of meaningful rituals, which as a specific form of spiritual care also contribute to women's health (Peng-Keller 2021; Kühn 2021). - Creation of meaning through structured rituals and spiritual practice generally have a positive effect on coping with difficult life situations. An example from the Christian context is the anointing of the sick, formerly understood as comfort through the sacraments of the dying.

Such and other forms of coping also have a positive effect in increasingly secularized societies. In this context, spirituality can be understood as every person's connection with the universe and can be distinguished from specific forms of religious identity and identification. In other words: promoting mental health through suitable forms of spiritual practice can also have positive effects if a person does not consider themselves religious.

An example from the field of women's health is mastectomy or hysterectomy. Such interventions inevitably lead to questions about one's own body image and self-worth. Where religions credibly convey that neither professional performance nor the fulfillment of fertility and beauty ideals determine a person's value, they can reduce mental burdens and make an effective contribution to the mental and ultimately also physical health of affected women.

The influence of religions on women's health is, as mentioned above, generally underestimated to this day. This is particularly true when the inherent logic of a religion in the broader context of comprehensive self- and world interpretation is not recognized or even actively ignored.

From a medical and civil society perspective, it is particularly worthwhile to understand religions as allies in the interest of women's health and the enforcement of human rights. This also applies when certain sociocultural practices appear questionable and could possibly be disrupted with a view to a new religious interpretation.

World religions in particular are fundamentally highly adaptable and themselves actors of social and religious change. What is required is not only a willingness to change within religions, but also a public that is capable of religion, which brings a minimum level of expertise and understanding for the societal relevance of religions. Future generations of girls and women will thank those involved in such beneficial and humane changes.

Answers to the Initial Questions

1. C. Christianity and Islam
2. D. Christianity and Islam
3. All answers are correct

References

Aschmann B (2021) Liebe und tu, was du willst? Die „Pillenenzyklika" Humanae Vitae von 1968 und ihre Folgen. Brill-Schöningh, Paderborn

Bar S (2021) Death by stoning in the Hebrew Bible and in post-Biblical traditions. Old Testament Essays 34:789–805

Brauer S (2020) Glaube und Rituale im medizinischen Kontext. Theologischer Verlag, Zürich

Eckenrode J (1991) The social context of coping. Plenum Press, New York

Goffman E (1974) Frame analysis. An essay on the organization of experience. Northeastern University Press, Boston

Gräve M, Johannemann H, Klein M (Hrsg) (2021) Katholisch und queer. Bonifatius, Paderborn

Grützmann TT (2015) Interkulturelle Kompetenz in der klinisch-ethischen Praxis. LIT, Münster

Halbhuber-Gassner L, Pravda G (Hrsg) (2013) Frauengesundheit im Gefängnis. Lambertus, Freiburg im Breisgau

Heiler F (1977) Die Frau in den Religionen der Menschheit. De Gruyter, Berlin

Hemel U (Eds) (2019a) Weltethos für das 21. Jahrhundert. Herder, Freiburg im Breisgau

Hemel U (2019b) Mentale Architektur und Wirtschaftsanthropologie – eine Zukunftsaufgabe. In: Kießig S, Kühnlein S (Eds) Anthropologie und Spiritualität für das 21. Jahrhundert. Festschrift für Erwin Möde. Pustet, Regensburg, p 335–350

Hemel U (2020) Kritik der digitalen Vernunft. Warum Humanität der Maßstab sein muss. Herder, Freiburg im Breisgau

Hemel U (2022) Wie gelingt gutes Zusammenleben der Religionen? „Gute religiöse Praxis" (SDG 18) als Ziel der globalen Zivilgesellschaft. In: Braun K, Ratzinger G, Zörb R (Eds) Zum 95. Geburtstag, Festschrift der Gesellschaft zur Förderung christlicher Verantwortung e. V. für den Heiligen Vater em. Benedikt XVI. GcV, Rohrbach, p 126–146

Höpflinger AK, Jeffers A, Pezzoli-Olgiati D (Hrsg) (2021) Handbuch Gender und Religion, 2nd ed. V& R, Göttingen

Jütte R (2003) Lust ohne Last. Geschichte der Empfängnisverhütung von der Antike bis zur Gegenwart. C. H. Beck, München

Kühn L (2021) Liturgie im Krankenhaus. Plurale Feierformen in der Begleitung kranker und sterbender Menschen. Kohlhammer, Stuttgart

Kuschel KJ (2019) Weltreligionen im Dialog über Weltprobleme. Die Erklärung des Parlaments der Weltreligionen in Chicago. In: Hemel U (Eds) Weltethos für das 21. Jahrhundert. Herder, Freiburg im Breisgau, p 39–54

Lecso PA (1987) A buddhist view of abortion. J Relig Health 26:214–218

Leimgruber U (Eds) (2021) Catholic women. Menschen aus aller Welt für eine gerechtere Kirche. Echter, Würzburg

Levinson PN (1984) Sexualität in der jüdischen Religion. In: Klöcker M, Tworuschka U (Eds) Ethik der Religionen – Lehre und Leben, Bd 1: Sexualität. Kösel, München, p 12–31

Maguire D (Hrsg) (2003) Sacred rights. The case for contraception and abortion in world religions. Oxford University Press, Oxford

Mauer S (2009) Die Frau als besonderes Schutzobjekt strafrechtlicher Normen. Logos, Berlin

Peng-Keller S (2021) Klinikseelsorge als spezialisierte Spiritual Care. V&R, Göttingen

Poggendorf-Kakar K (2017) Hindu-Frauen zwischen Tradition und Moderne. Religiöse Veränderungen der indischen Mittelschicht im städtischen Umfeld. J. B. Metzler, Stuttgart-Weimar

Tworuschka M (1984) Sexualität im Islam. In: Klöcker M, Tworuschka U (Hrsg) Ethik der Religionen – Lehre und Leben, Bd 1: Sexualität. Kösel, München, p 119–147

Wolf G (2004) Erfahrungen und gesundheitliche Entwicklungen lesbischer Frauen im Coming-out-Prozess. Centaurus, Herbolzheim

Ziebertz HG (Hrsg) (2010) Menschenrechte, Christentum und Islam. LIT, Berlin

Women's Health, Culture, and Ethics—Anthropological and Socio-Ethical Aspects in Global Health

7

Walter Bruchhausen

Contents

Introductory Questions

1. Which of the following options do not apply? Social and cultural anthropology deals with:
   A. Patriarchal power relations with possible influence on women's health
   B. Customs and taboos of nutrition in pregnancy
   C. Institutions for the preservation and restoration of women's health
   D. Factors influencing health-relevant behavior of women
   E. Frequencies of women's diseases depending on the physical environment
2. In which area have international programs from the Global South been criticized as particularly patronizing and Eurocentric, even neocolonial?
   A. Family planning
   B. Antenatal care services
   C. Iron supplementation

W. Bruchhausen (✉)
Sektion Global Health, Institut für Hygiene und Public Health, Universitätsklinikum Bonn, Bonn, Germany
e-mail: walter.bruchhausen@ukbonn.de

J. Wacker et al. (eds.), *Global Women's Health*,
https://doi.org/10.1007/978-3-662-69700-9_7

D. Folic acid supplementation
E. Emergency cesarean section
3. What is not an area of medical anthropology in women's health?
F. Culture-dependent conceptions of pregnancy
G. Herbal and ritual means to accelerate childbirth
H. Social behavioral norms for the postpartum period
I. Positions of the fetus in the womb
J. Maternal birthing positions

The fact that human health depends not only on natural laws but also on man-made norms is hardly anywhere as obvious as in women's health. This applies to both the prevention and treatment of diseases. The enormous worldwide differences in dealing with pregnancy and childbirth show the sociocultural range, the perhaps even greater differences in maternal mortality demonstrate the unequal and thus also unjust distribution of personnel, technical and financial resources for a good outcome of pregnancy. This makes women's health an important and accordingly frequently studied area of social and cultural anthropology, especially its interface with medicine and health sciences in medical anthropology, and also social ethics, which, beyond individual ethical questions of possible prohibitions of certain actions, also deals with global justice. This article will focus on both culture and ethics as indispensable parts of the new interdisciplinary field of Global Health, which combines practice, study and research. Only when particular sociocultural norms and universal moral claims are simultaneously in view can the medical opportunities for improving women's health be applied in an appropriate manner. Anything else would not do justice to people as members of a particular society and of humanity.

7.1 Social and Cultural Anthropology and Women's Health

As interest in the health protection and healing measures of foreign peoples intensified during the early modern expansion of Europe to all continents, women's health was by no means at the forefront. This is because the ship crews were largely male, so obstetric expertise was not expected from their ship surgeons, and the Europeans accordingly had little exposure to the childbirths of indigenous women. The focus of interest was on medicinal plants for the threatening febrile diseases out of self-interest and on the exotic healing rituals, often from perhaps a more religious perspective. Only with increasing numbers of missionaries, mission doctors and nurses, and colonial doctors in the colonial imperialism of the late 19th century do reports on the indigenous handling of pregnancy and childbirth become more frequent. Given the central importance of reproduction for human development, it is not surprising that the "armchair anthropologists", who mostly wrote their works from the reports sent to them without their havin been to the tropics themselves, also asked about and dealt with conceptions and practices around childbirth. Not least, birthing chairs were of ethnographic interest.

Beyond the topic of birth, the observations on the status of women in society in older anthropological works are also interesting for women's health. It can be observed that a stronger social position of women can lead to more attention to their medical care. Some matrilineal or matrilocal societies, in which property, leadership roles or residence are passed on through the female line, but not necessarily to women themselves, point in this direction. A true matriarchy, which would be a counterpart to the known patriarchal structures, hardly exists despite occasional female rulers. However, if women can separate from their husbands at any time because they are economically independent of them due to matrilineal property relations (Moser 1997) or their own success as market women, they can also make decisions about expenditures for medical treatment and other measures for their own health.

Closely linked to the position of girls and women in a society is the highly health-relevant question of sexual relationships. If women are sufficiently self-determined here or determined by authoritarian structures to protect premarital virginity and marital fidelity, unwanted or unprotected sexual intercourse with the consequences of sexually transmitted diseases, injuries from sexualized violence and pregnancies is rather prevented. On the other hand, if there is strong economic or social dependence, e.g. on male teachers, superiors and family members, the chances of girls and women to enforce their sexual self-determination are very limited.

The outstanding role that fertility, pregnancy and birth play for the survival of a group has led to numerous female initiation rituals, which have some parallels to the customs for the males. These rituals are usually the task of older women, many of whom also act as birth attendants, and in some places involve intrusive, painful, dangerous and consequential manipulations of the genitals, which are the subject of another contribution in this volume as female genital mutilation (FGM). Overall, the rituals serve to prepare the girls at or around the time of their sexual maturity or immediately before marriage for their role as wifes and mothers, which can include information, warning, cleansing, and protective measures. The latter is particularly important after the onset of pregnancy, as this, together with birth and the postpartum period, is perceived as a particularly dangerous phase of life. Taboo violations and curses, such as the evil eye, can allegedly harm the child before birth or cause the mother to die during childbirth and require corresponding renunciations and countermeasures. If, for example, eatings an egg before or during pregnancy is supposed to lead to baldness of the child or the consumption of certain animals to corresponding malformations such as a cleft lip, this can exacerbate protein deficiency. Therefore, relevant knowledge of local customs is also important from a nutritional medical point of view.

An important recent branch of anthropology from a Global Health perspective is development anthropology, which examines planned and politically promoted change processes in societies and their institutions (Bierschenk 2014). Even from this perspective, women's education and emancipation represent a significant factor, as the classic role of the woman as the caregiver of the family leads to her greater attention to basic needs, including health. Women are therefore often seen as the key to development. If they are convinced of the importance of certain procedures, such as in the education or health sector, and empowered to do so, these procedures are more likely to be implemented in households. Health competence, as "health literacy" is increasingly translated instead of health maturity, has an impact far beyond the individual, especially in women.

7.2 Medical Anthropology and Women's Health

The anthropological interest in childbirth has already been mentioned. Even though birth is a physiological process in the vast majority of cases and thus not a subject of medicine, medical anthropology, like European medicine since the early modern period, has intensively dealt with pregnancy, childbirth, postpartum period, and child care, focusing primarily on the culturally different concepts and practices (Sich 1980; Schievenhövel 1995; Binder-Fritz 2003, p. 99–102). Medical anthropology has been developed as an interdisciplinary field between social and cultural anthropology and medicine or health sciences since the 1950s. The small German-speaking community in this field has extensive parallels in its research on dealing with disease and healing to the much larger Medical Anthropology in the Anglophone world.

Just as gynecology has only slowly evolved from obstetrics in academic European medicine, it is also difficult to identify a separate area of women's diseases beyond pregnancy and childbirth in the so-called traditional medicine of other continents. Complaints that would lead to a gynecologist in Germany can therefore be treated by both traditional midwives and general healers of various kinds.

One area of women-specific problems that receives the most attention in traditional medicine, however, is infertility. A woman's inability to have children can result in her not permanently getting a male partner, i.e., either not marrying ceremonially at all or being left by the husband. Male infertility, i.e., Impotentia generandi, as a reason for childlessness in couples is much less often assumed, except of course in the obvious case of Impotentia coeundi. In societies with dia- or synchronous polygamy, men can prove their respective ability, but in various societies, women also often try to escape their misfortune by having intercourse with other men.

Childlessness is such a great misfortune that its cause gives rise to many speculations. For the woman, it would be particularly bad if she were suspected of having broken a taboo or angered ancestral spirits, i.e., being to blame for this fate herself. More often, there is suspicion of witchcraft or cursing, i.e., that envious fellow human beings, e.g., co-wives and angry mothers-in-law, have deliberately or unintentionally caused this condition with secret powers. These ideas, also common in European folk medicine or religion, usually lead to attempts to identify the supposed culprits and neutralize them with public or secret means.

Experts for the treatment of female infertility are therefore in high demand and expensive. They do not need to be traditional, but in Asian or African metropolises, they can be experts for modern reproductive medicine including in-vitro fertilization (Hörbst 2012). In my field research region in rural southeastern Tanzania, a survey in over a hundred households on the accessibility of treatment in general revealed that of all health problems and therapy offers, the treatment of infertility by a Muslim scholar would be the most expensive (Bruchhausen 2006, p. 264).

Given the central role that maternal mortality plays in missionary and colonial medicine, later in Primary Health Care (PHC) and International Health, the so-called traditional midwives have also received special attention in medical anthropology. Corresponding studies have proven enormous differences in the degree of professionalization and accordingly in the knowledge of these women, ranging from non-formally learned neighborhood assistance with perhaps one or two childbirths per year to several years of apprenticeship with subsequent almost professional activity. Despite these very different prerequisites,personnel from traditional practice were integrated into PHC with the goal of "health for all" in many countries. These women were trained as so-called "Traditional Birth Attendants" (TBA). The term is intended to distinguish them from the "Midwives", often further trained enrolled nurses, as biomedically educated employees of the health system. Their training consisted particularly in hygiene measures in the management of physiological births as well as recognition of lacking birth progress and birth-impossible child positions for timely transfer to the hospital (Bruchhausen 2006, p. 512–518). Accordingly, they can be recognized both by biomedical attributes such as gloves or scissors for cutting the umbilical cord and by carrying out the local rituals in the various phases of pregnancy, childbirth, and postpartum period, as the following depiction by a Tanzanian painter shows (Fig. 7.1).

Although the TBA programs can be seen as a great success in terms of the retention of trained women in their villages and acceptance in the population, thus fulfilling the health system evaluation criterion "Responsiveness (to people's non-medical expectations)" (World Health Report 2000, p. 25) to a high degree, their future contribution to reducing maternal mortality remains too limited. This is because most causes of death occur unexpectedly during delivery and can therefore only be controlled in health facilities, not during home deliveries. Therefore, WHOand UNICEF, together with UNFPA and the World Bank, did not endorse the continuation of the programs for independent childbirth management (WHO/UNFPA/UNICEF/World Bank 1999).

Other important topics in medical anthropology related to women's health and especially to the temporal environment of childbirth are the introduction of new science-based technologies and the challenges from migration. The former has also arisen internally in Western societies and has been intensively discussed and partially criticized under terms such as "medicalization of pregnancy, childbirth and menopause" (Pfleiderer 1997). Both, new techniques and new contexts, arise particularly in the migration of people, methods and material around the globe, driven by globalization. Today, measures for the preparation, conduct and follow-up of childbirth are shaped everywhere in the world by the encounter of international with local or various national expectations and practices. Thus, ethnographic studies examined how the transfer of prenatal ultrasound to East Africa

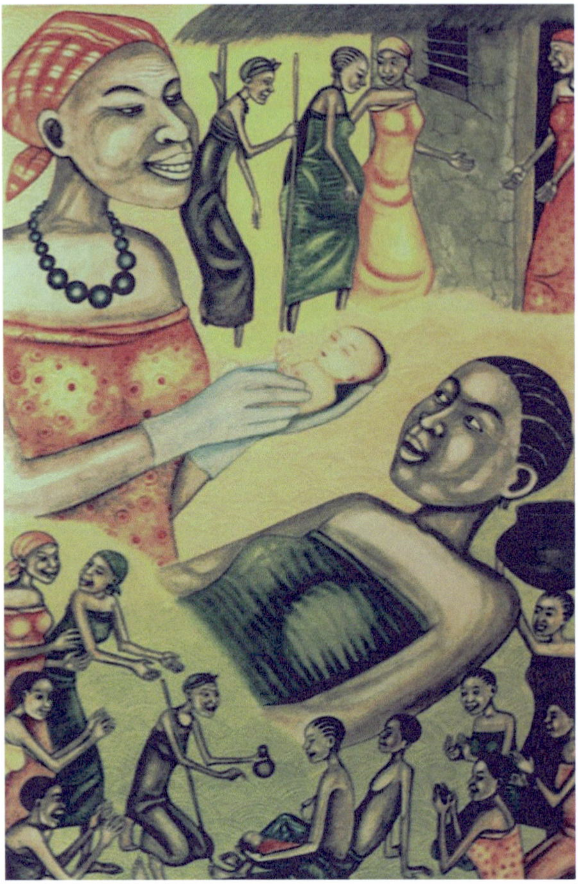

Fig. 7.1 "Traditional Birth Attendant" with modern hygiene equipment and traditional initiation rituals during pregnancy, childbirth, and postpartum period (painting by Steve Malolo, Tanzania, 2001)

(Müller-Rockstroh 2010) or the delivery of Chinese women in a German hospital (Kotte 2010) change the experiences of pregnancy and postpartum period.

7.3 Social Ethics and Women's Health

The question of what ethical justification and possibly even obligation exists to intervene in culturally established conditions and practices that can be harmful to women's health has been very controversial. Here, differences between male and increasingly numerous female anthropologists were evident, for example, in the case of FGM, demonstrating the great importance of one's own societal positioning for anthropological perspectives.

In the moral philosophical debate, a dispute arose between absolutist universalism, which dominates in both consequentialist-utilitarian and deontological conceptions and favors worldwide uniform norms, and more relativisticly arguing particularism on the other hand. The latter focuses more on the realization of normativity in concrete and thus very different living conditions. The feminist care ethics (Gilligan 1993), which has identified rigid adherence to universal duties as a characteristic of the white, male Protestant in the USA and places personal relationships more in the foreground than purely abstract obligations, belongs to the latter direction. The fact that this emphasis on relationship also corresponds to many moral concepts of groups and societies that are regarded as traditional warns against hasty classifications and partisanship in the sense of a supposedly clear dichotomy between tradition and modernity.

Since the two directions argue at quite different levels, they do not have to remain irreconcilable, but have entered into a mutual learning process (Bruchhausen 2003). Universalism can learn how it must take into account different life worlds, e.g., of genders and ethnic groups, in order not to become potentially counterproductive—a decision must always be in line with "justice and equity", not only correct in terms of the wording of a rule. And every particularism must constantly measure actually effective norms against the general demands of common humanity, e.g., universal women's rights. Thus, the debate in social ethics has largely moved from mere obligations to the corresponding claims in the form of rights.

Even though the legal equity of women in Western societies is only slowly being established, it is now an internationally recognized prerequisite for the rule of law, which is also found in constitutions in the Global South. In Europe and North America—as common in democracies—the moral demand usually preceded the legal implementation, while at the same time in various societies around the world the prevailing morality often lags behind the legal claim. Women's health has to deal with such strong discrepancies between legal norm and social reality of the situation of women.

Internationally, the most important normative instrument for improving women's health is probably the human right to the highest attainable standard of health, as formulated after the Second World War in the preamble to the Constitution of the World Health Organization and in the Universal Declaration of Human Rights. Particularly influential is now the legally binding Comment No. 14 on the right to health from the year 2000, because it addresses possible tensions between different types of claims quite clearly: It is about respect for the culture of individuals and groups and for all age groups and genders, so one cannot simply be played off against the other (CESCR 2000).

The human rights approach is always particularly necessary where it concerns weak and vulnerable groups, because socially strong individuals can assert their interests even without such protection. Accordingly, vulnerable groups include women and children, as their physical, social, and economic inferiority is often glaring. Thus, the provision of the commentary stating that health facilities must respect the culture of groups and individuals, explicitly also states that this must not impair gender and age-related rights. Therefore, the health claims of women and children must not be sacrificed to cultural customs. Traditional rules that men can decide on treatment and health protection for their wives and parents for their children against their will and interests are thus questioned by the right to health. How this should look in a specific case is to be decided each time. Human rights, as abstract norms, are not detailed instructions, but binding claims that must be realized under respective conditions, not in a never-existing vacuum.

In addition to the necessity of concretization, which every norm has, the particular challenge of human rights is the orientation towards the best possible. Often it is not the lack of will, but the lack of possibility, that prevents what is medically necessary in gynecology and obstetrics. This is particularly strongly felt in medical missions abroad. The safest anesthesia and monitoring methods are often not available, hygienic conditions and lack of staff qualifications pose additional risks. However, simply doing nothing because the best possible standards cannot currently be met would be cynical and certainly not in the interest of those affected. But to permanently accept enormous, life-threatening differences in standards would be just as cynical.

Further ethical challenges for global women's health lie in the tensions between European and respective local values. For in the evaluation of fertility and number of children, there are—or at least were—clear differences, not least because of the continuing significant inequalities in the survival chances of born children and old-age care. The higher number of children in various African, Asian, and indigenous Latin American societies is by no means only unwanted, i.e., due to lack of access to hormonal or mechanical contraceptives. Even in Western Europe, the number of children began to decline before the introduction of scientifically developed contaceptives already with the start of pension insurance and declining child mortality around 1900. The conflict of interest became clear in 1974 at the World Population Conference in Bucharest, when the accusation from the Global South was that the North wanted to prevent the poor rather than poverty, i.e., to eliminate what other countries are richer in, namely children. This tension was formally resolved in 1994 at the follow-up conference in Rome, where—instead of state and international pressure—access to contraceptives was formulated as a right. But the suspicion of European interests remains, as the recurring rumor, most recently in northern Nigeria, shows that vaccines are mixed with infertility-inducing agents. It is now often shortened to the claim, also common in Europe, that vaccinations cause infertility.

7.4 Conclusion and Implications

In the preceding explanations and observations, it has repeatedly become apparent how much women's health requires a global and also sociocultural perspective. Comprehensive health care, as required by the human right to health, demands both, action on the determinants of health and functioning healthcare services. In the determinants of health, the living situation of women, which in turn is determined by social structures and cultural norms, plays a decisive role. From an ethical perspective, in the global comparison of such "hard" data as maternal mortality, ratio of qualified personnel and health facilities per capita, or number of institutional births, we are far from global justice and equality ("health equity"). In the healthcare services, the cultural and social anthropological issues of every day behaviour may be less crucial than gross inequity from social structures. In comparison, the devastating effects of poverty, underfunding and brain drain in many countries could be the higher hurdles for the use of health facilities and better survival chances of pregnant women and their children. However, socio-cultural aspects will become more important with increasing "availability", "accessability" and "quality" of healthcare services. For the right to health (according to this "AAAQ approach") explicitly includes, in addition to these three conditions for health facilities, as a fourth, the "acceptability", i.e., the adaptation of healthcare services to the socioculturally determined expectations, needs, and opportunities of people.

Answers to the Initial Questions

At the latest against the background of these explanations, the correct answers to the questions asked at the beginning should hopefully have become clear: **1E, 2A and 3D**. As a discipline in humanities and social science, social and cultural anthropology deals with the factors of health in the sociocultural environment, not with the scientifically investigable properties of pathogens and other physical causes of disease, and also not with biological processes in the human body. In the debates about the adoption of Western measures in former colonial territories, medical measures that directly protect the life of the mother and child during pregnancy and childbirth were largely uncontroversial. The argument, however, that fewer births through family planning measures ("spacing of births") improve the health of the mother and children was initially critically to negatively received as European paternalism in various societies of different religious orientation and ethnic composition.

References

Bierschenk T (2014) Entwicklungsethnologie und Ethnologie der Entwicklung: Deutschland, Europa, USA = Arbeitspapiere des Instituts für Ethnologie und Afrikastudien der Johannes Gutenberg-Universität Mainz 150. Ifeas, Mainz. http://www.ifeas.uni-mainz.de/Dateien/AP_150.pdf. Accessed 11 Mar 2023

Binder-Fritz C (2003) Gender, Körper und Kultur. Ethnomedizinische Perspektiven auf Gesundheit von Frauen. In: Lux T (Hrsg) Kulturelle Dimensionen der Medizin – Ethnomedizin, Medizinethnologie, Medical Anthropology. Reimer, Berlin, pp 89–121

Bruchhausen W (2003) Wider naiven Relativismus und vorschnellen Universalismus: Ethik in der Ethnomedizin. In: Lux T (Hrsg) Kulturelle Dimensionen der Medizin – Ethnomedizin, Medizinethnologie, Medical Anthropology. Reimer, Berlin, pp 328–349

Bruchhausen W (2006) Medizin zwischen den Welten. Vergangenheit und Gegenwart des medizinischen Pluralismus im südöstlichen Tansania. v&r/Bonn University Press, Göttingen
CESCR (Council for Economic, Social and Cultural Rights) (2000) General comment no. 14: the right to the highest attainable standard of health (art. 12)
Gilligan C (1982) In a different voice. Psychological theory and women's development. Harvard University Press, Cambridge/MA, 2nd edition
Hörbst V (2012) Assisted reproductive technologies in Mali: asymmetries and frictions. In: Knecht M, Beck S (Hrsg) IVF as global form. Ethnographies of knowledge, practices, and transnational encounters. Campus, New York, pp 120–148
Kotte G (2010) Wochenbetterfahrungen chinesischer Migrantinnen in Berliner Krankenhäusern. In: Dilger H, Hadolt B (Hrsg) Medizin im Kontext. Krankheit und Gesundheit in einer vernetzten Welt. Peter Lang, Frankfurt/Main, pp 121–138
Moser R (1997) Der Mann als Bettler. Geschlechterbeziehungen bei den mutterrechtlichen Mwera von Südtanzania. In: Völger G (Hrsg) Sie und Er. Frauenmacht und Männerherrschaft im Kulturvergleich, vol 1. Rautenstrauch-Joest-Museum, Cologne, pp 381–386
Müller-Rockstroh B (2010) Ultraschall in Tansania. Ethnographische Explorationen in den Transfer von Medizintechnologie. In: Dilger H, Hadolt B (Hrsg) Medizin im Kontext. Krankheit und Gesundheit in einer vernetzten Welt. Peter Lang, Frankfurt/Main, pp 35–52
Pfleiderer B (1997) Zur Konstruktion biomedizinischen Tuns und Wissens. In: Pfleiderer B, Greifeld K, Bichmann W (Hrsg) Ritual und Heilung. Eine Einführung in die Ethnomedizin. Reimer, Berlin., 2nd completely revised edition of „Krankheit und Kulture", pp 163–198
Schievenhövel W (Hrsg) (1995) Gebären – ethnomedizinische Perspektiven und neue Wege , 3rd edition, VWB, Berlin
Sich D (1980) Mutterschaft und Geburt im Kulturwandel. Ein Beitrag zur transkulturellen Gesundheitsforschung aus Korea, Diss. med., Heidelberg
WHO/UNFPA/UNICEF/World Bank (1999) Reduction of maternal mortality. A Joint WHO/UNFPA/UNICEF/World Bank Statement, WHO, Geneva
WHO (2000) World Health Report 2000, WHO, Geneva

8 Maternal Mortality: Status, Progress, and Outlook

Claudia Hanson and Ali Saidi

Contents

Introductory Questions

1. Maternal mortality (Maternal Mortality Ratio) refers to the number of maternal deaths during pregnancy, childbirth, and the six weeks thereafter, relative to the:
   A. Total population of the respective country

C. Hanson (✉)
Department of Global Public Health, Karolinska Institutet, Stockholm, Sweden
e-mail: claudia.hanson@ki.se

A. Saidi
Muhimbili National Hospital, Muhimbili University of Health and Allied Health Science (MUHAS), Dar-es-Salam, Tanzania

J. Wacker et al. (eds.), *Global Women's Health*,
https://doi.org/10.1007/978-3-662-69700-9_8

B. Number of women of childbearing age
C. Number of live births in the same time and area
2. Which combinations of factors lead to the highest maternal mortality rates?
A. Asia and oppression of women
B. Africa and poverty
C. America and restrictive abortion laws
D. Conflicts, poverty, and non-functioning health systems
3. Which strategy is currently seen as most important to significantly reduce maternal mortality?
E. Improvement of the quality of obstetric care
F. Improvement of access routes to the respective maternity clinics
G. Better education of pregnant women

8.1 Introduction: Maternal Mortality

Deaths during pregnancy, childbirth, and the six weeks of the postpartum period—so-called maternal deaths—continue to be one of the most urgent and shameful problems of our time. In 2017, the last year for which we currently have data (March 2022), 295,000 women (Uncertainty Interval [UI]: 279,000 to 340,000) died during pregnancy, childbirth, or the postpartum period. The global maternal mortality ratio was estimated at 211 per 100,000 live births in 2017—with very large regional differences: Africa had a maternal mortality ratioof 542 (UI 498 to 649) south of the Sahara in 2017. In comparison: The subregion of southern Asia had a ratio of 157 per 100,000 births. This was a decrease from 384 to 157 in the 17 years since 2000, an improvement of 5.3% per year (WHO et al. 2019) (Fig. 8.1)!

In absolute numbers, Nigeria and India have the most maternal deaths to report, about a third of all global deaths: 67,000 and 35,000 cases respectively occurred in these two countries in 2017 according to estimates (WHO et al. 2019).

But there is also positive news: The global risk of a 15-year-old girl dying during pregnancy, childbirth, and the postpartum period has dropped from 1 in 100 to 1 death among 190 girls between the years 2000 and 2017.

8.2 Main Causes of Maternal Mortality

The main causes of maternal mortality are bleeding before and after childbirth (27% of deaths), hypertensive diseases (14%), sepsis (11%), and abortions (miscarriages and terminations of pregnancy, (8%), embolism (3%) and other direct causes (10%). In addition, there are so-called indirect causes such as malaria or HIV infections or anemia (Say et al. 2014). The main causes have changed little in recent years. Pre-existing conditions, often due to the mother's older age, play a larger role in wealthier countries, but bleeding remains the main cause of death (Graham et al. 2016).

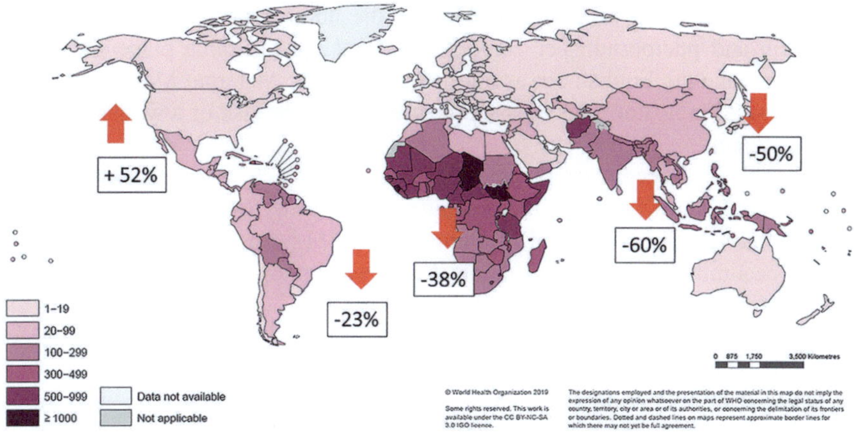

Fig. 8.1 Maternal mortality 2017 and progress since 2000, adapted WHO map 2019 (CC-BY-NC-SA 3.0 License). Map legend: North America (+52%), Latin America and the Caribbean (−23%), Africa south of the Sahara (−38%), central and southern Asia (−60%) and East Asia (−50%). (Courtesy of WHO)

8.3 How is Maternal Mortality measured?

All maternal mortality data are rough estimates, so they are published with the so-called uncertainty interval. The uncertainty must be distinguished from the confidence intervals known from epidemiology. The uncertainties go beyond the known 95% confidence uncertainties that come from samples: Most studies in poor countries use indirect methods such as the so-called Sisterhood or Siblings Sister Method. Here, sisters or siblings are asked about the survival of sisters in household studies under the assumption that sisters maintain contact throughout their lives and can provide information (WHO and UNICEF 1997).

Direct methods, for example the direct household method, which asks mothers about child and newborn deaths in household studies, are also difficult for maternal mortality measurements: Firstly, there are fortunately fewer maternal than infant deaths—so direct measurements would require very large samples, and secondly, households often dissolve when a mother dies. In countries in Europe, Australia, the USA and other wealthier countries, the data come from the state birth and death registers. These are also not complete, but provide much more accurate data than the indirect measurements. It is therefore important to always view maternal deaths as estimates and never as absolute valid numbers (Hanson 2011).

There are three indicators that should be distinguished, even though this is difficult in some languages, such as German, because rate and ratio are not differentiated. In principle, a "rate" refers to deaths within a period of time—while a ratio is a simple quotient.

The **maternal mortality ratio (MMR)**, the number of deaths in pregnancy, childbirth and puerperium per *100,000 live births* at the same place and at the same time take the English out as not needed(English: Maternal Mortality Ratiois the most used indicator. This measurement describes the risk of a woman dying if she is pregnant.

Then there is a second **maternal mortality rate**, which also measures deaths in pregnancy, childbirth and puerperium, but refers these to *100,000 women of child-bearing age* (English: Maternal Mortality Rate, MM-rate). This rate measures the risk of becoming pregnant *and* dying during pregnancy, childbirth and puerperium. Therefore, this rate often decreases quickly when family planning reduces the number of pregnancies per woman.

A third measurement is the **lifetime risk**, which often indicates the risk of a 15-year-old dying during pregnancy, childbirth and puerperium. This also measures the number of pregnancies as well as the risk of dying during pregnancy, childbirth and puerperium.

8.4 A Brief Historical Perspective: From the Beginnings in 1980 to the End of the Millennium Development Goal Period in 2015

While family planning and child health have had a firm place in international discussion and development cooperation since the 1960s, the problem of global maternal mortality first came onto the international agenda in 1987 with the first international conference in Nairobi (Moller et al. 2019). Here, for the first time, the goal was set to reduce maternal mortality, a goal which was emphasized again at the World Population Conference in Cairo in 1994 (United Nations 1994): The halving of maternal mortality within 15 years (Moller et al. 2019).

At the beginning of the 1990s, maternal mortality was estimated at about 850 per 100,000 live births in Africa and 410/100,000 in Southeast Asia. In most poor countries, less than 40% of women gave birth in health facilities and only 1–2% had a cesarean section. These data clearly showed that many women with complications were not reached.

In 1994, the World Health Organization published an initial strategy document, the Mother-baby Package (Mother-baby Package). This paper defined four main pillars for the care of women and their newborns: i) family planning, ii) prenatal care, iii) clean and adequate home birth assistance, mostly provided by village midwives, and iv) access to obstetric care for complications, including cesarean sections (WHO 1996). These four pillars were integrated into the *Primary Health Program* (WHO 1978), which the World Health Organization has been proposing since 1978 to improve health.

In the 1990s, many programs supported training of village midwives. Prenatal care was introduced or expanded. The provision of family planning was also expanded in many countries with comprehensive international aid to give women the opportunity to prevent unwanted pregnancies. In addition, family planning allows for the avoidance of high-risk pregnancies: pregnancies at a very young or old age, following too rapid a succession of births, or in multiparous women (Royston and Armstrong 1990). Family planning programs were very successful in Asia. In most countries in Asia, the number of pregnancies per woman is now just slightly above two children.

By the end of the 1990s, however, village midwives and prenatal care programs were increasingly seen as not sufficiently goal-oriented, as the maternal mortality did not decrease as hoped. The idea of the Mother-Baby Package was based on the assumption that high-risk pregnancies could be identified with sufficient certainty. Women without risk were then recommended a home birth with a Traditional Birth Attendant (TBA), who could ideally apply basic hygiene measures. This included the use of an unused, disinfected razor blade for cutting the umbilical cord, soap for hand washing, and a clean pad. High-risk pregnancies should only take place in a hospital. However, this principle reached its limits, as it was difficult to precisely identify high-risk pregnancies (Jahn et al. 1998). For example, most twin births could not be filtered out, as there was no ultrasound and clinical methods were too imprecise (Hanson et al. 2019). Simple risk factors such as first birth and many previous births have a low predictive power for the occurrence of complications. The principle of risk identification thus proved to be unsuitable for reducing maternal deaths on a larger scale.

By the end of the 1990s, several studies were published that examined how countries in Europe reduced maternal mortality in the last century, such as in Sweden (Högberg 1985). These studies pointed out that village midwives bring too little experience and training to reduce maternal mortality. Only when fully trained midwives took over obstetric care did maternal mortality decrease (De Brouwere et al. 1998; Högberg and Wall 1986; Loudon 1992). This was then included in the so-called Millennium Goals as a main indicator. In addition to reducing maternal mortality by 75% between 1990 and 2015, the most important goal was now to enable all women to give birth with a trained professional (United Nations 2015). This led to a strong expansion of training programs. However, the professionals were often only trained for one to two years and therefore cannot be considered fully trained midwives (Adegoke et al. 2012; Utz et al. 2013). Since the programs were often integrated into basic health programs, even nurses with only 6 months of obstetric training were often hired (Fig. 8.2).

At the same time, there were important voices calling for improved access to obstetric emergency care. The term "obstetric emergency care" focused primarily on the main causes of maternal mortality such as post-partum bleeding, eclampsia, infections and abortions (WHO et al. 2009). Many programs since the early 2000s have tried primarily to create better access to care for complications, i) by training health personnel to offer cesarean sections in all hospitals, ii) improved provision of essential drugs such as oxytocin for the prevention and treatment of bleeding after birth and magnesium sulfate for the treatment of (pre-)eclampsia and iii) training in the management of complications.

As a third pillar, antenatal prenatal carewas redesigned—away from the primary goal of risk detection to a greater focus on initiating important preventive

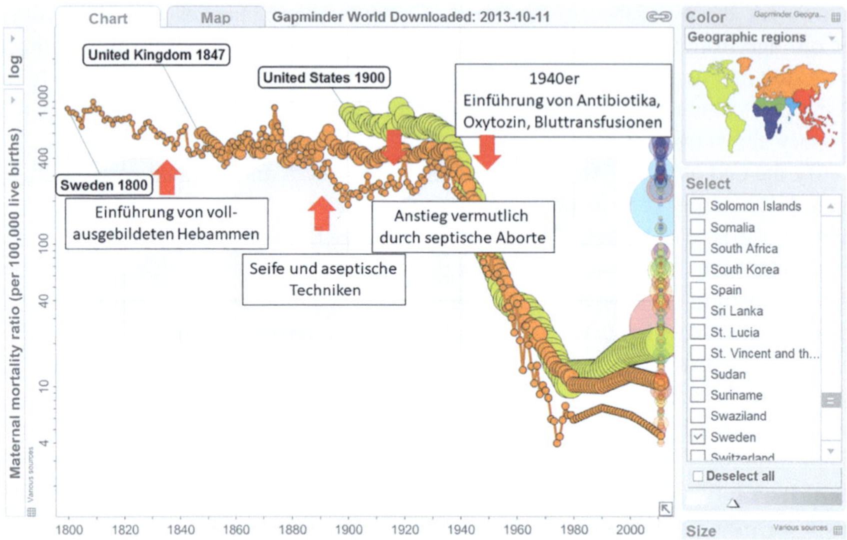

Fig. 8.2 Timeline of successes with midwifery training in Sweden compared to other countries. (Graphic produced with Gapminder: Sweden introduced midwifery nationwide in the early 19th century. This reduced maternal mortality from about 800 to 500 deceased women per 100,000 live births. After the studies by Semmelweis, aseptic measures were also introduced, which further reduced maternal mortality. There were very large differences between Sweden on the one hand and the UK and the USA on the other, which prefer a more clinical obstetric care by doctors. After the turn of the century, maternal mortality also increased in Sweden, probably due to a high number of septic abortions. In the further course, maternal mortality in all three countries then dropped drastically. Modern medicine with antibiotics, oxytocin for the treatment of bleeding, and blood transfusions among other things showed success here). (Source: Gapminder World, download on 11.10.2013)

measures such as the administration of preventive malaria drugs and mosquito nets. At the same time, HIV prevention measures were intensified and testing every pregnant woman for HIV became standard. Initially, drugs were given that were intended to reduce the risk of transmission to the child at birth; later, simple therapy was initiated during pregnancy. Today, many countries have begun to initiate lifelong preventive HIV therapy during pregnancy to reduce the virus to a maximum. This has greatly reduced the transmission of HIV during birth.

8.5 Stocktaking at the end of the Millennium Development Goal period

The global maternal mortality stood at 216 (UI 206 to 249) per 100,000 live births in 2015 (WHO et al. 2015). This was a decrease of 44% between 1990 and 2015—far below the target of a 75% decrease, or 5.5% per year, as proposed in the

Millennium Development Goals. Furthermore, 99% of deaths occurred in low- or middle-income countries. Overall, 66% of deaths occurred in sub-Saharan Africa. The Central African Republic, Chad, Nigeria, South Sudan, Somalia, Liberia, Burundi—all countries with internal political instability—had the highest maternal mortality ratios, over 700 per 100,000 live births (WHO et al. 2015).

The strategies to improve access to trained professionals were indeed successful: The number of deliveries accompanied by trained professionals began to rise steeply around 2010. Montagu calculated in a paper published in 2017 that births in health facilities in rural Africa had increased by an average of 15% between approximately 2005 and 2015 (Montagu et al. 2017). Some rural areas, such as in southern Tanzania, even showed a doubling, an increase from 40 to 80% of all births in health facilities (Hanson et al. 2015). However, it is important to bear in mind that this increase often took place in poorly equipped primary health care facilities with only limitedly trained staff (Straneo et al. 2021).

The cesarean section rates showed a divided success in 2015: In middle-income countries, such as Iran, Brazil, the Dominican Republic and many others, cesarean section rates shot up to over 30%. However, in rural Africa, they often remained below 5% (Betrán et al. 2016). This trend of a strong increase in cesarean section rates continues almost unabated. Especially in Latin America and the Caribbean, over 40% of women give birth by cesarean section. But many areas and countries in Asia also had growth rates of 30–40% in the last 30 years (Betran et al. 2021). This analysis by Betran et al. also points to the expected negative consequences of high cesarean section rates on the health of mothers as well as on the costs for health systems.

8.6 Challenges Today: Utilizing the Time of Sustainable Development Goals (SDGs)

The era of the Millennium Development Goals up to the year 2015 can be characterized as two decades in which improved access to obstetric facilities was primarily in focus. In 2015—also against the backdrop of the lingering hope for a significant reduction in maternal mortality—a period began in which the improvement of quality is at the center. In a much-cited publication, Kruk and co-authors suggest that more deaths today are due to lack of quality care compared to problems accessing health services (Kruk et al. 2018). For example, many women die because a hypertensive disease during pregnancy was not detected, even though they have taken advantage of prenatal care.

Many programs have tried to improve the quality of obstetric care through improved training and education methods (Alwy Al-beity et al. 2019; Ameh et al. 2019), quality management (Quality of Care Network 2021; Waiswa et al. 2017) and the established auditing of maternal and newborn deaths.

8.7 Midwifery Education and Improvement of Maternal and Newborn Health

The training of health workers in obstetric care, as already mentioned, is at the center of efforts to reduce maternal mortality. The 2018 formulated definition of a "skilled birth attendant" not only defines aspects of knowledge and competencies, but also defines a supportive work environment (WHO et al. 2018). This has also initiated a discussion about whether births should take place in primary health facilities or only in well-equipped hospitals (Hanson and Schellenberg 2019; Hanson et al. 2020; Nimako et al. 2021). The discussion raises open questions: Can women in rural areas of Africa and also Asia now afford a trip to the hospital 15–20 km away due to good economic developments? Do they arrive in time? Can we offer prenatal care in 2020 with ultrasound so that multiple births take place in the hospital?

A concept of a midwife-led delivery room, located between primary health services and hospitals, could be an alternative. But in such a concept, a functioning risk history and examination must be possible, so that, for example, women with hypertensive diseases or multiple births are referred early enough. In addition, cooperation with the hospitals must work, ambulances need sufficient equipment. The Lancet paper in the series on maternal health from 2016 also discusses this (Campbell et al. 2016).

Another international discussion is whether further nurses with additional training in the obstetric field should be trained or specifically midwives. In high-income countries, there are many different training programs and midwifery is often a specialization after a nursing education. This means that a midwife is first fully trained as a nurse, and then does a special training to become a midwife. However, this leads to long training periods and high costs. In Sweden, for example, there is consideration of creating a midwifery education as a stand alone education .

In any case, it can be seen internationally in recent years that many programs have now started to offer *dedicated* training programs for midwives (UNFPA 2021). But this requires larger investments, not only in training programs, but also regulation and certification. In countries like India, where obstetrics often takes place in the private sector, this encounters great difficulties (Mayra et al. 2021).

8.8 Respectful Obstetric Care

In the last 5–10 years, the problem of disrespectful treatment during childbirth, such as shouting, hitting, kicking, but also leaving alone, has increasingly come onto the international agenda (Bohren et al. 2015, 2019). The WHO, but also the International Organization for Gynecology and Obstetrics (FIGO), have published policy and strategy papers to end these unacceptable forms of treatment (Homer et al. 2014; Lalonde et al. 2019). It is also important in this context that over- and under-supply often occur simultaneously: Late, incorrectly indicated and not internationally standard cesarean sections often occur together with unnecessary obstetric interventions (Miller et al. 2016). Communication and education is not good enough to give women the feeling of being well cared for, and that they understand what is happening to them (Kwezi et al. 2021).

8.9 Auditing Maternal and Neonatal Deaths and Quality Improvement

Discussing maternal deaths in health facilities has a long tradition. Since maternal deaths do not occur daily even where we still see high numbers, discussing causes and factors in a round with everyone involved is a good management component for quality improvement. The first book on this was published by the WHO as early as 2004 (AbouZahr et al. 2004). Meanwhile, there are many more books and guidelines from WHO and FIGO, which have incorporated years of experience in poor countries (WHO et al. 2013). It is important that today not only maternal deaths but also neonatal deaths should be discussed and the system should ideally also be used for *counting* maternal and perinatal mortality within the Maternal and Perinatal Death Surveillance and Response, MPDSR program (World Health Organization 2021). Important in this now published guide is that it is increasingly pointed out that quality really improves only when the developed improvement suggestions are also implemented. In several publications in recent years, it has been stated that auditing itself does not lead to improved implementation (Said et al. 2021a, b).

Parallel to the auditing of deaths, other quality improvement concepts have also been increasingly introduced in many countries. The best known is certainly the WHO and UNICEF supported "*Quality of Care network*", which is active in many countries in Africa (Tanzania, Malawi, Uganda etc.) (Quality of Care Network 2021). The principle is based on the "Plan-Do-Study-Act-Cycle". Various evaluations have pointed to the potential, but also to difficulties in implementation (Waiswa et al. 2017; Zamboni et al. 2021).

8.10 A Brief Excursion to Perinatal Health

A chapter on maternal mortality, without pointing out the still equally shameful perinatal mortality, is incomplete: **The most urgent health problem is the many stillbirths**, which are still not registered in any international numbers. Every year, it is estimated that over 2 million babies are born dead (Hug et al. 2021). In addition, it is assumed that around 2.4 million newborns die each year in the first 28 days of life. The main reasons are prematurity and complications during birth (Perin et al. 2021; UN Inter-agency Group for Child Mortality Estimation 2021). The negative effects on mothers and their families of this often unnecessary death are far too rarely pointed out (Heazell et al. 2016; Lawn et al. 2016). It is important that programs to reduce maternal mortality finally also strongly consider comprehensive quality improvements during pregnancy and birth. Pediatricians have introduced the very successful "Helping Babies Breathe" program in many countries (Dol et al. 2018), now it is time for antenatal care and obstetric care to focus more on reducing stillbirths and neonatal deaths.

Answers to the Initial Questions

1. C. Number of live births at the same time and area
2. D. Conflicts, poverty and non-functioning health systems
3. A. Improvement of the quality of obstetric care

References

AbouZahr, C., De Bernis, L., Guidotti, R., Van Look, P., & Zupan, J. (2004). Beyond the numbers. Reviewing maternal deaths and complications to make pregnancy safer. WHO, Genf

Adegoke A, Utz B, Msuya SE, van den Broek N (2012) Skilled birth attendants: who is who? A descriptive study of definitions and roles from nine Sub Saharan African countries. PLoS One 7(7):e40220. https://doi.org/10.1371/journal.pone.0040220

Alwy Al-beity F, Pembe A, Hirose A, Morris J, Leshabari S, Marrone G, Hanson C (2019) Effect of the competency-based Helping Mothers Survive Bleeding after Birth (HMS BAB) training on maternal morbidity: a cluster-randomised trial in 20 districts in Tanzania. BMJ Glob Health 4(2):e001214. https://doi.org/10.1136/bmjgh-2018-001214

Ameh CA, Mdegela M, White S, van den Broek N (2019) The effectiveness of training in emergency obstetric care: a systematic literature review. Health Policy Plan 34(4):257–270. https://doi.org/10.1093/heapol/czz028

Betrán AP, Ye J, Moller A-B, Zhang J, Gülmezoglu AM, Torloni MR (2016) The increasing trend in caesarean section rates: global, regional and national estimates: 1990–2014. PLoS One 11(2):e0148343. https://doi.org/10.1371/journal.pone.0148343

Betran AP, Ye J, Moller AB, Souza JP, Zhang J (2021) Trends and projections of caesarean section rates: global and regional estimates. BMJ Glob Health 6(6). https://doi.org/10.1136/bmjgh-2021-005671

Bohren MA, Vogel JP, Hunter EC, Lutsiv O, Makh SK, Souza JP, Aguiar C, Saraiva Coneglian F, Diniz ALA, Tunçalp Ö, Javadi D, Oladapo OT, Khosla R, Hindin MJ, Gülmezoglu AM (2015) The mistreatment of women during childbirth in health facilities globally: a mixed-methods systematic review. PLoS Med 12(6):e1001847. https://doi.org/10.1371/journal.pmed.1001847

Bohren MA, Mehrtash H, Fawole B, Maung TM, Balde MD, Maya E, Thwin SS, Aderoba AK, Vogel JP, Irinyenikan TA, Adeyanju AO, Mon NO, Adu-Bonsaffoh K, Landoulsi S, Guure C, Adanu R, Diallo BA, Gülmezoglu AM, Soumah A-M et al (2019) How women are treated during facility-based childbirth in four countries: a cross-sectional study with labour observations and community-based surveys. Lancet 394(10210):1750–1763. https://doi.org/10.1016/S0140-6736(19)31992-0

Campbell OMR, Calvert C, Testa A, Strehlow M, Benova L, Keyes E, Donnay F, Macleod D, Gabrysch S, Rong L, Ronsmans C, Sadruddin S, Koblinsky M, Bailey P (2016) The scale, scope, coverage, and capability of childbirth care. Lancet:2193–2208. https://doi.org/10.1016/S0140-6736(16)31528-8

De Brouwere V, Tonglet R, Van Lerberghe W (1998) Strategies for reducing maternal mortality in developing countries: what can we learn from the history of the industrialized West? Tropical Med Int Health 3:771–782

Dol J, Campbell-Yeo M, Murphy GT, Aston M, McMillan D, Richardson B (2018) The impact of the Helping Babies Survive program on neonatal outcomes and health provider skills: a systematic review. JBI Database System Rev Implement Rep 16(3):701–737. https://doi.org/10.11124/jbisrir-2017-003535

Graham W, Woodd S, Byass P, Filippi V, Gon G, Virgo S, Chou D, Hounton S, Lozano R, Pattinson R, Singh S (2016) Diversity and divergence: the dynamic burden of poor maternal health. Lancet 388(10056):2164–2175. https://doi.org/10.1016/S0140-6736(16)31533-1

Hanson C (2011) Documentation for data on maternal mortality. Historical information compiled for 14 countries (up to 200 years). Gapminder. Retrieved 1 April 2022 from https://www.gapminder.org/documentation/documentation/gapdoc010.pdf

Hanson C, Schellenberg J (2019) Redesigning maternal health services: is centralisation the answer in low-resource settings? BMJ Glob Health 4(3):e001488. https://doi.org/10.1136/bmjgh-2019-001488

Hanson C, Manzi F, Mkumbo E, Shirima K, Penfold S, Hill Z, Shamba D, Jaribu J, Hamisi Y, Soremekun S, Cousens S, Marchant T, Mshinda H, Schellenberg D, Tanner M, Schellenberg J (2015) Effectiveness of a home-based counselling strategy on neonatal care and survival: a cluster-randomised trial in six districts of rural Southern Tanzania. PLoS Med 12(9):e1001881. https://doi.org/10.1371/journal.pmed.1001881

Hanson C, Munjanja S, Binagwaho A, Vwalika B, Pembe AB, Jacinto E, Chilinda GK, Donahoe KB, Wanyonyi SZ, Waiswa P, Gidiri MF, Benova L (2019) National policies and care provision in pregnancy and childbirth for twins in Eastern and Southern Africa: a mixed-methods multi-country study. PLoS Med 16(2):e1002749. https://doi.org/10.1371/journal.pmed.1002749

Hanson C, Waiswa P, Pembe A, Sandall J, Schellenberg J (2020) Health system redesign for equity in maternal and newborn health must be codesigned, country led, adapted to context and fit for purpose. BMJ Glob Health 5(10):e003748. https://doi.org/10.1136/bmjgh-2020-003748

Heazell AEPD, Siassakos DMD, Blencowe HM, Burden CMD, Bhutta ZAP, Cacciatore JP, Dang NRM, Das JMBA, Flenady VP, Gold KJMD, Mensah OKB, Millum JP, Nuzum DB, O'Donoghue KP, Redshaw MP, Rizvi AM, Roberts TP, Toyin Saraki HEL, Storey CBA, Downe SP (2016) Stillbirths: economic and psychosocial consequences. Lancet (British Edition) 387(10018):604–616. https://doi.org/10.1016/S0140-6736(15)00836-3

Högberg U (1985) Maternal mortality in Sweden university of Umeå. Umeå

Högberg U, Wall S (1986) Secular trends in maternal mortality in Sweden from 1750 to 1980. Bull World Health Organ 64(1):79–84

Homer CSE, Friberg IK, Dias MAB, ten Hoope-Bender P, Sandall J, Speciale AM, Bartlett LA (2014) The projected effect of scaling up midwifery. Lancet 384(9948):1146–1157. https://doi.org/10.1016/S0140-6736(14)60790-X

Hug L, You D, Blencowe H, Mishra A, Wang Z, Fix MJ, Wakefield J, Moran AC, Gaigbe-Togbe V, Suzuki E, Blau DM, Cousens S, Creanga A, Croft T, Hill K, Joseph KS, Maswime S, McClure EM, Pattinson R, Alkema L (2021) Global, regional, and national estimates and trends in stillbirths from 2000 to 2019: a systematic assessment. Lancet (British Edition) 398(10302):772–785. https://doi.org/10.1016/S0140-6736(21)01112-0

Jahn A, Kowalewski M, Kimatta S (1998) Obstetric care in southern Tanzania: does it reach those in need? Trop Med Int Health 3(11):926–932

Kruk ME, Gage AD, Joseph NT, Danaei G, García-Saisó S, Salomon JA (2018) Mortality due to low-quality health systems in the universal health coverage era: a systematic analysis of amenable deaths in 137 countries. Lancet 392(10160):2203–2212. https://doi.org/10.1016/S0140-6736(18)31668-4

Kwezi HA, Mselle LT, Leshabari S, Hanson C, Pembe AB (2021) How communication can help women who experience a maternal near-miss: a qualitative study from Tanzania. BMJ Open 11(11):e045514. https://doi.org/10.1136/bmjopen-2020-045514
Lalonde A, Herschderfer K, Pascali-Bonaro D, Hanson C, Fuchtner C, Visser GHA (2019) The international childbirth initiative: 12 steps to safe and respectful MotherBaby–Family maternity care. Int J Gynecol Obstet 146(1):65–73. https://doi.org/10.1002/ijgo.12844
Lawn JEP, Blencowe HM, Waiswa PP, Amouzou AP, Mathers CP, Hogan DP, Flenady VP, Frøen JFP, Qureshi ZUBM, Calderwood CBM, Shiekh SM, Jassir FBM, You DP, McClure EMP, Mathai MP, Cousens SP (2016) Stillbirths: rates, risk factors, and acceleration towards 2030. Lancet (British Edition) 387(10018):587–603. https://doi.org/10.1016/S0140-6736(15)00837-5
Loudon I (1992) Death in childbirth. An international study of maternal care and maternal mortality 1800–1950. Clarendon Press, Oxford
Mayra K, Padmadas SS, Matthews Z (2021) Challenges and needed reforms in midwifery and nursing regulatory systems in India: implications for education and practice. PLoS One 16(5):e0251331. https://doi.org/10.1371/journal.pone.0251331
Miller S, Abalos E, Chamillard M, Ciapponi A, Colaci D, Comandé D, Diaz V, Geller S, Hanson C, Langer A, Manuelli V, Millar K, Morhason-Bello I, Castro CP, Pileggi VN, Robinson N, Skaer M, Souza JP, Vogel JP, Althabe F (2016) Beyond too little, too late and too much, too soon: a pathway towards evidence-based, respectful maternity care worldwide. Lancet 388(10056):2176–2192. doi: 2110.1016/S0140-6736(2116)31472-31476. Review. https://doi.org/10.1016/S0140-6736(16)31472-6
Moller AB, Patten JH, Hanson C, Morgan A, Say L, Diaz T, Moran AC (2019) Monitoring maternal and newborn health outcomes globally: a brief history of key events and initiatives. Tropical Med Int Health 24(12):1342–1368. https://doi.org/10.1111/tmi.13313
Montagu D, Sudhinaraset M, Diamond-Smith N, Campbell O, Gabrysch S, Freedman L, Kruk M, Donnay F (2017) Where women go to deliver: understanding the changing landscape of childbirth in Africa and Asia. Health Policy Plan (May 25). https://doi.org/10.1093/heapol/czx1060. [Epub ahead of print]
Nimako K, Gage A, Benski C, Roder-DeWan S, Ali K, Kandie C, Mohamed A, Odeny H, Oloo M, Otieno JTB, Wanzala M, Okumu R, Kruk ME (2021) Health system redesign to shift to hospital delivery for maternal and newborn survival: feasibility assessment in Kakamega County, Kenya. Glob Health Sci Pract 9(4):1000–1010. https://doi.org/10.9745/ghsp-d-20-00684
Perin J, Mulick A, Yeung D, Villavicencio F, Lopez G, Strong KL, Prieto-Merino D, Cousens S, Black RE, Liu L (2021) Global, regional, and national causes of under-5 mortality in 2000–19: an updated systematic analysis with implications for the Sustainable Development Goals. Lancet Child Adolesc Health. https://doi.org/10.1016/s2352-4642(21)00311-4
Quality of Care Network (2021) National Quality of Care Network. Retrieved 1 April from https://www.who.int/groups/Quality-of-care-network
Royston E, Armstrong S (1990) La prévention des décès maternels. WHO, Genf
Said A, Pembe AB, Massawe S, Hanson C, Malqvist M (2021a) Maternal death surveillance and response in Tanzania: comprehensiveness of narrative summaries and action points from maternal death reviews. BMC Health Serv Res 21(1):52. https://doi.org/10.1186/s12913-020-06036-1
Said A, Sirili N, Massawe S, Pembe AB, Hanson C, Malqvist M (2021b) Mismatched ambition, execution and outcomes: implementing maternal death surveillance and response system in Mtwara region, Tanzania. BMJ Glob Health 6(5). https://doi.org/10.1136/bmjgh-2021-005040
Say L, Chou D, Gemmill A, Tunçalp O, Moller A, Daniels J (2014) Global causes of maternal death: a WHO systematic analysis. Lancet Glob Health 2. https://doi.org/10.1016/s2214-109x(14)70227-x
Straneo M, Benova L, Hanson C, Fogliati P, Pembe AB, Smekens T, van den Akker T (2021) Inequity in uptake of hospital-based childbirth care in rural Tanzania: analysis of the 2015–16

Tanzania Demographic and Health Survey. Health Policy Plan 36(9):1428–1440. https://doi.org/10.1093/heapol/czab079
UN Inter-agency Group for Child Mortality Estimation (2021) Levels and trends in child mortality: report 2021. Retrieved 1 March from https://childmortality.org/reports
UNFPA (2021) The State of the World's Midwifery, 2021. UNFPA. Retrieved 1 April from https://www.unfpa.org/sowmy
United Nations (1994) International Conference on Population and Development (ICPD). The final programme of action agreed to in Cairo. Retrieved 1 April from https://www.unfpa.org/resources/cairo-declaration-population-development.
United Nations (2015) The millennium development goals report 2015. United Nations. Retrieved 1 April from http://www.un.org/millenniumgoals/2015_MDG_Report/pdf/MDG%202015%20rev%20%28July%201%29.pdf
Utz B, Siddiqui G, Adegoke A, van den Broek N (2013) Definitions and roles of a skilled birth attendant: a mapping exercise from four South-Asian countries. Acta Obstet Gynecol Scand 92(9):1063–1069. https://doi.org/10.1111/aogs.12166
Waiswa P, Manzi F, Mbaruku G, Rowe AK, Marx M, Tomson G, Marchant T, Willey BA, Schellenberg J, Peterson S, Hanson C (2017) Effects of the EQUIP quasi-experimental study testing a collaborative quality improvement approach for maternal and newborn health care in Tanzania and Uganda. Implement Sci 12(1):89. https://doi.org/10.1186/s13012-017-0604-x
WHO (1978) Declaration of Alma-Ata. International Conference on Primary Health Care, Alma-Ata, USSR, 6–12 September 1978. Retrieved 1 April from https://www.who.int/publications/almaata_declaration_en.pdf
WHO (1996) Mother-baby-package. Maternal Health and Safe Motherhood Programme, WHO
WHO, FIGO, UKaid, E4A, UNFPA, CDC, ICM (2013) Maternal death surveillance and response. Technical guidance. Information for action to prevent maternal death. http://apps.who.int/iris/bitstream/10665/87340/1/9789241506083_eng.pdf?ua=1. Accessed 31 Mar 2022
WHO, UNFPA, UNICEF, AMMD (2009) Monitoring emergency obstetric care: a handbook. WHO.
WHO, UNFPA, UNICEF, ICM, ICN, FIGO, IPA (2018) Definition of skilled health personnel providing care during childbirth. The 2018 joint statement by WHO, UNFPA, UNICEF, ICM, ICN, FIGO, IPA. http://www.who.int/reproductivehealth/publications/statement-competent-mnh-professionals/en/
WHO, UNICEF (1997) The sisterhood method for estimating maternal mortality: guidance notes for potential users. Division of Reproductive Health, WHO
WHO, UNICEF, UNFPA, World Bank Group, United Nations (2015) Trends in maternal mortality: 1990–2015. Estimates by WHO, UNICEF, UNFPA, World Bank Group and the United Nations Population Division. http://www.who.int/reproductivehealth/publications/monitoring/maternal-mortality-2015/en/
WHO, UNICEF, UNFPA, World Bank Group, United Nations Population Division (2019) Maternal mortality: levels and trends 2000 to 2017. https://apps.who.int/iris/handle/10665/327595. Zugegriffen am 11.12.2019
World Health Organization (2021) Maternal and perinatal death surveillance and response: materials to support implementation. WHO
Zamboni K, Singh S, Tyagi M, Hill Z, Hanson C, Schellenberg J (2021) Effect of collaborative quality improvement on stillbirths, neonatal mortality and newborn care practices in hospitals of Telangana and Andhra Pradesh, India: evidence from a quasi-experimental mixed-methods study. Implement Sci 16(1):4. https://doi.org/10.1186/s13012-020-01058-z

Important Tropical Diseases with Relevance for Women's Health and Obstetrics

9

Camilla Rothe and Jürgen Wacker

Contents

C. Rothe (✉)
Consultant in Tropical Medicine, LMU University Hospital Centre, Institute of Infectious Diseases and Tropical Medicine, Munich, Germany
e-mail: camilla.rothe@med.uni-muenchen.de

J. Wacker
Retired Head of Frauenklinik Bruchsal, Bruchsal, Germany
e-mail: wacker@menschenfuerfrauen.de

J. Wacker et al. (eds.), *Global Women's Health*,
https://doi.org/10.1007/978-3-662-69700-9_9

Introductory Questions

1. What impact does malaria have on pregnancy?
   A) The pregnant woman has an increased risk of severe malaria.
   B) The rate of premature births is increased.
   C) Mother and child suffer from anemia.
   D) All are correct.
2. What complications does urogenital schistosomiasis cause for the woman?
   A) Cervical cancer
   B) Increased rate of twin pregnancies
   C) Chronic lower abdominal pain
   D) Severe embryonic malformations
3. What complications can a Zika virus infection have during pregnancy?
   A) Severe disease progression in the mother
   B) Microcephaly in the child
   C) Preeclampsia
   D) Increased risk of placenta praevia

9.1 Introduction

The following chapter introduces three tropical diseases that have particular significance for global women's health and obstetrics: Malaria is the most important parasitic infection in humans, it can endanger both pregnant women and unborn children. Schistosomiasis causes a variety of gynecological complaints in millions of women in Africa and is still extremely underestimated in its importance. Zika virus infection can cause severe fetal developmental disorders.

9.2 Malaria

9.2.1 Introduction and Epidemiology

Malaria is a potentially serious parasitic infection transmitted by mosquitoes.

Around 249 million people worldwide contracted malaria in 2022, more than 608,000 people died from it. About 95% of all malaria cases and deaths occur in

Sub-Saharan Africa; the majority of malaria deaths are children under 5 years old (WHO 2023).

Malaria during pregnancy can have negative effects on the health of both the mother and child. Around 12.7 million pregnancies in Africa were exposed to a malaria risk in 2022. The proportion was highest in West and Central Africa at around 40% (WHO 2023).

Malaria also exists in Asia, Oceania, and Latin America, but the number of cases in many of these regions is declining.

9.2.2 Pathogen and Transmission of Malaria

Malaria parasites are single-celled organisms of the genus Plasmodium. They are transmitted from dusk till dawn by female Anopheles mosquitoes. The most dangerous form of malaria is known as falciparum malaria. It is caused by the pathogen Plasmodium (P.) falciparum.

After being injected into the body, the malaria plasmodia first travel through the liver, where they multiply exponentially. After about a week, the parasites are released into the blood. They infect the red blood cells (erythrocytes). Inside the erythrocytes, they continue to multiply, the infected cells disintegrate and release parasites into the blood, which infect further red blood cells. The infected erythrocytes carry features (antigens) on their surface. With these, they attach to surface structures of numerous cells. This causes complex inflammatory reactions. The smallest blood vessels are blocked by the parasitized blood cells. This endangers the blood supply to vital organs including the placenta during pregnancy.

9.2.3 Clinical Course of Malaria

The incubation period of falciparum malaria is approximately 7–30 days, but it can also be longer (Ashley et al. 2018). Fever is the key symptom. In addition, chills, headaches, body aches, and diarrhea may occur. If malaria is not treated in a timely manner, there will be a rapid deterioration in health status (so-called severe malaria) in people without partial immunity (see below) after a few days. Patients with severe malaria may fall into a coma and develop multi-organ failure. The lethality is high.

9.2.4 Immunity to Malaria

Residents of high-risk malaria areas are usually confronted with the disease from childhood, many die from it. If they survive several episodes of malaria thanks to timely therapy, a so-called partial immunity to the disease develops over time (White et al. 2014). "Partially immune" means that an infection with malaria pathogens is still possible, but severe disease courses do no longer occur.

9.2.5 Malaria in Pregnancy

Pregnant women suffer more mosquito bites and therefore have an increased risk of malaria. Partial immunity to malaria is not effective in the first two pregnancies (Rogerson et al. 2018). Therefore, pregnant women are more likely to suffer from severe malaria. The risk of severe courses decreases in the course of further pregnancies. An immunity to pregnancy-specific antigens of the parasite develops.

In addition, malaria in pregnancy causes anemia in mother and child. This often exacerbates an existing anemia, which can be caused by malnutrition and helminth infections. Malaria in pregnancy endangers the blood supply to the placenta and thus the supply of the child with oxygen and nutrients. The affected children often have a low birth weight. Growth delays can also persist after birth (Fig. 9.1).

Due to the reduced transfer of antibodies through the placenta, the children have an increased susceptibility to infection and respond to vaccinations with a reduced immune response.

The neonatal and infant mortality of the affected children is increased (Chua et al. 2021; Rogerson et al. 2018). In the case of malaria in pregnancy, the rate of miscarriages and stillbirths is also increase. Premature births are more common,

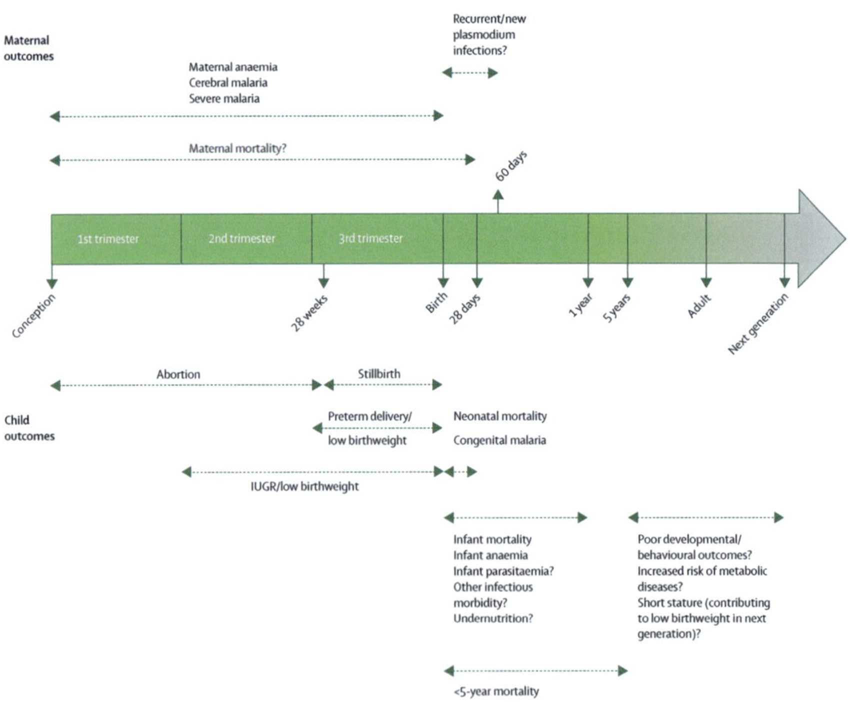

Fig. 9.1 Influence of malaria on pregnancy and on the health of mother and child. (From: Rogerson et al. 2018)

which is particularly problematic against the background of limited neonatal care in many countries of the global South.

9.2.6 Malaria Diagnostics

The gold standard for malaria diagnosis is the microscopy of a stained drop of blood to detect the parasites inside the red blood cells. Molecular biological methods such as the polymerase chain reaction (PCR) are also used in diagnostics.

In Africa, rapid malaria tests are preferably used today. The tests detect proteins of the pathogen in the blood. Rapid diagnostic tests for malaria have revolutionized malaria diagnosis in the global South, as they are very easy to perform. No electricity, no water, no laboratory, and no specialists are needed. The malaria diagnostics in pregnant women do not differ from the tests used in non-pregnant women (WHO 2022).

9.2.7 Malaria Therapy

Malaria is easily treatable, provided it is diagnosed early. The longer the diagnosis is delayed, the worse the result. This is particularly true for people without partial immunity (small children and primigravidae in malaria areas, travelers).

The therapy is carried out according to WHO with so-called artemisinin combination preparations (ACT).These are administered as tablets over a period of three days. They are highly effective and very well tolerated. Severe malaria with organ failure is acutely life-threatening. It is primarily treated with intravenous antimalarial drugs and patients should, if possible, be cared for in an intensive care unit. This is often not possible in most high-risk malaria areas due to the very low number of available intensive care beds.

In pregnancy, malaria is treated in the same way as in non-pregnant women: ACTs can be administered during the entire pregnancy (WHO 2022).

9.2.8 Malaria Prevention

Protection against malaria for people in malaria-endemic areas is based on the use of insecticide-treated bed nets (ITNs) and early treatment of malaria.

For pregnant women in endemic areas, the repeated preventive intake of antimalarial drugs is also recommended ("intermittent preventive treatment in pregnancy", IPTp) (WHO 2022).

Pregnant women who do not live in malaria regions should refrain from (holiday) travel to malaria risk areas (Rothe et al. 2021a). Travel is usually elective, the risk of malaria in pregnancy unnecessarily large. In addition, two of the three drugs recommended in Germany for chemoprophylaxis of malaria are contraindicated in pregnancy. The only available one, Mefloquine, potentially causes severe neuropsychiatric side effects.

For children in malaria endemic areas, the WHO has recommended vaccination against malaria since 2021, which reduces the risk of infection (Alonso and O'Brien 2022). In the context of travel medicine, the vaccination is not recommended, not even for malaria prevention in pregnancy. However, research is currently being conducted on specific vaccines against malaria in pregnancy (Chua et al. 2021).

9.3 Schistosomiasis (Bilharzia)

9.3.1 Introduction

Schistosomiasis is a tropical helminth disease of great importance for women's health. The disease was discovered by the German parasitologist Theodor Bilharz, hence it is also referred to as "Bilharzia". Schistosomiasis is caused by so-called paired flukes (schistosomes) that live in the venous blood vessels of humans. The eggs of the parasites cause a chronic inflammatory reaction in the tissue (Colley et al. 2014). Schistosomiasis of the urogenital tract can lead to a variety of gynecological problems.

9.3.2 Schistosomiasis—Epidemiology

More than 230 million people worldwide are infected with schistosomiasis. About 40–50 million women suffer from urogenital schistosomiasis (Bustinduy et al. 2022). It is caused by Schistosoma (S.) haematobium. This parasite is native only to Africa, the Arabian Peninsula and, for a few years now, also to Corsica (Holtfreter et al. 2014; Rothe et al. 2021b). Schistosomiasis is also one of the most important tropical diseases amongst migrants from Africa (Buonfrate et al. 2018). Despite its importance, it is considered one of the neglected tropical diseases (neglected tropical diseases, NTDs).

9.3.3 Life Cycle of Schistosomes

Infection occurs through contact with freshwater, e.g., when bathing, fishing, or fetching water, which is a daily task for many women and girls in Africa without access to running water. In the water, there are schistosome larvae (so-called cercariae; Fig. 9.2). These penetrate the skin. In the human body, they reach the lungs through the bloodstream and from there into the circulatory system. The parasites mature; male and female parasites live as pairs in the venous plexus of the liver and urogenital tract. The female lays many thousands of eggs per day. The eggs

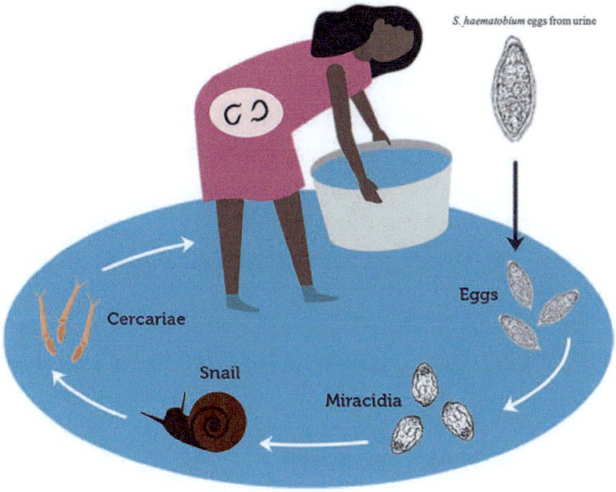

Fig. 9.2 Life cycle of Schistosoma haematobium, the causative agent of urogenital schistosomiasis. (From: Bustinduy et al. 2022)

are excreted with the urine, in other forms of schistosomiasis also in the stool. Some eggs cause an inflammatory reaction on their way through the body. This can lead to tissue remodeling and loss of organ function (see below).

The life cycle of the parasite can only close if human urine or feces enter freshwater unfiltered, where other people bathe. Therefore, regions where people live in extreme poverty are often affected (Hotez et al. 2019a).

9.3.4 Clinical presentation and Importance for Women's Health

Bloody urine often appears as an early symptom of urogenital schistosomiasis. Chronic schistosomiasis can lead to bladder carcinoma and kidney failure.

The schistosome eggs can be deposited in the vagina, uterus, cervix, and ovaries. The local inflammatory reaction leads to abdominal pain, dyspareunia, bleeding during intercourse, fertility impairments, vaginal discharge, ectopic pregnancies, and irregular menstrual bleeding.

There is evidence that women with genital schistosomiasis have an increased risk of HIV infection. Pregnant women who suffer from HIV and schistosomiasis also have an increased risk of transmitting the HIV infection to the child (Hotez et al. 2019b).

It is estimated that 33–75% of women and girls with schistosomiasis have urogenital complaints, around 40–50 million in total. Thus, urogenital Schistosomiasisis one of the most common gynecological disorders in Africa (Hotez et al. 2019a).

9.3.5 Diagnosis of Urogenital Schistosomiasis

The schistosome eggs can be detected microscopically in the urine. Inflammatory changes and calcifications of the tissue can be detected during a cystoscopy, colposcopy, or laparoscopy. Schistosome eggs and the typical inflammatory reaction can also be detectable in biopsies of affected tissues (Colley et al. 2014; Kjetland et al. 1996). However, inflammation foci may not be visible or easily accessible.

Serological blood tests can provide evidence of a current or past schistosomiasis infection.

In reality, many women in tropical schistosomiasis areas have no access to a diagnosis of the infection. Their complaints are often misinterpreted or ignored.

9.3.6 Treatment of Schistosomiasis

Currently, there is only one drug available to treat schistosomiasis: Praziquantel (Biltricide). Praziquantel kills the adult flukes, but the eggs and their inflammatory reaction cannot be eliminated by the drug. Chronic changes are therefore not reversible. The therapy is therefore only promising if it is carried out early.

In areas with a high disease burden of schistosomiasis, school children are ideally treated once or twice a year with praziquantel as part of a treatment programme.

Children and adolescents who do not (yet or any longer) go to school miss this therapy. Beyond the campaigns, access to the health system is often difficult. This explains why many millions of women worldwide suffer from chronic health problems as a result of urogenital schistosomiasis.

9.4 Zika

9.4.1 Introduction

Zika is a flu-like viral infection that is predominantly transmitted by mosquitoes. Zika made headlines when it became known that a Zika infection during pregnancy can lead to severe damage to the fetal nervous system.

9.4.2 Pathogen and Epidemiology of Zika

The Zika virus(ZIKV) was first described in 1947 in the Zika forest in Uganda. The virus spread in the decades after its discovery in Asia and the Pacific region. Initially, Zika was not given much attention as it was considered a harmless febrile disease. In 2015, there was the first major Zika outbreak in the Western Hemisphere. For the first time, it was observed that transmission from mother to child occurs and this can lead to the most severe child malformations. Today, Zika circulates in many countries in the tropics and subtropics, occasionally leading to outbreaks.

9.4.3 Transmission Routes of Zika

The Zika virus is primarily transmitted by the "tiger mosquito" (Aedes aegypti). Unusually for such a virus , Zika can also be transmitted from mother to child (see below) and is also sexually transmitted (Musso et al. 2019): Infectious virus particles are detectable in semen for about 30 days (Musso et al. 2019). Transmission from women to men is comparatively rare. Zika virus transmissions through blood transfusions have been described (Chen and Hamer 2018). Although ZIKV is detectable in breast milk, transmission through breastfeeding has not been documented so far (Eppes et al. 2017; Musso et al. 2019).

9.4.4 Clinical course of Zika Virus Infection and Importance for Women's Health

The incubation period for Zika is 3–14 days. Only 20–50% of those infected develop symptoms. Zika usually manifests as a mild flu-like infection with fever, a rash, body aches, headaches, and conjunctivitis. The symptoms are short-lived.

In 2015, during a Zika outbreak in Brazil, it became known that transmission from mother to child occurs a which may lead to severe fetal malformations: In 4–7% there is a miscarriage or stillbirth, 5–14% of children show a congenital Zika virus syndrome with microcephaly (Musso et al. 2019). About 70–90% of infected newborns initially show no symptoms, with medium or long-term damage such as neurocognitive developmental delays, epileptic seizures, hearing damage, eye damage or swallowing disorders often only being diagnosed later.

Mother-to-child transmission of Zika virus can occur in any trimester of pregnancy, with the risk being highest in the first trimester. The disease does not progress more severely in pregnant women than in non-pregnant women. The transmission is independent of whether the mother herself is symptomatic.

9.4.5 Diagnosis of Zika

The virus can be detected in the blood for about 2–10 days using PCR. It can be detected in the urine on average 2 weeks longer than in the blood (Eppes et al. 2017). A serological detection of Zika virus is usually possible 2–12 weeks after the onset of symptoms. Since the Zika viremia is short, even a negative result of an amniocentesis does not rule out the infection. An amniotic fluid examination to detect a Zika infection is therefore not primarily recommended. However, it can serve to exclude other causes of malformations in the child (e.g. other infections, genetic causes). Regular ultrasound checks by an experienced examiner are an essential part of prenatal care in the case of a Zika infection in the mother (Eppes et al. 2017).

9.4.6 Zika Diagnosis for Couples Planning to Have Children

Couples often wish to exclude Zika after returning from a trip to the tropics before a planned conception. Unfortunately, there is currently no test to definitively rule out a recent Zika virus infection. Preconception screening for couples planning to have children after one or both partners have stayed in an area with Zika virus circulation is therefore not recommended.

Instead, men should refrain from unprotected sex for at least 3 months after traveling to Zika areas, women for at least 8 weeks (Chen and Hamer 2018).

9.4.7 Precaution of Pregnant Women after Possible Zika Exposure

Pregnant women should be tested for a Zika infection after returning from an area with current Zika cases, even if they have no symptoms themselves. A PCR test from blood or urine and an antibody test are recommended. In addition, close ultrasound monitoring every 3–4 weeks is recommended (Musso et al. 2019).

9.4.8 Zika Therapy

Treatment is symptomatic. Newborns and infants with congenital Zika virus syndrome require the care of a multidisciplinary team, which accompanies the child and can recognize and possibly treat neurocognitive developmental delays early. Support offers for affected families play an important role in the care of the children (Musso et al. 2019).

9.4.9 Zika Prevention

There is currently no vaccine against Zika. Vaccines are being researched, but it is not foreseeable whether and when they will be marketed . Mosquito protection is therefore the most important prevention. Pregnant women or couples planning to have children from non-endemic areas should avoid traveling to tropical or subtropical areas.

Answers to the Initial Questions

1. D. All are correct.
2. C. Chronic lower abdominal pain
3. B. Microcephaly in the child

References

Alonso PL, O'Brien KL (2022) A malaria vaccine for Africa – an important step in a century-long quest. N Engl J Med 386(11):1005–1007. https://doi.org/10.1056/NEJMp2116591

Ashley EA, Pyae Phyo A, Woodrow CJ (2018) Malaria. Lancet 391(10130):1608–1621. https://doi.org/10.1016/S0140-6736(18)30324-6

Buonfrate D, Gobbi F, Marchese V, Postiglione C, Badona Monteiro G, Giorli G, Bisoffi Z (2018) Extended screening for infectious diseases among newly-arrived asylum seekers from Africa and Asia, Verona province, Italy, April 2014 to June 2015. Euro Surveill 23(16). https://doi.org/10.2807/1560-7917.ES.2018.23.16.17-00527

Bustinduy AL, Randriansolo B, Sturt AS, Kayuni SA, Leustcher PDC, Webster BL, Gyapong M (2022) An update on female and male genital schistosomiasis and a call to integrate efforts to escalate diagnosis, treatment and awareness in endemic and non-endemic settings: the time is now. Adv Parasitol 115:1–44. https://doi.org/10.1016/bs.apar.2021.12.003

Chen LH, Hamer DH (2018) Zika virus and sexual transmission: updated preconception guidance. J Travel Med 25(1). https://doi.org/10.1093/jtm/tay095

Chua CLL, Hasang W, Rogerson SJ, Teo A (2021) Poor birth outcomes in malaria in pregnancy: recent insights into mechanisms and prevention approaches. Front Immunol 12:621382. https://doi.org/10.3389/fimmu.2021.621382

Colley DG, Bustinduy AL, Secor WE, King CH (2014) Human schistosomiasis. Lancet 383(9936):2253–2264. https://doi.org/10.1016/S0140-6736(13)61949-2

Eppes C, Rac M, Dunn J, Versalovic J, Murray KO, Suter MA, Aagaard KM (2017) Testing for Zika virus infection in pregnancy: key concepts to deal with an emerging epidemic. Am J Obstet Gynecol 216(3):209–225. https://doi.org/10.1016/j.ajog.2017.01.020

Holtfreter MC, Mone H, Muller-Stover I, Mouahid G, Richter J (2014) Schistosoma haematobium infections acquired in Corsica, France, August 2013. Euro Surveill 19(22). https://doi.org/10.2807/1560-7917.es2014.19.22.20821

Hotez PJ, Engels D, Gyapong M, Ducker C, Malecela MN (2019a) Female Genital Schistosomiasis. N Engl J Med 381(26):2493–2495. https://doi.org/10.1056/NEJMp1914709

Hotez PJ, Harrison W, Fenwick A, Bustinduy AL, Ducker C, Sabina Mbabazi P, Floerecke Kjetland E (2019b) Female genital schistosomiasis and HIV/AIDS: reversing the neglect of girls and women. PLoS Negl Trop Dis 13(4):e0007025. https://doi.org/10.1371/journal.pntd.0007025

Kjetland EF, Poggensee G, Helling-Giese G, Richter J, Sjaastad A, Chitsulo L, Feldmeier H (1996) Female genital schistosomiasis due to Schistosoma haematobium. Clinical and parasitological findings in women in rural Malawi. Acta Trop 62(4):239–255. https://doi.org/10.1016/s0001-706x(96)00026-5

Musso D, Ko AI, Baud D (2019) Zika virus infection – after the pandemic. N Engl J Med 381(15):1444–1457. https://doi.org/10.1056/NEJMra1808246

Rogerson SJ, Desai M, Mayor A, Sicuri E, Taylor SM, van Eijk AM (2018) Burden, pathology, and costs of malaria in pregnancy: new developments for an old problem. Lancet Infect Dis 18(4):e107–e118. https://doi.org/10.1016/S1473-3099(18)30066-5

Rothe C, Veit O, Rosenbusch D, Bühler S, Feldt T, , Frühwein M, Boecken G (2024) Empfehlungen zur Malariaprophylaxe. Flug u Reisemed 31(4):165–206

Rothe C, Zimmer T, Schunk M, Wallrauch C, Helfrich K, Gultekin F, Boissier J (2021b) Developing endemicity of schistosomiasis, Corsica, France. Emerg Infect Dis 27(1). https://doi.org/10.3201/eid2701.204391

White NJ, Pukrittayakamee S, Hien TT, Faiz MA, Mokuolu OA, Dondorp AM (2014) Malaria. Lancet 383(9918):723–735. https://doi.org/10.1016/S0140-6736(13)60024-0

WHO (2023) World Malaria report 2022. https://www.who.int/teams/global-malaria-programme/reports/world-malaria-report-2023. Accessed 13 Sep 2024

WHO (2022) WHO Guidelines for Malaria, 25 November 2022. https://apps.who.int/iris/handle/10665/364714. Accessed 13 Mar 2023

Pandemics

10

Camilla Rothe and Laeticia Nwaeburu

Contents

C. Rothe (✉)
Consultant, LMU Hospital Centre Munich, Institute for Infectious Diseases and Tropical Medicine, Munich, Germany
e-mail: camilla.rothe@med.uni-muenchen.de

L. Nwaeburu
Ingolstadt Hospital, Department of Gynecology and Obstetrics, Ingolstadt, Germany

J. Wacker et al. (eds.), *Global Women's Health*,
https://doi.org/10.1007/978-3-662-69700-9_10

Introductory Questions

1. What percentage of people with HIV live in resource-limited countries?
   A. 5%
   B. 25%
   C. 50%
   D. 95%
2. What is the risk of mother-to-child transmission of HIV if no precautions are taken?
   A. <1%
   B. Approx. 5%
   C. Approx. 45 %
   D. Approx. 100%
3. Risk factors for a severe course of COVID-19 in pregnancy include:
   A. Maternal age <18 years
   B. Mother's obesity with Body Mass Index >30
   C. Multiple pregnancy
   D. Mother's pre-existing epilepsy

10.1 Introduction – Pandemics: Definition and History

An epidemic is an increase in the number of cases of a disease beyond the expected level. A pandemic is an epidemic that has spread across several continents. Humanity has been repeatedly plagued by pandemics throughout history. An overview is provided in Table 10.1.

In the third decade of the 21st century, two pandemics were preoccupying the world: HIV/AIDS and COVID-19, both viral infections that most likely originated from the animal kingdom.

HIV/AIDS entered human consciousness in 1981 and quickly spread around the world. It probably originated several decades earlier in Central Africa. From 2020-2023, the COVID-19 pandemic restricted access to the health system in most countries of the world. The collateral damage for patient care, health systems, but also for the global economy and ecology, was e considerable. We will look at the significance of the two major pandemics for global women's health in this chapter.

10.2 HIV/AIDS

10.2.1 History of the HIV Pandemic

In 1981, medical journals first reported clusters of unusual infectious diseases and tumors in homosexual men in the USA and Europe. The patients showed a significant deficiency of CD4-T-helper cells, which are important for infection defense.

Table 10.1 Major pandemics in human history. (Sampath et al. 2021).

Pandemic	Period	Pathogen	Region of Origin	Deaths
Justinian Plague	541–543	Yersinia pestis	Egypt	approx. 30–50 million
The "Black Death"	1347–1351	Yersinia pestis	Central Asia	approx. 200 million
Cholera (7 pandemics)	1817–present	Vibrio cholerae	India	approx. 40 million
"Spanish Flu"	1918-1920	Influenza H1N1	USA	approx. 20–50 million
HIV[1]	1981[2]–present	HIV	Central Africa	approx. 36 million
"Swine Flu"	2009/2010	Influenza H1N1	Mexico	approx. 150,000–250,000
SARS[3]	2002–2003	SARS-Coronavirus	China	approx. 800
COVID-19	2019–2023t	SARS-Coronavirus-2 (SARS-CoV2)	China	>6.8 million[4]

[1] HIV = Human Immunodeficiency Virus, [3] SARS = Severe Acute Respiratory Syndrome, [4] As of March 2023; [2] first cases were reported in 1981, the pandemic likely began several decades earlier

At that time, it was not yet clear that the cases of the novel disease that seemed to affect a then socially stigmatized fringe group were instead an expression of an already advanced pandemic. A pandemic that would not only cost the lives of many homosexual men, but also of many millions of women and children, a pandemic whose end is still not in sight more than forty years later.

Soon after, cases of an unknown immunodeficiency syndrome were also reported from Zaire (today's Democratic Republic of Congo). This time women and men were affected alike. The African patients also had noticeably few CD4-T-helper cells in their blood (Piot et al. 1984). The number of patients was large, the lethality high.

In 1983, a French and an American research group identified the cause of the immune deficiency phenomenon: a retrovirus, which was later referred to as the Human Immunodeficiency Virus (HIV) (Barre-Sinoussi et al. 1983).

Genetic analyses revealed that HIV originated in Central Africa and spilled over from the animal kingdom. It is closely related to the primate virus SIV (Simian Immunodeficiency Virus). Hunters in Central Africa with close contact to primates were most probably the humans first infected.

10.2.2 Epidemiology of HIV

Approximately 39 million people were infected with HIV worldwide in 2022. 95% lived in resource-limited countries, two-thirds in Africa alone (UNAIDS 2023).

About half of the people with HIV worldwide are women. In countries of the global North, however, women make up only a small proportion of people living with HIV. In Germany, for example, in 2023 only just above 20% of the approximately 96,700 people with HIV were female (Heiden et al. 2023).

This is because the transmission routes of HIV differ in different regions of the world. In Europe, North America, and Japan, the main route of transmission is sex between men (men having sex with men, msm).

In Africa, where the majority of people with HIV live, the main route of transmission is heterosexual intercourse (Fig. 10.1). Women and men are equally affected there. Risk groups are found only among certain professions: among prostitutes (Sex Workers) as well as in professions characterized by high mobility, such as long-distance truck drivers, fishermen, police, and military.

In particular, young women aged 15–24 are significantly more affected by HIV infections in the high prevalence regions in Africa than men of the same age. The causes for this are complex. One reason is that young women are significantly more exposed to sexual assaults than young men. Subtle economic dependencies on older men ("Sugar Daddies") also play a role (Wyrod et al. 2011).

10.2.3 Transmission of HIV and Special features in Women

The most common mode of HIV transmission worldwide is unprotected sexual intercourse. HIV is also transmitted through IV drug use with the exchange of injection equipment ("Needle Sharing").

Mother-to-child transmission has become extremely rare in the global North, but is still significant in Africa (Sect. 10.2.7). Transmission through blood products is rare today. For medical personnel, needlestick injuries are a possible source of infection, as well as mucous membrane contact with blood from HIV-positive patients.

In unprotected sexual intercourse, women have a higher risk of becoming infected with HIV than men. This is because the exposed mucosal surface of the female genitalia is larger than in men. In addition, small lesions often occur on the female genital mucosa during sexual contact, which facilitate the penetration of the virus. The virus concentration in semen is also higher than in female vaginal fluid.

Sexual practices prevalent in Sub-Saharan Africa such as "Dry Sex" further promote HIV infection. In this practice, the vagina is kept dry by inserting, for example, leaves, thereby increasing the frictional resistance and supposedly the pleasure for the man during intercourse. This results in painful injuries to the vaginal mucosa. These injuries make women more susceptible to HIV and other pathogens (Schwandt et al. 2006).

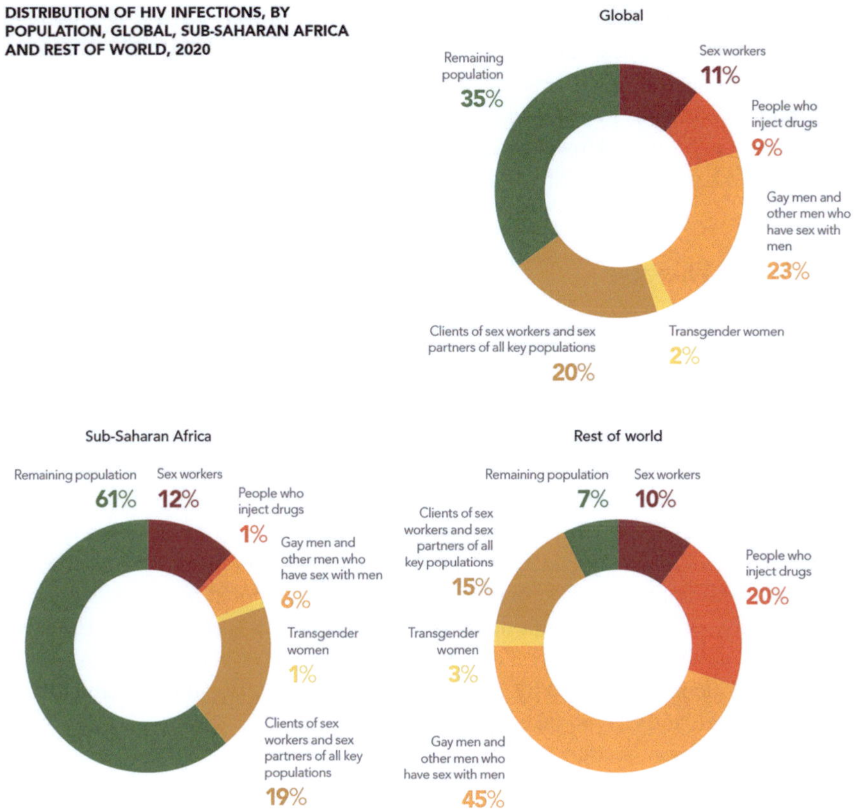

Fig. 10.1 Risk groups for HIV transmission compared between Sub-Saharan Africa and the rest of the world. Homosexual men, transgender people, or IV drug addicts make up a small proportion of people with HIV in Sub-Saharan Africa. The dominant "remaining population" in Africa are heterosexual men and women as well as children of HIV-positive mothers (with kind permission: Joint United Nations Programme on HIV/AIDS 2021, p. 12., UNAIDS 2021)

10.2.4 Clinical Course of HIV Infection

The HIV virus infects human T-helper cells (CD4 cells), the number of which decreases over the course of the infection. As the number of CD4 cells decreases, the body's ability to defend itself against certain infections and tumors decreases. People with HIV do not become ill from the virus itself, but from the diseases that result from the immune deficiency. The advanced stage of HIV infection is referred to as "Acquired Immunodeficiency Syndrome", AIDS. The time between initial HIV infection and the onset of AIDS is very variable and usually lasts several years without treatment. With timely therapy, the onset of AIDS can be completely prevented.

An untreated HIV infection in women progresses differently than in men. Hormonal factors appear to play a role: Directly after an initial HIV infection, women generate a stronger inflammatory response than men. Therefore, the viral load in the blood does not increase as much, and the CD4 cells do not decrease as significantly as in men. However, in the further course, women show a faster progression into the AIDS stage (Addo and Altfeld 2014).

10.2.5 HIV Therapy

HIV is now well treatable, but not curable. It has become a chronic disease. The antiretroviral Therapy (ART) usually consists of three drugs. These can now be administered as a fixed drug combination in one tablet. Alternatively, injectable antiretroviral therapies with depot effect are increasingly available.

A highly effective HIV combination therapy has existed since 1996. Only about 10 years later, antiretroviral therapy gradually became available for people in the global South. Major initiatives by international donors were decisive for this. Without these donor consortia, comprehensive care for HIV patients with medication would still not be possible in many countries of the global South today.

Originally, only people with advanced HIV infection were treated. However, since 2015, the principle of "Test and Treat" has been in effect: Every person with HIV worldwide should start ART as soon as possible after diagnosis. Today's ART is well tolerated and easy to take.

About three months after starting antiretroviral therapy, the viral load is below the detection limit and the affected person is considered no longer infectious. This is also crucial for preventing mother-to-child transmission of HIV (see below).

10.2.6 HIV Prevention

Women still do not have self-determination over their bodies in many places and are exposed to men and their needs. Against this background, those methods of HIV prevention that can be used autonomously are attractive to women.

Condoms protect against HIV and other sexually transmitted diseases; they also serve family planning. However, women depend on the cooperation of the male partner for their use.

Microbicides are substances that neutralize HIV and other pathogens. They are usually applied locally as vaginal gels, lubricants, diaphragms, or vaginal rings. They can therefore be applied autonomously by women. The WHO recommends, for example, a vaginal ring coated with an antiretroviral drug. However, study results on the effectiveness of microbicides are generally rather disappointing. Microbicides should therefore always be used in combination with other HIV prevention measures.

Two concepts have proven to be groundbreaking for HIV prevention in recent years:

Treatment as Prevention, (TasP) is based on the finding that infectivity correlates with the HIV viral load, i.e., the number of virus copies in the blood. About three months after the start of antiretroviral therapy, the HIV viral load is usually below the detection limit. A low viral load results in a low probability of transmission. An HIV-negative woman with a successfully treated and therapy-adherent HIV-positive partner therefore has a very low risk of HIV infection thanks to TasP, and an HIV-positive mother has a good chance of not infecting her baby with HIV under effective antiretroviral therapy (see Sect. 10.2.7).

Antiretroviral therapy has thus become the most important pillar of HIV prevention.

HIV Pre-Exposure Prophylaxis ("PrEP"), describes the intake of antiretroviral drugs (ARVs) by HIV-negative people for their own protection against HIV.

The introduction of PrEP has ensured that the rate of new HIV-infections among msm in the Global North has significantly decreased (Nwokolo et al. 2017)

PrEP strategy would also potentially be attractive for women, especially in high-risk areas in Sub-Saharan Africa, as a method of self-determined HIV prevention.

Studies on oral PrEP in African women have so far produced rather disappointing results (Van Damme et al. 2012). Low adherence among study participants was presumably the cause. Female oral PrEP requires daily pill intake. In men, intermittent intake before and after sexual intercourse is also possible, as the drugs reach a higher concentration in the anal mucosa than in the vaginal mucosa. Therefore, a PrEP using an injectable long-acting antiretroviral drug (Cabotegravir), which has a depot effect lasting two months, could potentially be promising. In one study, the administration of Cabotegravir reduced the risk of HIV infection by 89% compared to taking oral PrEP (Delany-Moretlwe et al. 2022).A newer drug seems even more promising: Lenacapravir, has only to be given twice a year and can be administered subcutaneously (Bekker LG, 2024).

HIV Post-Exposure Prophylaxis (PEP), describes the intake of antiretroviral drugs after a high-risk exposure (e.g., rape by an HIV-positive person, needlestick injury). The antiretroviral drugs must be taken as soon as possible after exposure, preferably within the first 72 hours and for a duration of 4 weeks (WHO 2021). A vaccine against HIV is being intensively researched, but is still not available four decades after the first description of HIV.

10.2.7 HIV in Pregnancy

HIV-discordant couples, that is, couples where one partner is HIV-positive, can have children together. It is important that the HIV-positive partner is taking effective antiretroviral therapy and the viral load is below the detection limit. The HIV-negative partner can additionally protect themselves with PrEP.

If an expectant mother is HIV-positive herself, it is of crucial importance to prevent the transmission of HIV to the child. Without any protective measures, up to

45% of children become infected with HIV (Bailey et al. 2018). Transmission can occur in utero, during birth, or through breastfeeding (Knapp 2022).

The most important measure to prevent mother-to-child transmission of HIV is the successful antiretroviral therapy of the mother. With effective ART during pregnancy and childbirth, and abstaining from breastfeeding, the transmission rate in industrialized nations is less than 1%. In countries of the Global South, where HIV-positive mothers are advised to breastfeed (see below), the transmission rate under optimal conditions is about 5% (WHO 2018), but under real-life conditions it is much higher in many countries (UNAIDS 2021).

HIV therapy should ideally be started before conception (Mandelbrot et al. 2015). In that case, a normal vaginal delivery is very well possible. Pregnant women who do not take antiretroviral therapy or who do not have suppressed viral load under therapy are advised to deliver by cesarean section. During childbirth, the mother may be given additional antiretroviral drugs. For newborn children of HIV-positive mothers, the intake of antiretroviral drugs is recommended, usually for a duration of 4-6 weeks (DAIG 2020; Knapp 2022; WHO 2021).

Breastfeeding recommendations differ between countries of the Global North and South. Even successfully treated mothers are advised against breastfeeding here, as there is a small residual risk of HIV transmission through breast milk (DAIG 2020).

However, breastfeeding is essential for the child's health in many countries with lower socioeconomic standards, without access to safe drinking water and with limited offers of breast milk substitutes. Non-breastfed children are clearly disadvantaged in this environment, so a residual risk of HIV transmission is accepted. Breast milk also contains antibodies and thus protects the child from infections.

Mothers who both breastfeed and use formula milk (so-called "mixed feeding") have an approximately 6-fold higher risk of HIV transmission than mothers who exclusively breastfeed. Therefore, the WHO recommends women in the Global South to exclusively breastfeed for 6 months.

10.2.8 Global Therapy Goals

"90-90-90" was issued by the UN organization UNAIDS as a global treatment goal for the year 2020: 90% of all people with HIV should know their status, of whom 90% should be taking antiretroviral therapy and 90% should have a viral load below the detection limit.

Many countries in the world, especially in southern Africa, have already achieved this goal (UNAIDS 2021). The new goal for 2030 is "95-95-95".

Women perform better at reaching "90-90-90" than men. One reason for this could be the fact that in many countries of the world, and especially in Africa, pregnancies provide women with important contact with the health system. As part of prenatal care, women receive an HIV test and possibly immediate antiretroviral therapy. The goal of not transmitting HIV to the child could be an additional incentive for the woman to take HIV medication regularly. Men do not have comparable access to preventive measures. Therefore, they often present later than women, only in the AIDS stage, when therapy becomes complicated and the prognosis is poor.

10.3 COVID-19

10.3.1 Course of SARS-CoV2 Infection in Pregnancy

A significant proportion of SARS-CoV-2 infections in pregnancy are asymptomatic.

The symptoms of COVID-19 infection in pregnant women are comparable to those in non-pregnant women of childbearing age (Table 10.2). Persistent symptoms and sequelae can occur (Zollkau et al. 2022).

However, there is evidence that COVID-19 infection in pregnancy often has a more severe course than in non-pregnant individuals. Risk factors for severe disease progression in pregnant women include maternal age >35 years, obesity with a BMI >30, chronic hypertension, pre-existing diabetes, gestational diabetes, preeclampsia, and the presence of a high-risk pregnancy (Allotey et al. 2020)

The exact pathomechanisms that explain the severe course of SARS-CoV-2 infection in some patients are not yet fully understood. However, there is increasing evidence that the virus causes endothelial damage in the end-organs with activation of coagulation (Varga et al. 2020). Decidual arteriopathies and increased intervillous thromboses have been detected in the placenta (Shanes et al. 2020).

10.3.2 Impact of COVID-19 on Pregnancy

Pregnant women with COVID-19 have a higher rate of preterm birth. The rate of newborns from mothers with COVID-19 who had to be cared for in a neonatal intensive care unit is also increased (Allotey et al. 2020).

Table 10.2 Symptoms of COVID-19 disease in pregnancy. (Elshafeey et al. 2020)

Symptom	Frequency
Fever	67%
Cough	66%
Dyspnea	7%
Sore throat	7%
Fatigue	7%
Myalgia	6%
Moderate liver enzyme elevation	5%
Thrombocytopenia	1%
Smell/taste disorders	64–89%

A SARS-CoV-2 infection in pregnancy may also be associated with an increased incidence of preeclampsia and more frequent thromboembolic events (Jering et al. 2021)

10.3.3 Mother-to-Child Transmission of SARS-CoV2

In light of increased antibody and cytokine levels in the blood of newborns of SARS-CoV-2-positive mothers and COVID-typical histopathological placental changes, the possibility of transplacental virus transmission was discussed (Dong et al. 2020).

The vaginal mucosa does not appear to be involved in virus transmission or replication. However, viral RNA has been detected in stool samples; this must be considered as a possible source of contamination during vaginal delivery. The risk of newborn infection with SARS-CoV-2 is low, the outcome is usually favorable; also, the transmission risk does not seem to be increased if the newborn stays in the mother's room instead of being cared for in a separate room. It is unclear whether postpartum transmission depends on the severity of the maternal infection.

Separation of mother and healthy child is not necessarily required in the case of SARS-CoV-2 infection or COVID-19 disease, provided hygiene rules and measures to prevent virus transmission are adhered to: Skin-to-skin contact between mother and child should be allowed while adhering to hygiene rules and measures. (Hand disinfection, face mask, no mucous membrane contact, among others, no kissing)

The risk of transmission of SARS-CoV-2 through breast milk is very low when hygiene recommendations are followed. The main route of transmission of the virus to the newborn during breastfeeding is maternal droplet or aerosol formation (Williams et al. 2020). Practical guidance on the specific hygiene rules and measures during breastfeeding is mandatory. In addition to the known benefits of breastfeeding, passive immune protection through breastfeeding is also conceivable.

10.3.4 Covid-19 Vaccination during Pregnancy

The German Standing Committee on Vaccination (STIKO) recommends vaccination against COVID-19 during pregnancy from the second trimester with an mRNA-based vaccine.

Postpartum and breastfeeding women as well as their close contacts should also be vaccinated against COVID-19 (RKI 2021). A breastfeeding pause or refusal is not necessary. An accidental vaccination against COVID-19 in the first trimester or periconceptionally is not an indication for termination of pregnancy.

Maternal antibodies formed by vaccination represent a potential infection protection for the infant. Maternal IgG antibodies after SARS-CoV-2 infection also correlate positively with the antibody levels of their newborns.

Virus-specific antibodies were detected in the breast milk of women with active or past SARS-CoV-2 infection during pregnancy (Gao et al. 2020). Whether these provide maternal passive immunity is currently unclear.

Studies on the side effect profile after vaccination with an mRNA vaccine of women of childbearing age showed that menstrual disorders were frequently reported. However, COVID-19 immunization in pregnancy and lactation showed no increased or deviating side effects. By trend, both local and systemic vaccine reactions were even less common in pregnant women than in non-pregnant women. Complaints were pain at the injection site, fatigue, headache, myalgia, and chills. There is no evidence to date that the COVID-19 vaccination negatively affects pregnancy and childbirth or even leads to birth complications (Leik et al. 2021).

However, resistance to COVID-19 vaccination has developed in many countries (Schmelz and Bowles 2021). A German survey among pregnant women showed only a vaccination willingness of 11% compared to 64% strict vaccination refusal. Gynecologists should work on the vaccination readiness of pregnant women or women of childbearing age, as an infection with SARS-CoV-2 during pregnancy is a risk factor for severe diseases and complications of the mother (see above).

Education and informed counseling on COVID-19 vaccination during pregnancy of a mother who lacks basic immunity to COVID can help improve the relatively low acceptance of vaccination by the mother.

It is crucial to take the concerns and fears of women seriously and to provide targeted information.

10.3.5 Collateral Damage from COVID-19?

The collateral damage caused by the COVID-19 pandemic is difficult to quantify. However, it is assumed to be significant. Particularly in African countries, where the pandemic overall seems to have been much less severe than elsewhere, it is assumed that the sometimes drastic lockdown measures have caused greater economic, social, and medical damage than COVID-19 itself.

The pandemic has led to a deterioration in patient care in most countries around the world, due to lockdowns, fear of infection when in contact with medical facilities, blocked hospital beds, overloaded intensive care units, postponement of elective procedures, and staff shortages and reassignments. For example, a German study showed a decrease in the number of oncology inpatients by 6% (Griewing et al. 2022). In contrast, the number of births increased by 11%. As a result of the local "Stay at home policy", a higher rate of stillbirths and ruptured ectopic pregnancies was reported from Israel. A higher rate of surgical deliveries and postpartum complications was reported from Austria.

The full medical, social, economic, and ecological implications of the pandemic will only be able to be conclusively assessed in a few years' time.

Answers to the Initial Questions

1. D
2. C
3. B

References

Addo MM, Altfeld M (2014) Sex-based differences in HIV type 1 pathogenesis. J Infect Dis 209(Suppl 3):S86–S92. https://doi.org/10.1093/infdis/jiu175

Allotey J, Stallings E, Bonet M, Yap M, Chatterjee S, Kew T et al (2020) Clinical manifestations, risk factors, and maternal and perinatal outcomes of coronavirus disease 2019 in pregnancy: living systematic review and meta-analysis. BMJ 370:m3320. https://doi.org/10.1136/bmj.m3320

Bailey H, Zash R, Rasi V, Thorne C (2018) HIV treatment in pregnancy. Lancet HIV 5(8):e457–e467. https://doi.org/10.1016/S2352-3018(18)30059-6

Barre-Sinoussi F, Chermann JC, Rey F, Nugeyre MT, Chamaret S, Gruest J et al (1983) Isolation of a T-lymphotropic retrovirus from a patient at risk for acquired immune deficiency syndrome (AIDS). Science 220(4599):868–871. https://doi.org/10.1126/science.6189183

DAIG (2020) Deutsch-Österreichische Leitlinie zur HIV-Therapie in der Schwangerschaft und bei HIV-exponierten Neugeborenen. https://www.awmf.org/uploads/tx_szleitlinien/055-002l_S2k_HIV-Therapie-Schwangerschaft-und-HIVexponierten_Neugeborenen_2020-10_01.pdf. Accessed 30.03.2022

Delany-Moretlwe S, Hughes JP, Bock P, Ouma SG, Hunidzarira P, Kalonji D et al (2022) Cabotegravir for the prevention of HIV-1 in women: results from HPTN 084, a phase 3, randomised clinical trial. Lancet. https://doi.org/10.1016/S0140-6736(22)00538-4

Dong Y, Chi X, Hai H, Sun L, Zhang M, Xie WF, Chen W (2020) Antibodies in the breast milk of a maternal woman with COVID-19. Emerg Microbes Infect 9(1):1467–1469. https://doi.org/10.1080/22221751.2020.1780952

Elshafeey F, Magdi R, Hindi N, Elshebiny M, Farrag N, Mahdy S et al (2020) A systematic scoping review of COVID-19 during pregnancy and childbirth. Int J Gynaecol Obstet 150(1):47–52. https://doi.org/10.1002/ijgo.13182

Gao X, Wang S, Zeng W, Chen S, Wu J, Lin X et al (2020) Clinical and immunologic features among COVID-19-affected mother-infant pairs: antibodies to SARS-CoV-2 detected in breast milk. New Microbes New Infect 37:100752. https://doi.org/10.1016/j.nmni.2020.100752

Griewing S, Wagner U, Lingenfelder M, Heinis S, Schieffer B, Markus B (2022) Impact of the COVID-19 pandemic on delivery of gynecology and obstetrics services at a maximum care university hospital in Germany. Geburtshilfe Frauenheilkd 82(4):427–440. https://doi.org/10.1055/a-1687-9674

an der Heiden M, Marcus U, Kollan C, Schmidt D, Koppe U, Gunsenheimer-Bartmeyer B, Bremer V: HIV 2022 und 2023. Epid Bull 2024;(28):3-20 . DOI https://doi.org/10.25646/12212

Jering KS, Claggett BL, Cunningham JW, Rosenthal N, Vardeny O, Greene MF, Solomon SD (2021) Clinical characteristics and outcomes of hospitalized women giving birth with and without COVID-19. JAMA Intern Med 181(5):714–717. https://doi.org/10.1001/jamainternmed.2020.9241

Knapp KM (2022) Prevention of mother-to-child human immunodeficiency virus transmission in resource-limited countries. Pediatr Clin N Am 69(1):1–18. https://doi.org/10.1016/j.pcl.2021.08.007

Leik NKO, Ahmedy F, Guad RM, Baharuddin DMP (2021) Covid-19 vaccine and its consequences in pregnancy: brief review. Ann Med Surg (Lond) 72:103103. https://doi.org/10.1016/j.amsu.2021.103103

Mandelbrot L, Tubiana R, Le Chenadec J, Dollfus C, Faye A, Pannier E et al (2015) No perinatal HIV-1 transmission from women with effective antiretroviral therapy starting before conception. Clin Infect Dis 61(11):1715–1725. https://doi.org/10.1093/cid/civ578

Nwokolo N, Hill A, McOwan A, Pozniak A (2017) Rapidly declining HIV infection in MSM in central London. Lancet HIV 4(11):e482–e483. https://doi.org/10.1016/S2352-3018(17)30181-9

Piot P, Quinn TC, Taelman H, Feinsod FM, Minlangu KB, Wobin O et al (1984) Acquired immunodeficiency syndrome in a heterosexual population in Zaire. Lancet 2(8394):65–69. https://doi.org/10.1016/s0140-6736(84)90241-1

RKI (2021) Impfungen bei Schwangeren, Stillenden und bei Kinderwunsch. https://www.rki.de/SharedDocs/FAQ/COVID-Impfen/FAQ_Liste_Impfung_Schwangere_Stillende.html

Sampath S, Khedr A, Qamar S, Tekin A, Singh R, Green R, Kashyap R (2021) Pandemics throughout the history. Cureus 13(9):e18136. https://doi.org/10.7759/cureus.18136

Schmelz K, Bowles S (2021) Overcoming COVID-19 vaccination resistance when alternative policies affect the dynamics of conformism, social norms, and crowding out. Proc Natl Acad Sci U S A 118(25). https://doi.org/10.1073/pnas.2104912118

Schwandt M, Morris C, Ferguson A, Ngugi E, Moses S (2006) Anal and dry sex in commercial sex work, and relation to risk for sexually transmitted infections and HIV in Meru, Kenya. Sex Transm Infect 82(5):392–396. https://doi.org/10.1136/sti.2006.019794

Shanes ED, Mithal LB, Otero S, Azad HA, Miller ES, Goldstein JA (2020) Placental pathology in COVID-19. Am J Clin Pathol 154(1):23–32. https://doi.org/10.1093/ajcp/aqaa089

UNAIDS (2023) UNAIDS Data 2023 Geneva. Accessed 14.09.2024

Van Damme L, Corneli A, Ahmed K, Agot K, Lombaard J, Kapiga S et al (2012) Preexposure prophylaxis for HIV infection among African women. N Engl J Med 367(5):411–422. https://doi.org/10.1056/NEJMoa1202614

Varga Z, Flammer AJ, Steiger P, Haberecker M, Andermatt R, Zinkernagel AS et al (2020) Endothelial cell infection and endotheliitis in COVID-19. Lancet 395(10234):1417–1418. https://doi.org/10.1016/S0140-6736(20)30937-5

WHO (2018) HIV Diagnosis and ARV Use in HIV-exposed infants: a programmatic update. Geneva https://apps.who.int/iris/bitstream/handle/10665/273155/WHO-CDS-HIV-18.17-eng.pdf

WHO (2021) Consolidated guidelines on HIV prevention, testing, treatment, service delivery and monitoring. Recommendations for a public Health approach. In WHO (Hrsg), p 592

Williams J, Namazova-Baranova L, Weber M, Vural M, Mestrovic J, Carrasco-Sanz A et al (2020) The importance of continuing breastfeeding during coronavirus disease-2019: in support of the World Health Organization statement on breastfeeding during the pandemic. J Pediatr 223:234–236. https://doi.org/10.1016/j.jpeds.2020.05.009

Wyrod R, Fritz K, Woelk G, Jain S, Kellogg T, Chirowodza A et al (2011) Beyond sugar daddies: intergenerational sex and AIDS in urban Zimbabwe. AIDS Behav 15(6):1275–1282. https://doi.org/10.1007/s10461-010-9800-2

Zollkau J, Hagenbeck C, Hecher K, Pecks U, Schlembach D, Simon A et al (2022) Recommendations for SARS-CoV-2/COVID-19 during pregnancy, birth and childbed – update November 2021 (Long Version). Z Geburtshilfe Neonatol 226(1):e1–e35. https://doi.org/10.1055/a-1688-9398

Care during labour and childbirth

11

Anne Fritz, Grace Komuhangi, Anne-Katrin Klotzsch, Madeleine Da, Ramata Edvige Ilboudo, Margret Bauer and Jürgen Wacker

Contents

A. Fritz (✉)
Akademie für Gesundheitsberufe gGmbH, Heidelberg, Germany
e-mail: Anne.Fritz@med.uni-heidelberg.de

G. Komuhangi
Duisburg, Cham, Germany

A.-K. Klotzsch
Hebamme, Bachelor of Science in International Midwifery Studies, Berlin, Germany

M. Da · R. E. Ilboudo
Hebammenschule Saint-Edvige, Ouagadougou, Burkina Faso

M. Bauer
Frauenklinik, Fürst-Stirum-Klinik Bruchsal, Bruchsal, Germany
e-mail: Margret.Bauer@rkh-kliniken.de

J. Wacker
ehemaliger Chefarzt der Frauenklinik Bruchsal, Bruchsal, Germany

J. Wacker et al. (eds.), *Global Women's Health*,
https://doi.org/10.1007/978-3-662-69700-9_11

Introductory Questions

1. The number of children born globally per year is:
   A. 140 million
   B. 14 million
   C. 1.4 million
   D. Other number
2. On which continent most children are born globally each year?
   A. Asia
   B. Africa
   C. America
   D. Europe
   E. Australia
3. What percentage of registered births globally are attended by midwives? (Figures in %)
   F. 81%
   G. 75%
   H. 60%
   I. 50%

11.1 Introduction

The birth of a child is described as one of the fundamental experiences in a woman's life, and the aim of any care before, during, and after birth should be to maintain and strengthen the health of mother and child. This aim should be the measure of all actions taken by those involved in the birth process (Bundesministerium für Gesundheit 2017). Midwifery is crucial for the health of mother and child, because a large part of maternal mortality and morbidity could be prevented if women had unrestricted access to skilled care by midwives, as well as medical and in some countries specially trained nursing staff, during pregnancy, labour and birth, and the postnatal period (UNFPA/United Nations Populations Fund 2021).

The skilled care in a sensitive phase of a woman´s life is reflected in the professional titles of midwives. The English term *Midwife* means *to be with woman* and emphasizes the support for the expectant mother. The French term *sage-femme*, the wise woman, highlights the knowledge of midwives. The German term Hebamme comes from the Old High German term *hevianna = the ancestress, who lifts/holds the child,* and older midwifery texts describe that the task of the midwife is to assist women in their hour of need (Burger 1996; Grabrucker 1989).

This chapter focuses on care during labour and childbirth, starting with respectful maternity care, as well as the partograph, intermittent auscultation of the fetal heart rate, the WHO Safe Childbirth Checklist, and obstetric personnel. After that, experiences and implementations of the above-mentioned topics will be illustrated using the examples of Uganda and The Gambia, before finally addressing the cooperation between midwives, doctors, and traditional birth attendants.

11.2 Respectful Maternity Care

Due to high maternal mortality in emerging and developing countries, international organizations such as the WHO and national health systems have long focused solely on providing basic and emergency care in obstetrics, without adequately considering the quality of care and the working and living conditions of the staff providing maternity care. However, studies conducted worldwide have found that a large proportion of women experience various forms of violence and disrespect in health facilities. The following forms of disrespect and violence were identified: physical abuse, deep humiliation and verbal insult, imposed or medical interventions carried out without explicit consent (including sterilization), disregard of confidentiality, non-compliance with obtaining fully informed consent, withholding of pain relief, gross violation of privacy, refusal of admission to medical facilities, neglect of women during childbirth, which has led to life-threatening, avoidable complications in these women, as well as the detention of women and their newborns in obstetric facilities after birth, if they were unable to pay fees (Bohren et al. 2019; Bowser and Hill 2010; Sheferaw et al. 2017; World Health Organization 2015a). Particularly affected groups include adolescents, unmarried women, women of low socio-economic status, women belonging to an ethnic minority, women with a migration background and women infected with HIV (Bowser and Hill 2010). It is important to emphasize that this is a global problem affecting both rich and poor countries, as the causes of disrespect and violence being discussed affect many countries, such as high workload with low pay, inadequate supply and equipment of maternity wards with material and medication, difficult and often unsafe working conditions especially for women, rigid hierarchies and little appreciation of midwifery work (World Health Organization 2016a). The World Health Organization (WHO) therefore published the declaration "Prevention and elimination of disrespect and mistreatment during childbirth in obstetric facilities" in 2015 and named criteria by which, among other things, respectful health care during childbirth can be measured, such as social support by a companion chosen by the woman, mobility, access to food and drink, observance of confidentiality and privacy, obtaining fully informed consent, informing women about their rights, compensation mechanisms after violations of their rights and ensuring a high professional standard in clinical care (World Health Organization 2015a).

Some points of this declaration will also be addressed with regard to training and further education.

11.2.1 Choice of birth partner

The presence of a birth partner protects women in labor from assaults (Sheferaw et al. 2017) and has been and is being made possible in many obstetric facilities during the current Corona pandemic despite stricter hygiene regulations and social distancing rules. The person of trust who accompanies the woman in labour can stand up for her when she can no longer do so due to strong contractions. However, the attending midwife should also focus on "advocacy", which means standing up for the interests of the woman and protecting mother and child especially during the vulnerable period of labour and childbirth. Advocacy should be an integral part of midwifery training courses and awareness for advocacy issues can be raised through regulary reflecting on student´s experiences while caring for women in labour. The following Fig. 11.1 shows a woman in labour with her partner standing upright.

11.2.2 Maternal positions and Mobility During Childbirth

Mobility during childbirth and giving birth in upright birthing positions is more successful when appropriate rooms and facilities such as easily adjustable beds or birthing stools are available. But even without these, positions such as the all-fours position or standing upright can be chosen for coping with contractions or giving birth. However, supporting women in upright birthing positions not only has to be taught during midwifery training, but it also needs to be practiced regularly so that the attending midwife feels confident in delivering babies in upright birthing positions. In this respect, practical tips can be helpful, such as that in the all-fours position the foetal head has to be lifted first and then lowered for the delivery of the anterior shoulder, i. e. it is exactly the opposite of delivering in the supine position. When giving birth standing upright it is advisable to let the woman kneel down after delivering the head , in order to shorten the distance to the ground and to cushion it best with pillows etc. or to have a second pair of hands available that can support the baby´storso in order to be able to deliver the baby safely onto a clean, soft surface.

11.2.3 Debriefing of the Birth

In critical situations that require quick action during birth, there is often very little to no time to inform women about the actions taken or to obtain the aforementioned comprehensive informed consent, which can be disturbing for the birthing woman or perceived as violent. In this case, the postnatal debriefing has proven to be effective, to help the mother better understand the birth experience and clarify any questions (Deutscher Hebammenverband e. V. 2021a). This debriefing should ideally be done by staff that was present during labour and delivery, but if this is not possible any skilled obstetric staff can talk with the mother about her birth

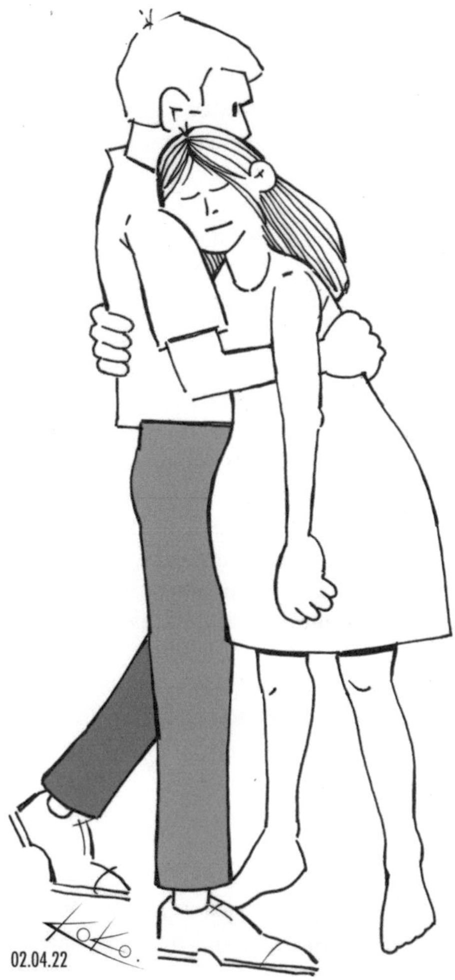

Fig. 11.1 Woman in labor with partner standing upright. (© Diethard Kokoska)

experience. This aspect of midwifery care should be taught during midwifery training and can be practiced , e.g. while caring for mothers in the early postnatal period.

11.2.4 One-To-One Care

Ensuring a high professional standard in clinical care must go hand in hand with improvements in the working conditions of health personnel, who can only exploit theirfull potential when working in a safe, supportive, and appreciative environment (World Health Organization 2016a). This is not the case even in many industrialized nations, where quite a number of midwives leave clinical work in labour units due to a high workload which forces them to regularly care for 3-4 labouring women simultaneously and that prevents them from giving the care they want to give. (Deutscher Hebammenverband e. V. 2021b).

One-to-one care allows midwives to respond to the needs of the birthing woman and quickly recognize complications, and increases the satisfaction of mothers and midwives (Deutscher Hebammenverband e. V. 2021b). Due to the global shortage of midwives of approximately 900,000 midwives (UNFPA/United Nations Populations Fund 2021), continuous one-to-one care is often not possible and it will take a long breath from a health and professional political perspective to implement this. Nevertheless, this goal should be pursued further.

Under the motto "A midwife for every woman", Dr. Catherine Hamlin, the world-renowned expert for the treatment of birth-related fistulas, founded the "Hamlin College of Midwives" in Ethiopia in 2007. The midwifery students, who are specifically selected from rural areas and sent back to their home region after a thorough midwifery training with a high practical training component, have made a significant contribution to reducing maternal morbidity and mortality in rural areas. The success of their work is also due to the fact that newly trained midwives are always sent to a rural maternity units in pairs, can consult with a gynaecologist and an experienced midwife at any time, and have access to an ambulance for transfers (Hamlin Fistula Ethiopia 2011, 2021).

11.3 The Partograph for Rapid Detection of Obstructed Labour

The partogram partograph is a graphical display of the progress of labour, in which the dilatation of the cervix and the descent of the presenting part of the child are plotted on a timeline. Other aspects that can be documented include the fetal and maternal vital signs, the frequency and strength of contractions, rupture of membranes, and the assessment of amniotic fluid. The partograph was developed in Zimbabwe to provide midwives with a simple but effective tool to detect obstructed labour in a timely manner and to quickly transfer the woman in labour to a health facility where augmentation of labour with measures such as the administration of oxytocin could be performed (Hofmeyr et al. 2021; Wacker 2021). The introduction of an alert and action line made it possible to recognize at a glance whether the woman in labour and the course of labour required increased attention or active support from the obstetric staff. This is particularly important in regions where the journey to the nearest health facility is long and transport means are not continuously available and free of charge, and therefore take significantly longer when compared to industrialized nations.

Partographss come in different versions, adapted to the needs of the respective health system. However, all have in common that correct completion must not only be taught but also be practiced, e.g., by writing birth reports during training, which the student midwives prepare in addition to the labour ward reports and for which they receive feedback from the teaching staff.

In 2021, the World Health Organization (WHO) fundamentally revised the traditional partograph (Hofmeyr et al. 2021). The Labour Care Guide no longer contains an alert and action line, but evidence-based time limits for each centimeter of cervical dilatation to account for individual labor duration have been included instead. The active first stage of labour is defined here from 5 cm cervical dilatation onwards. In addition, a section for more intensive monitoring in the second stage of labour was added, as well as columns for important aspects of respectful maternity care such as birth companion, pain relief, oral fluid intake, and birthing positions. Deviations from normal and treatment thereof can now also be documented here (Hofmeyr et al. 2021).

A modification of a round partograph (sun partograph) is shown in the following Fig. 11.2.

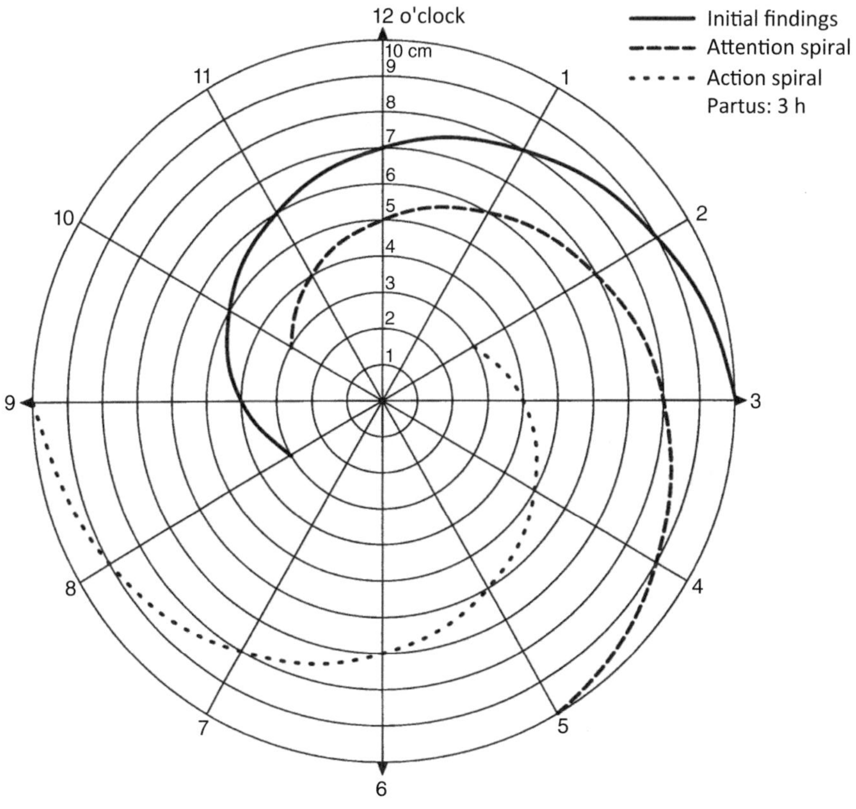

Fig. 11.2 The sun partograph. The individual circles correspond to the dilatation of the cervix. Upon admission of the woman in labour, a mark is made at the actual time on the circle corresponding to the current cervical finding. The start of the "alert spiral" is marked in color on the same circle, offset by 2 hours. This moves outward at a speed of 1 cm/h per hour. An action spiral starts on the same circle offset by another 4 hours. (From: Wacker 1994)

11.4 Auscultation of the Fetal Heart Rate

The new S3 guideline Vaginal Birth at Term (Deutsche Gesellschaft für Gynäkologie und Geburtshilfe und Deutsche Gesellschaft für Hebammenwissenschaft 2020) describes that structured intermittent auscultation of the fetal heart rate offers more advantages in low-risk births than monitoring with the cardiotocogram (CTG), the heart rate contraction recorder. However, the following conditions must be met:

- One-to-one care from the active first stage of labour onwards (cervical dilation approximately 4–6 cm or admission to the delivery room)
- Obstetric staff trained and experienced in auscultation.
- Careful, complete documentation of the fetal heart rate and other relevant obstetric findings.

The guideline recommends that the fetal heart rate should be auscultated with a Pinard stethoscope or a Doppler ultrasound device for one minute after a contraction, while simultaneously measuring the mother's pulse to ensure differentiation between the two. Auscultation should occur every 15–30 minutes during the first stage of labour and every 5 minutes during the second stage of labour.

In industrialized nations, it has been common for decades to monitor the fetal heart rate with the CTG in clinical obstetrics, often for forensic reasons. Therefore, hospital staff here often have little routine in auscultating the fetal heart rate, and implementing the guideline would require training and support for hospital staff, whereas in emerging and developing countries, staff generally have a lot of experience and routine with auscultation. However, what they both have in common is that staff shortages often make the above-mentioned one-to-one care impossible.

11.5 The WHO Safe Childbirth Checklist

The World Health Organization (World Health Organization 2015b) has developed the Safe Childbirth Checklist to provide healthcare professionals worldwide with an easily manageable tool, regardless of the type of health facility, to ensure that crucial measures are carried out safely at critical points during labour and delivery. The list includes measures that have been proven to protect mother and child from serious complications. The obstetric staff should pause at four points ("pause points") during and after birth, go through the checklist and carry out the appropriate measures. The four points are admission to a health facility, directly before the second stage of labour or before caesarean section, in the first hour after birth, and before discharge from the health facility.

The checklist for the second stage of labour includes the possible need for antibiotics in case of signs of infection and magnesium sulfate for high blood pressure, as well as the provision of essential materials for birth. For the mother, these are gloves, hand disinfectant, clean water, and oxytocin 10 IU, and for the child, a clean towel, umbilical cord band or clamp, a sterile blade to cut the umbilical cord, a suction device, and a resuscitation bag with mask. The checklist recommends active management of the third stage of labour with rapid administration of oxytocin and rapid delivery of the placenta, as well as massage of the uterus until it is well contracted. However, uterine massage is no longer routinely recommended in the 2018 recommendations (World Health Organization 2018b). In the first hour after the birth of the child, the corresponding checklist includes, in addition to possibly necessary administration of antibiotics and magnesium sulfate, checking the bleeding in the mother and the assessing the condition of the baby, with particular attention to skin-to-skin contact with the mother and support for early breastfeeding (World Health Organization 2015b).

11.6 Obstetric Staff

Care during labour and delivery should be carried out by skilled staff in the field of maternal and child health, who are trained and regulated according to national and international standards (World Health Organization 2018a). Midwives predominantly undertake this task in cooperation with medical staffl from the fields of gynecology, pediatrics, and anesthesia. In some countries, however, specially trained nursing staff are also responsible for maternity care. Although the midwifery profession is a predominantly female profession, there is a higher proportion of male midwives in many countries. This seems to contradict many cultures in which men are traditionally not involved during pregnancy, childbirth, and the postnatal period. However, the author herself has had good experiences with male midwives abroad who empathetically cared for the birthing women under difficult circumstances. Particularly noteworthy here was that the original career aspiration of the male midwives had partly been nursing. They could not implement this career aspiration because training places in the various health professions were centrally allocated, without the applicants being able to influence this. From the author's private correspondence, it emerged that women put more emphasis on the professional competence of the staff, than on their gender They also exoressed the hope that the great efforts of women during labour and childbirth will be more appreciated in society if male midwives are part of the obstetrics team too. Figure 11.3 shows a midwife's bag with important instruments for monitoring a birth: Pinard stethoscope, sphygmomanometer, and adult stethoscope.

11.7 Health Services for Obstetrics and Gynecology in Uganda

The following chapter aims to address important aspects of obstetric care, using Uganda as an example. Uganda has a high maternal mortality rate of 336 per 100,000 live births due to obstetric emergencies (Ssebagereka et al. 2021). The direct causes for this are bleeding (34%), followed by hypertension (19%),

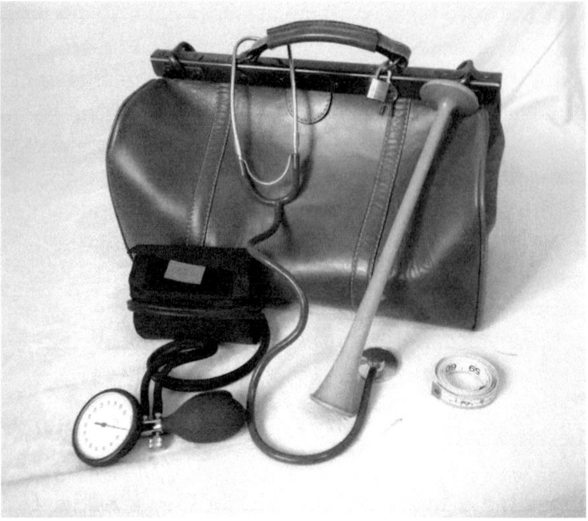

Fig. 11.3 Midwife's bag

abortions (9%), sepsis (8%), and indirect causes such as malaria, anemia, HIV (Human Immunodeficiency Virus), and other infections (18%). In accordance with the Sustainable Development Goal (SDG) 3.1, measures have been taken to reduce the mortality rate to 70% by 2030. These primarily include a program for national safe motherhood and the revival of family planning, improved access to prenatal care, and the improvement of access to emergency obstetric care.

These measures require sufficient staff. However, there is a significant shortage of nurses and midwives. The nurse/midwife to patient ratio of 6:100,000 illustrates the general lack of medical personnel in Uganda, which is low compared to the World Health Organization's (WHO) recommendations of 2.5:1000 (Kumakech et al. 2020). Midwives, on the other hand, have played a crucial role in reducing maternal and neonatal mortality in Uganda, as they provide the majority of maternal and neonatal care. In Uganda, there are several paths to becoming a midwife. These include both diploma and bachelor's degree programs for basic care, as well as bachelor's and master's degree programs for advanced care, which also include the management of difficult births (Copestake et al. 2020; Edwards et al. 2018; Isangula et al. 2021; Kemp et al. 2018; Kumakech et al. 2020; Telfer et al. 2021).

Midwives in Uganda also care for numerous refugee women from neighboring countries, who are often affected by FGM/FGC (= female genital mutilation or female genital cutting), which is one of the main causes of birth complications, such as postpartum haemorrhage due to perineal tears. Ugandan midwives developed a birthing position where the mother is in a supine position, with one leg bent and the other straight, at the time of birth when the longest diameter of the baby's head is to pass through the birth canal. This would reduce the likelihood of perineal tears and thus preserve more women from vaginal and perineal tears.

However, there is no evidence for this yet. If a risk for perineal tears is identified during birth, most midwives in various facilities across the country apply this method.

Adherence to SPIC (Standard Precautions for Infection Control) is crucial for preventing perinatal infections in mothers in all health facilities (Abdulraheem et al. 2012; Bedoya et al. 2017). The WHO (2016b) strongly recommends asepsis in six areas, including a clean birthing surface, clean hands of the obstretric staff, a clean perineum of the mother, a clean umbilical cord cutting instrument, a clean umbilical cord ligature, and clean umbilical cord care. In Uganda, most deliveries are conducted by midwives in lower health facilities, and all are required to adhere to WHO and national guidelines for infection prevention and control. All pregnant women in Uganda receive a delivery package, often referred to as "Mama-Kit". The delivery package includes a sterile delivery set that the mothers must bring with them when they want to give birth in a health facility. The sterile delivery set consists of about four pairs of sterile gloves, umbilical cord ligatures, a razor blade, a sterile towel, a rubberized pad, and a piece of soap. This is also intended as a back up for emergencies, such as when labor starts at home or on the way to the health facility.

Another important measure to reduce birth complications caused be obstructed labour is the use of a partograph. The Ugandan Ministry of Health adapted the World Health Organization's partograph in 1990 (Ogwang et al. 2009) and modified it to meet local needs. The change included the introduction of a code for the elimination of mother-to-child HIV transmission (EMTCT), which serves as an indicator of the mother's HIV serostatus. These codes indicate whether the mother has been counseled, tested, and started on highly active antiretroviral therapy (HAART). In this way, all attending midwives can quickly recognize which precautions to take during the birthing process. In addition, the Ministry of Health added letter codes for the mother's nationality to ensure traceability, as well as an additional page for details on care during labour and delivery.

11.8 Importance of Obstetrics in Humanitarian Aid Using the Example: Gambia

11.8.1 Definition of Humanitarian Aid

Worldwide, there are conditions in which people experience suffering due to natural disasters, crises, and conflicts. As part of humanitarian aid, support options are created to cope with these emergencies and to ensure people's safety, prospects, and improvements in a dignified way. Despite challenges and difficulties, such as rapidly changing political situations on the ground, humanitarian aid should always follow the principles of independence, neutrality, and impartiality and avoid unwanted side effects (do-not-harm principle) as much as possible (Auswärtiges Amt 2020).

11.8.2 The Country of The Gambia

In the example of The Gambia, there is currently no acute crisis, yet problems such as poverty, hunger, drought, economic instability, high unemployment, or diseases like malaria are omnipresent. The Gambia, like so many other emerging and developing countries, is suffering significantly from the Corona pandemic.

The smallest country on the African mainland, with its 2.2 million inhabitants, located on the west coast and enclosed by Senegal, ranks 172 out of 189 in the UN Human Development Index. On average, a woman is estimated to have 3.13 children and is20.7 years old at the birth of her first baby. 597 mothers per 100,000 live births die around the time of birth (worldwide rank 13); 35.9 infants per 1000 live births do not survive their first birthday (The World Factbook 2022). 75.7% of women aged 15–49 are affected by FGM/C (female genital mutilation/cutting) and 44% of women believe in continuing this practice (28 Too Many 2018).

11.8.3 Obstetric Aspects in Humanitarian Aid

All these facts, even if only estimates, underline the necessity to focus on obstetrics and women's health. There are over 100 registered NGOs (Non-Governmental Organizations) that are involved on the ground, among other things, in the medical field. The focus of support and need varies greatly. While in the urban area around the capital Banjul there are hospitals and a few modern private clinics, people living further east do not even have access to drinking water and electricity in their settlements.

To minimize maternal and infant mortality, the primary goal is to ensure access to medical care . This includes establishing a system for providing antenatall care that includes all basic examinations as well as the possibility of diagnosing and treating chronic diseases, such as diabetes or high blood pressure, which could negatively affect a pregnancy. For the labour and delivery, it is important to create a safe and especially hygienic environment in order to give birth attended by skilled staff. In rural areas, care is currently still dominated by traditional birth attendants, who are very experienced in supporting the labouring woman emotionally, but do not have a medical education. Long and inadequately managed labour not only increases complications for the unborn child but also the maternal risk for obstetric finstulas fistula formation with complex and protracted gynecological consequences such as incontinence (Siebenkotten-Branca 2020). birth After the delivery anybirth injuries should be correctly and hygienically treated, especially in the sense of not continuing to practice FGM/C. Before a woman is discharged , which usually happens a few hours after birth, she must receive basic information about deviations from normal during the postnatal period and hygiene recommendations and she should be informed about when a medical facility should be consulted again. Counselling on family planning can also take place here. Breastfeeding is usually the first choice of infant nutrition . It is recommended to discuss any open questions at this point.

To simplify the execution of all tasks, important organizations such as Médecins Sans Frontières(MSF), the World Health Organization (WHO), and also the national Ministry of Health have published practical and easily accessible guidelines, recommendations, and documents. An important document is, among others, "The WHO Partograph", a written report of labour progress that helps to recognize obstructed labour in a timely manner. for tg., mun), As English as international language cannot always be expected and because there are high illiteracy rates in certain areas, visualization is often used to aid medical staff to care for their patients (e.g, medication that needs to be taken in the morning is marked with the rising sun).

Another significant aspect of care includes information and education on topics such as FGM/C, hygiene, vaccination or immunization programs, violence against women, choice of contraception, early (forced) marriage, and polygamy.

11.8.4 The Role of the midwife in the field

The potential roles for midwives in the field are diverse. The activities just described can be fulfilled through active participation and the contribution of one's own experiences. It should be emphasized that in countries like The Gambia, certain tasks are taken on across the interprofessional team. Thus, as a midwife working in humanitarian programs, it is possible to take over typical g tasks of a nurse, such as wound car and to works, or assisst in the pharmacy with the dispensing of medication.

Midwives from Germany and other European countries have the opportunity to work for a certain period of time in various health facilities on behalf of NGOs or other official institutions on site. The longer the deployment, the more beneficial the result for the country. Short-term deployments should increasingly be critically examined in respect to their benefit. While the humanitarian actors do get a first impression of life in another country, a change of perspective, and gain personal enrichment; the benefit for the local population is rather insignificant. Short-term deployments carry the risk of the business model of helper tourism, which can even cause extensive damage. Long-term projects are to be preferred. Advantages of a longer deployment include mutual acquaintance, the opportunity to build trust and it guarantees cooperation and networking opportunities as well as further developments.

11.8.5 Important Principles in Humanitarian Work

One of the most important principles in humanitarian work relates to cooperation with national staff in the field and the promotion of local health personnel through training and other further education opportunities. However, when transferring knowledgefe, an exclusive and one-sided teaching attitude should not be adopted. The aim should be to establish a mutual basis of trust first in order to jointly work on the international state of knowledge,to reflect on it and then to adapt it to the local culture and resources.

Humanitarian work involves providing sustainable and long-term support with the aim of making the respective country independent of external aid and respecting the country's own individual aspirations. The exchange between all participants should always take place on an equal level. An important aspect is to communicate criticism or suggestions for improvement extremely sensitively and to work on them together in a reflective manner. For example, it was observed that the national midwives exclusively used the supine position as the birthing position during labour and delivery, although current evidence proves the advantages of an upright birthing position (World Health Organization 2018b).

To emphasize the importance of global women's health and international collegial exchange, this contribution should conclude with a quote from a Gambian midwife who has significantly influenced me in our joint work: "I am Fatou Gaye, a nurse midwife. The education of girls inspired me to dedicate my life to care for women and their children. Because: If you educate a boy, you will educate an individual; but if you educate a girl, you will educate a nation!"

11.9 Collaboration between Midwives, Doctors, and Traditional Birth attendants

It is no coincidence that many of the former development workers of the German Development Service (DED) chose the field of gynecology and obstetrics after completing their development service. This is certainly not solely due to the importance of obstetrics in a district hospital in rural Africa, but is based on factors such as the efficiency of manual interventions, which do not require large technical devices and can even function without electricity. For this reason, we were able to gain many practical experiences in our daily work, which we could apply back in the German delivery rooms. We have described these possibilities of obstetrics under simple conditions, of Obstetrics unplugged, in two manuals (Wacker et al. 1994, 2020). Working without electricity or with significantly less electricity to save energy is also becoming increasingly important in European countries in terms of sustainability (Wacker 2021).

Even with simple methods, we can perform a Caesarean section, in a district hospital in rural Africa in a timely, correct manner and without increased complications, even for fetal indications (Wacker 2008, 2009). To inspire the local midwives to use the partograph, we developed a modified, more understandable "sun partograph" (Wacker 2009)

We internalized the art of correct indication right from the beginning and were thus able to keep the caesarean section rate within a reasonable, justifiable framework (Wacker 1994, 2010, 2020).

The following methods and measures helped us:

- Monitoring of fetal heart rate (Pinard stethoscope; Dopton)
- Use of a partograph ('sun partograph')
- Hand vacuum device with a manual suction pump; Naegele forceps

- Spinal anaesthesia
- Misgav-Ladach caesarean section technique without wound drains

The collaboration with the midwives in the respective delivery rooms was impressive. It is therefore no coincidence that the former leading midwives of the Maternité in Dori in 1986–1988, Mrs. Ramata Edvige Ilboudo, and Madeleine Da, the former head of the children's ward at CHU Yalgado Ouedraogo in Ouagadougou are co-authors of this chapter. The trusting cooperation with the village midwives (Traditional Birth Attendants), who accompanied the labouring women from the remote villages to our Maternité, was crucial for the success of inpatient obstetrics. We trained these Traditional Birth Attendants in numerous further training courses, which we continued to conduct almost annually even after the end of my service in Dori in 1988. Topics of the further training courses were: management of the postnatal period, preeclampsia with introduction to blood pressure measurement, recognition of obstructed labour, criteria for the transferral to hospital, abolition of FGM, recognition of patients with vesicovaginal fistula in case of urinary incontinence etc.

For further reading, we recommend the sources in the bibliography and the chapters in this book on caesarean section, preeclampsia and birth injuries.

Answers to the Initial Questions

1. A. 140 million. (https://ourworldindata.org/births-and-deaths)
2. A. Asia (https://ourworldindata.org/births-and-deaths)
3. A. 81% increase by 64% since 2000–2006 (https://www.who.int/data/gho/data/indicators/indicator-details/GHO/births-attended-by-skilled-health-personnel-(-)

References

Abdulraheem IS, Amodu MO, Saka MJ, Bolarinwa OA, Uthman MMB (2012) Knowledge, awareness and compliance with standard precautions among health workers in north eastern Nigeria. J Community Med Health Educ 2(3):1000131

Auswärtiges Amt (2020) Grundlagen der humanitären Hilfe. https://www.auswaertiges-amt.de/de/aussenpolitik/themen/humanitaere-hilfe/huhi/205108. Accessed 7 Mar 2022

Bedoya G, Dolinger A, Rogo K, Mwaura N, Wafula F, Coarasa J, Das J (2017) Observations of infection prevention and control practices in primary health care, Kenya. Bull World Health Organ 95(7):503

Bohren MA, Mehrtash H, Fawole B, Maung Maung T, Balde MD, Maya E, Thwin SS, Aderoba AK, Vogel JP, Irinyenikan TA, Adeyanju AO, Mon NO, Adu-Bonsaffoh K, Landoulsi S, Guure C, Adanu R, Diallo BA, Gülmezoglu AM, Soumah A-M, Sall AO, Tunçalp Ö (2019) How women are treated during facility-based childbirth in four countries: a cross-sectional study with labour observations and community-based surveys. Lancet. Published Online October 8, 2019. https://doi.org/10.1016/S0140-6736(19)31992-0

Bowser D, Hill K (2010) Exploring evidence for disrespect and abuse in facility-based childbirth: report of a landscape analysis. Bethesda, MD: USAID-TRAction Project and Harvard School of Public Health. https://www.hsph.harvard.edu/wp-content/uploads/sites/2413/2014/05/Exploring-Evidence-RMC_Bowser_rep_2010.pdf. Accessed 16 Mar 2023

Bundesministerium für Gesundheit (2017) Nationales Gesundheitsziel Gesundheit rund um die Geburt. Nationales Gesundheitsziel (bundesgesundheitsministerium.de)

Burger L (1996) Mit Zwillingen fing es an. Erzählungen einer Hebamme. Weißes Kreuz GmbH Ahnatal/Kassel

Copestake J, Theuss M, Brownie S, Davies G, Burke E, Mukuru M, Edwards G (2020) Recently graduated midwives in Uganda: self-perceived achievement, wellbeing and work prospects. Midwifery 82:102596

Deutsche Gesellschaft für Gynäkologie und Geburtshilfe und Deutsche Gesellschaft für Hebammenwissenschaft (2020) S3-Leitlinie Vaginale Geburt am Termin. AWMF online, AWMF 015-083 015-083l_S3_Vaginale-Geburt-am-Termin_2021-03.pdf (awmf.org)

Deutscher Hebammenverband e. V. (2021a) Zukunft der Geburtshilfe. Deutscher Hebammenverband e. V., Karlsruhe

Deutscher Hebammenverband e. V. (2021b) Unsere Hebammen. Fakten und Infos. Hebammenarbeit. Geburtshilfe. https://www.unsere-hebammen.de/fakten-infos/hebammenarbeit/. Accessed 3 Feb 2022

Edwards G, Hellen K, Brownie S (2018) Developing a work/study programme for midwifery education in East Africa. Midwifery 59:74–77

Grabrucker M (1989) Vom Abenteuer der Geburt. Die letzten Landhebammen erzählen. Fischer, Frankfurt

Hamlin Fistula Ethiopia (2011) The Hamlin College of Midwives. Hamlin Fistula Ethiopia, Addis Ababa

Hamlin Fistula Ethiopia (2021) Our midwives. https://hamlinfistula.org/our-midwives/. Accessed 3 Feb 2022

Hofmeyr GJ, Bernitz S, Bonet M, Bucagu M, Dao B, Downe S, Galadanci H, Homer CSE, Hundley V, Lavender T, Levy B, Lissauer D, Lumbiganon P, McConville FE, Pattinson R, Qureshi Z, Souza JP, Stanton ME, ten Hoope-Bender P, Vannevel V, Vogel JP, Oladapo OT (2021) WHO next-generation partograph: revolutionary steps towards individualised labour care. BJOG 128:1658–1662

Isangula K, Edwards G, Mwansisya T, Mbekenga C, Pallangyo E, Sarki A, Ndirangu-Mugo E (2021) Open and distance learning programs for nursing and midwifery education in East Africa: protocol for a scoping review. JMIR Res Protoc 10(1):e17765

Kemp J, Shaw E, Musoke MG (2018) Developing a model of midwifery mentorship for Uganda: the MOMENTUM project 2015–2017. Midwifery 59:127–129

Kumakech E, Anathan J, Udho S, Auma AG, Atuhaire I, Nsubuga AG, Ahaisibwe B (2020) Graduate midwifery education in Uganda aiming to improve maternal and newborn health outcomes. Ann Glob Health 86(1):52. https://doi.org/10.5334/aogh.2804

Ogwang S, Karyabakabo Z, Rutebemberwa E (2009) Assessment of partogram use during labour in rujumbura health Sub district, Rukungiri district, Uganda. Afr Health Sci 2009:9(2)

Sheferaw ED, Bazant E, Gibson H, Fenta HB, Ayalew F, Belay TB, Worku MM, Kebebu AE, Woldie SA, Kim Y-M, van den Akker T, Stekelenburg J (2017) Respectful maternity care in Ethiopian public health facilities. Reprod Health 14:60

Siebenkotten-Branca V (2020) Geburtshilfliche Fisteln – Relevanz für Hebammen in Deutschland. Die Hebamme 33:46–53. https://doi.org/10.1055/a-1159-4910

Ssebagereka A, Apolot RR, Nyachwo EB, Ekirapa-Kiracho E (2021) Estimating the cost of implementing a facility and community score card for maternal and newborn care service delivery in a rural district in Uganda. Int J Equity Health 20(1):1–13

Telfer M, Zaslow R, Nabirye RC, Mbalinda SN (2021) Review of midwifery education in Uganda: toward a framework for integrated learning and midwifery model of care. Midwifery 103:103145

The World Factbook (2022) Gambia, The. https://www.cia.gov/the-world-factbook/countries/gambia-the/. Accessed 7 Mar 2022

Too Many (2018) Prevalence of FGM. https://www.28toomany.org/country/the-gambia/. Accessed 7 Mar 2022

UNFPA/United Nations Populations Fund (2021) The state of the world's midwifery report. UNFPA; New York the state of the world's midwifery 2021 | United Nations Population Fund (unfpa.org)

Wacker J (2010) Kaiserschnitt vs. Natürliche Geburt. Geburtshilfe Frauenheilkd 840:843

Wacker J (2021) Nachhaltigkeit im Kreißsaal Die Hebamme 34:55–61

Wacker J, Baldé MD, Bastert G (1994) Geburtshilfe unter einfachen Bedingungen. Springer, Heidelberg

Wacker J, Baldé MD, Bastert G (2020) Obsterics unplugged, 3rd edn. im Regional-Verlag Ubstadt-Weiher

World Health Organization (2015a) Vermeidung und Beseitigung von Geringschätzung und Misshandlung bei Geburten in geburtshilflichen Einrichtungen. WHO_RHR_14.23_ger.pdf;sequence=22. Accessed 1 Feb 2022

World Health Organization (2015b) WHO Safe Childbirth Checklist Implementation Guide. Improving the quality of facility-based delivery for mothers and newborns. WHO/HIS/SDS/2015.26. www.who.int/patientsafety/implementation/checklists/childbirth/. Accessed 1 Feb 2022

World Health Organization (2016a) Midwives voices, midwives realities. Findings from a global consultation on providing quality midwifery care World Health Organization. ISBN 978 92 4 151054 https://www.whiteribbonalliance.org/wp-content/uploads/2019/02/MidwivesVoicesMidwivesRealities.pdf. Accessed 1 Feb 2022

World Health Organization (2016b) Guidelines on core components of infection prevention and control programmes at the national and acute health care facility level. ISBN 978-92-4-154992-9. World Health Organization, Geneva

World Health Organization (2018a) Definition of skilled health personnel providing care during childbirth: the 2018 joint statement by WHO, UNFPA, UNICEF, ICM, ICN, FIGO and IPA WHO-RHR-18.14-eng.pdf

World Health Organization (2018b) WHO recommendations Intrapartum care for a positive childbirth experience. https://apps.who.int/iris/bitstream/handle/10665/272447/WHO-RHR-18.12-eng.pdf. Accessed 7 Mar 2022

Further Reading

Dehne KL, Wacker J, Cowley J (1995) Training birth attendants in the Sahel. World Health Forum 16(415):419. Accessed 1 Feb 2022

Lindert J, Breitbach R, Sieben G, Tiemasse S, Coulibaly A, Wacker J (2011) Perinatal health in rural Burkina Faso. Gynecol Obstet:295–297

Wacker J, Breitkopf B (2008) Gebären – Gedeihen und Genesen, 50 Jahre Frauenklinik Bruchsal. Regionalkultur: Ubstadt – Weiher

Wacker J, Kantelhardt E (2009) Geburtshilfe und Gynäkologie in den Tropen. In Tropenmedizin in Klinik und Praxis (2009), 4th edn; Herausgeber: Thomas Löscher und Gerd-Dieter Burchard; Thieme, Stuttgart, pp 119–132

Wacker J, Unkels R, Dehne KL (1998a) Training birth attendants in the detection of preeclampsia/eclampsia. Int J Gynecol Obstet 62:287–288

Wacker J, Utz B, Kyelem M, Lankoandé JP, Bastert G (1998b) Introduction of a simplified round partogramm in rural maternity units: Seno province, Burkina Faso, West-Africa. Trop Dr 28:146–152

12 Treatment of Birth Injuries and Fistulas

Jürgen Wacker, Peggy Seehafer and Kees Waaldijk

Contents

Introductory Questions

1. Vaginal deliveries in Germany without birth injury:
   A. 70%
   B. 50%

J. Wacker (✉)
ehemaliger Chefarzt der Frauenklinik Bruchsal, Bruchsal, Germany
e-mail: prof.wacker@gmail.com

P. Seehafer
GynZone, Aarhus, Denmark
e-mail: peggy.seehafer@gynzone.dk

K. Waaldijk
HC Gennep, Netherlands

J. Wacker et al. (eds.), *Global Women's Health*,
https://doi.org/10.1007/978-3-662-69700-9_12

   C. 38%
   D. 18%
2. Factors that favor the occurrence of a birth injury include:
   A. Size and shape of the baby's head
   B. Height of the perineum
   C. Mother's birthing position
   D. Mother's psychological situation
3. Vesicovaginal fistulas occur more frequently in LIC (Africa) compared to rich countries:
   A. because first-time mothers are younger
   B. due to poor nutrition
   C. because of the limited and less competent support during childbirth
   D. because the cesarean section rate in poor countries (LIC) is too high

12.1 Introduction

Even with the best care of the birthing woman, birth injuries can occur. Thus, more than half of all women giving birth vaginally suffer an injury in the vulva and perineal area. The chance that the perineum and vagina remain intact depends on various factors. Until the leading part has passed through, it cannot be correctly assessed. Depending on the condition of the maternal tissue and depending on the course of birth, injuries to the soft birth canal can always occur. The following factors decide (Samuelsson et al. 2002; Fitzgerald et al. 2007; Meister et al. 2016):

- Size and shape of the child's head, especially in case of malpositions
- Passage speed of the child's head
- Shape of the pubic arch
- Height of the perineum
- Elasticity of the perineal tissue
- Birth position of the mother
- Psychological situation of the mother

The mother's age, body size, geographical origin, and genetic predispositions are influencing factors that are unchangeable.

With the spread of modern obstetrics and the nationwide establishment of obstetric departments—especially in rural areas—the occurrence of a vesicovaginal fistula has become rarer in Germany. In contrast, in the poor countries of Africa, the occurrence of a vesicovaginal fistula due to protracted birth courses and the simultaneous lack of intact obstetric facilities is still a significant gynecological problem.

The "birth fistula", whether it is a vesicovaginal or rectovaginal fistula, is as old as humanity and has always been a source of misery for the affected women.

Although obstetrically caused fistulas have almost disappeared in high-income countries due to the high standard of obstetrics, they are still widespread in middle and low-income countries where the obstetric system is patchy, and according to Kees Waaldijk, they represent a significant public health problem for which no sustainable solution has yet been found.

As already mentioned in Chaps. 8 (Maternal Mortality) and 13 (Preeclampsia), there are numerous other factors that can lead to the death and suffering of mothers. Postpartum hemorrhages (atony), as we have already published elsewhere, are one of the most common causes of maternal deaths (Bräuer et al. 2014).

This chapter is dedicated to the fate of the "unlucky survivors" among the often young mothers of Africa.

12.2 Definition and Classification of Birth Injuries and Fistulas

Spontaneous birth injuries occur on their own, with the acting birth factors contributing causally. These birth injuries include: vaginal tear, cervical tear, perineal tear, uterine rupture, labial tear, clitoral tear, levator tear, symphysis rupture, coccyx injuries.

Table 12.1 shows the classification of birth injuries.

The fistula is indeed the most visible and disturbing phenomenon, but it is only part of a much more complex obstetric trauma, **the complex obstetric trauma.**

The variety of obstetric fistulas within the complex obstetric trauma is immense and ranges from a tiny fistula with minimal tissue loss to the formation of a cloaca in an empty pelvis with extensive intrapelvic/vaginal lesions and (sub)total loss of intrapelvic soft tissues. This is accompanied by further extravaginal lesions, lesions induced by the constant discharge of urine, and neurological lesions caused by intrapelvic/vaginal pressure necrosis.

The episiotomy is an iatrogenic birth injury. It is used as an obstetric procedure in connection with a main diagnosis code and does not represent a diagnosis in itself (WHO 2022a). According to the classification according to the guidelines of the RCOG, it would be classified under JB09.1 birth injury 2nd degree.

12.3 Frequency of Birth Injuries and Fistulas

In Germany, births in hospitals nationwide are evaluated by the Institute for Quality Assurance and Transparency in Healthcare (IQTIG). They account for 98% of all births. No distinction is made between first-time and multiple births. The Society for Quality in Outpatient Obstetrics e. V. (QUAG) is responsible for the evaluation of outpatient births.

Table 12.2 shows the frequency of birth injuries in Germany.

As our working group found out in a study in Ouagadougou, there are no major, clinically relevant differences in the occurrence of perineal tears in large Burkinabe clinics in Ouagadougou and German clinics (Wacker et al. 2020). This is due, among other things, to the good training of midwives in Burkina Faso. In

Table 12.1 Classification (by Peggy Seehafer). All diagnoses in outpatient and inpatient care must be coded according to ICD-11. The diagnoses for pregnancy, childbirth, and puerperium can be found in Chap. 18. (WHO 2022b)

Code No.	Definition	Included	Excluded
JB09	Perineal injuries due to childbirth	Episiotomy with subsequent tearing	High vaginal tear (JB0A.4)
JB09.0	First degree birth injury	Injury, rupture or tear of the perineum (involving): • Frenulum labiorum pudendi • Skin • Labia • Vagina • Vulva Injury, rupture or tear of the periurethral tissue	Periurethral tear involving the urethra (JB0A.6)
JB09.1	Second degree birth injury	Injury, rupture or tear of the perineum, as indicated under JB09.0, also involving: • M. bulbocavernos • M. transversus perinei • Septum rectovaginale	Involvement of the sphincter ani (JB09.2)
JB09.2	Third degree birth injury	Injury, rupture or tear of the perineum, as indicated under JB09.1, also involving: • M. sphincter ani externus • M. sphincter ani internus	Involvement of the anal or rectal mucosa (JB09.3)
JB09.3	Fourth degree birth injury	Injury, rupture or tear of the perineum, as indicated under JB09.2, also involving: • Anal canal • Rectal mucosa	
JB09.Z	Perineal tear during childbirth, not further specified		
QA46.0	Spontaneous birth of a singleton	No or minimal obstetric measures Normal birth Spontaneous birth from cephalic presentation Spontaneous vaginal birth of a singleton	

contrast, in the rural regions of Africa, due to the significantly longer birth processes, even when birth stagnation has been determined, there are significantly more higher-grade birth injuries and obstetrically caused fistulas (Waaldijk 1994, Wacker et al. 2020). According to Kees Waaldijk and numerous other authors, the frequency of a vesico-/rectovaginal fistula in rural Africa is about 2–3/1000 births (Waaldijk 1994). From the figures of the Ministry of Health of Burkina Faso, a

Table 12.2 Birth injuries in vaginal births in clinical obstetrics, Germany 2020. *Source*: IQTIG (2021)

Birth Injuries	Frequency in Clinical Obstetrics	Frequency in Outpatient Obstetrics n = 15,412
Without	42%	44%
1st Degree	17.7%	19.9% (w/o LR, SR)
2nd Degree	22.2%	17.5%
Episiotomy	16.2%	3.2%
3rd Degree	1.7%	1.0%
4th Degree	0.1%	
Other Tears (LR, SR)		20.8%

frequency of 4–6 VVF per 1000 stillbirths results (Ministere de la Santé; Burkina Faso, 2012).

12.4 Diagnosis

12.4.1 Diagnosis of Birth Injuries

Midwives and obstetricians must be able to correctly assess the full extent of a birth injury. Current studies confirm the effectiveness of the four-eyes principle for the benefit of the woman SBU (2021) Förlossningsbristningar. Insufficiently treated birth injuries affect women and their families for the rest of their lives. Most women who have just given birth are very sensitive to touch in the genital area. It makes sense to provide the woman with adequate analgesia before the diagnosis in order to correctly diagnose the full extent of the injury. A buttock clenched in pain does not necessarily mean that the sphincter is intact. Trauma at this point of the perineum should not be underestimated (Garthus-Niegel et al. 2012).

To make a precise diagnosis after birth, both palpation and visual skills are needed. A systematic inspection of the vulva, vagina, and perineum from anterior to posterior has proven effective in not overlooking any injury (Kindberg and Seehafer 2022).

BU: Illustration of the areas to be palpated to ensure that the muscle substance is intact

Palpate the M. bulbocavernosus between 02:00 and 10:00 around the introitus with your thumb and index finger to ensure that you can detect muscle substance or a defect everywhere. After each vaginal birth, a rectal examination must ensure that the sphincter is intact and no injury has been overlooked. During the rectal examination, lift the ring muscle from the inside towards your thumb with your index finger and systematically palpate the thickness of the M. sphincter ani externus for substance loss between 10 o'clock and 2 o'clock. An intact external sphincter is about 0.5 cm thick. If the M. sphincter ani internus is intact (DR IIIb), it appears as a whitish shiny structure at the bottom of the wound (Kindberg and Seehafer 2022).

Deep cervical lacerations or a high vaginal tear can only be demonstrated instrumentally. Vascular injuries that lead to superficial or deeper, infralevator and supralevator hematomas, or tears or avulsions of levator muscles are not externally visible and require extensive diagnostics if necessary.

Good diagnostics are not only characterized by systematic inspection and secure classification of the injury. Good diagnostics also include the duration of the examination, the handling of the woman's tissue, the consideration of painlessness during the procedure, and appropriate communication with the woman.

12.4.2 Symptoms and Diagnosis of Fistulas (VVF/RVF)

The leading symptom of vesicovaginal fistula is constant and involuntary loss of urine. Most patients present at the age of 24–26 years due to their symptoms (urinary incontinence, skin changes in the genital area, and other complaints) in a fistula clinic (Kammerer 2007). In most patients, the vesicovaginal fistula occurred during the first pregnancy (Hancock 2005; Kammerer 2007). The time span between the clinical onset of fistula-related symptoms and presentation in a fistula clinic averages 6 years in Uganda according to Hancock (Hancock 2005).

The consequences of constant urinary loss, the urine-soaked clothes, and the rapidly spreading foul smell lead to the social exclusion of the affected women, which we have detailed elsewhere (Kammerer 2007).

On inspection of the external genitalia, many patients with vesicovaginal fistula have a "urine dermatitis". The changes in the skin in the genital area are due to the constant contamination of the affected skin areas with concentrated urine. According to Hancock, in a study in Uganda, no opening of the urethra was found in 2% of the examined patients due to complete destruction of the anterior vaginal wall.

During the gynecological examination, in addition to the length of the vagina, the size and location of the fistula, the size and condition of the cervix must also be described.

If a patient has involuntary urinary incontinence without a visible and palpable fistula opening, the following procedure is recommended: examination in lithotomy position, insertion of Sims/Auvard specula, cough stress test while simultaneously inspecting the anterior vaginal wall.

To exclude the smallest fistulas, the so-called Dye-Test ("Dye don't lie") is performed: placement of a Foley catheter and instillation of 50–100 ml of saline-diluted methylene blue or gentian violet solution into the urinary bladder. Before performing the test, 2–3 wet swabs are inserted into the vagina. If after the test the first swab is without blue coloration, but the second is blue, the presence of a fistula is proven (Wacker et al. 2009).

12.5 Treatment

12.5.1 Treatment and Care of Birth Injuries

Superficial, non-bleeding tears that do not involve muscle can heal without suturing, provided the wound edges come together anatomically correctly. Injuries that extend into the muscle should always be sutured. Although there are ongoing considerations to let perineal tears heal on their own, according to current results of meta-analyses, this is "probably ineffective or even harmful" (Frohlich and Kettle 2011).

The timing of suture care can be placed after the first bonding phase, which should not be disturbed (UNICEF, WHO 1992). Often it is necessary to stop bleeding, so the timing for this cannot be delayed. Before a birth injury is surgically treated, every woman should be offered adequate analgesia, the onset of which should definitely be awaited. Since pain perception varies greatly from individual to individual, it must be negotiated with each woman individually what form of analgesia is sufficient for her. The positioning must be comfortable for the woman and also allow the surgeon to approach the suture as relaxed as possible. For a long-term good result in wound healing, it is important that the surgeon can sew under calm conditions to correctly identify and adapt muscles and fasciae. It has proven advantageous to put the woman in the lithotomy position. It is more comfortable for the woman if she can put her legs in a leg holder instead of having to hold them up herself. The lithotomy position allows the extent of the wound area to be adequately represented and the injury to be correctly identified under optimal lighting conditions (Kindberg and Seehafer 2022).

Based on the existing study situation, there is no sufficient evidence for or against the suture care of minor birth injuries up to second-degree perineal tears. However, third and fourth degree perineal tears require appropriate suture care. Median episiotomies are anatomically equivalent to a second-degree perineal tear. Mediolateral episiotomies usually injure larger blood vessels, which makes suturing inevitable.

The following advantages of suturing were found in studies (Fleming et al. 2003):

- faster wound healing,
- a more cosmetically pleasing result;
- a possibly faulty diagnosis can be revised by suturing under appropriate conditions.

Whether suturing was done or not had no effect on possible urinary incontinence and the resumption of sexual activity (Langley et al. 2006). There are no studies yet on how unsutured muscle ends affect possible incontinence, sexual experience, posture, back pain, etc. several years after birth. Although the study situation is not clear, most obstetricians agree that every perineal injury should be sutured if muscles are involved. The muscles of the pelvic floor are under tension and, when they tear, they retract into their fascia. This means they do not adapt to each other on their own and can no longer grow together and rebuild the tension of the pelvic floor.

In the treatment of birth injuries, almost exclusively synthetic, resorbable material is used today, so the threads do not have to be pulled. The most suitable suture material dissolves exactly when the wound begins to heal, without causing inflammatory reactions. It is usually offered as a ready-made package and contains an atraumatic needle and the thread made of polyglactin, a synthetic sugar. Allergies to the suture material itself are very rare. Sometimes intolerances to the type of sterilization of the material are observed.

For the suture of a birth injury of the first degree, a synthetic, thin, quickly resorbable thread is suitable. This could be, for example, Velosorb fast^{TM} or Vicryl rapid^{TM} 3–0. For second-degree birth injuries, there are different opinions among clinical doctors about how much tensile strength is required in the suture material. Thread strengths between 2–0 and 0–0 are suitable. The predominantly used coated polyglactin 910 (e.g., VicrylTM, Novosyn$^{TM)}$) loses half of its thread strength within 21 days, is dissolved after 28 days, and is completely resorbed by the tissue after 57–70 days.

The most commonly used suture material for sphincter injuries is Vicryl^{TM} or PDS^{TM}, i.e., a slowly dissolving thread. A randomized study compared the two materials and found only minor clinical differences in terms of the need for secondary suturing, infection rates, or later incontinence. For the reconstruction of the M. sphincter ani externus, both monofilament suture materials such as polidioxanone (PDS^{TM}) and braided suture materials such as polyglactin (e.g., Velosorb^{TM}) can be chosen.

The Ipswich Childbirth Study from 1992–1994, with 1780 participating primiparous and multiparous women, demonstrated that a transcutaneous suture on the perineum leads to significantly more pain both in the short term and in the long term than a subcutaneous suture, and that due to the pain after a transcutaneous suture, sutures often have to be removed prematurely. While the continuous suture technique has proven effective for sutures that lie on the surface, in some cases it is advantageous to tie deeper sutures individually. Transcutaneous single-button sutures should be avoided. International guidelines prefer the continuous suture technique for the treatment of second-degree birth injuries because it is associated with less pain during the healing phase. However, with some tears, it can be difficult to oversee the wound area. In such cases, a mixed suture technique of single-button support sutures and a continuous suture may be more suitable. The vaginal epithelium is treated with a continuous suture, the muscle ends of M. bulbocavernosus and M. transversus perinei are adapted in pairs with single-button sutures, and the skin is then closed with a continuous subcutaneous suture. If a vaginal tear is very deep, the rectovaginal fascia may be injured. If it is torn, it must be treated with its own (continuous) suture before the vaginal epithelium is closed.

In the case of sphincter injuries, the end-to-end technique can be used, in which both sphincter ends are connected end-to-end with single-button sutures. The overlapping suture technique can only be used for a completely torn M. sphincter ani externus. For this, both sphincter ends are laid over each other and sewn together. In an international context, there is no evidence as to which suture technique is best suited for fourth-degree perineal tears Grades. The sutures are placed through the anorectal mucosa in such a way that the wound edges come to lie end-to-end directly next to each other. Whether to sew transmucosally or submucosally is decided by each surgeon based on their own skills and experiences. The M. sphincter ani internus is included in this continuous suture.

Wound infections after a sphincter injury can lead to the formation of fistulas or result in suture or wound dehiscence. For third and fourth degree perineal tears, the Green-top Guideline recommends the routine intra- and post-operative administration of broad-spectrum antibiotics to prevent wound infections and dehiscence. A Cochrane Review from 2014 did not find sufficient evidence for routine antibiotic prophylaxis for third and fourth degree birth injuries (Buppasiri et al. 2014).

The risk of a wound infection after a vaginal birth is 0.1–23.6% according to a systematic review from 2019. The risk of suture dehiscence triples with an episiotomy. Depending on the course and extent of the birth injury, larger accumulations of blood can occur in the wound gap. Smaller hematomas are broken down during the healing process. Larger hematomas, in addition to pressure pain, may lead to dehiscence and may need to be cleared out. About 1–2% of all sutures come apart (partially) before they have healed. A suture dehiscence can be treated with an early secondary suture in the first 14 to 21 days postpartum. For this, the wound area should be clean and without visible inflammation. Experience after more than 30,000 women examined in the early postpartum period and more than 350 secondary sutures at the University Women's Clinic Aarhus shows that early secondary sutures heal as well as primary sutures. The particularly good healing ability of the maternal body during the postpartum period is assumed to be the reason for this.

Women who have suffered major injuries during childbirth feel sustainably wounded. Many of them do not seek medical care for urinary and fecal incontinence unless they are explicitly pointed out. Therefore, it is recommended to routinely reappoint women with third and fourth degree birth injuries to a specially designated consultation with a pelvic floor specialist after three to six months. This makes it possible to react early to incontinence problems. All women should be given enough attention in the first three weeks of the birth injury so that in the case of dehiscence, an infection or unexplained pain, it can be immediately clinically clarified whether an early secondary suture—especially after a sphincter injury—is necessary. This can be ensured in Germany by home visits from the midwife.

Healing

In the case of clean and well-adapted wound edges, the formation of new connective tissue is minimal and primary wound closure occurs quickly and without complications postpartum. If the wound edges are gaping, there is a delayed, secondary wound healing, in which the tissue defect is filled by granulation tissue and extensive scar formation. Superficial birth injuries, such as labial tears, vaginal tears, and first-degree perineal tears, typically heal within a good week. Second-degree perineal tears are superficially healed after about two weeks. An episiotomy heals slower than a spontaneous injury. The incision damages more nerves and capillaries than a spontaneous tear. Therefore, an episiotomy often hurts more because larger hematomas and swellings occur around the episiotomy during the exudation phase (Jiang et al. 2017). Sphincter injuries take about four weeks to heal. It is normal for women to have swelling and a feeling of pressure as well as mild pain for several weeks after birth. By the follow-up examination six to eight weeks postpartum, the suture should be completely healed and pain-free. How long the muscles take to fully heal is not yet known (Soerensen et al. 2008; Kindberg and Seehafer 2022).

The short-term occurrence of pain in the perineum area and a burning sensation during urination are considered normal due to the strong stretching during birth. However, the larger a birth injury is, the more frequently and longer women suffer from pain after birth. The suture material completely dissolves over the course of one to two months.

▶ The immediate administration of 1 g of paracetamol supp. after the completion of the suture leads to less pain within the first 24 hours postpartum and to less use of painkillers within the first 48 hours after birth (Hedayati et al. 2003). It can therefore be recommended as a routine measure. If the woman still needs medication for pain relief, she can take up to 1 g of paracetamol and 3 × 400 mg of ibuprofen up to four times a day for some time.

12.5.2 Treatment and Surgical Management of Obstetric Fistulas

The surgical management of vesicovaginal fistulas is reputed to be demanding and technically challenging. Even the most experienced "fistula surgeons" cannot close every fistula; they report success rates between 90 and 95%, with about 10% of the procedures requiring 2 or 3 operations for definitive fistula closure (Hancock 2005).

About 25% of vesicovaginal fistulas are simple fistulas that any experienced gynecologist or surgeon can treat if they have attended a corresponding workshop—preferably in an African country—under expert guidance (Wacker et al. 2009).

The following are some operative principles of fistula surgery:

- The selection of instruments and their use in operations take into account the often simple conditions of the respective hospitals.
- The following instruments have proven useful to us: Allis clamps instead of Kocher clamps; dissection scissors, e.g., Metzenbaum scissors; self-retaining Auvard speculum, forceps, vascular clamps, scalpel, and metal probe. The metal catheter probe (Beniquet) is used to exclude bladder stones and to assess the length of the urethra.
- Before the operation begins, the following anatomical prerequisites must be clarified: determination of the location and size of the fistula, determination of the distance between the external urethral opening and the distal edge of the fistula; determination between the proximal edge of the fistula and the cervix.
- Anesthesia: Spinal anesthesia with hyperbaric bupivacaine is usually sufficient and lasts for the duration of the operation.
- Before the dissection begins, inject the tissue layers with physiological saline solution; the posterior dissection is continued until at least 1 cm behind the fistula edge is mobilized. This is followed by the anterior dissection.
- The closure of the fistula edges begins with the placement of two corner sutures. The fistula edges are closed with a single-layer, inverting (not including the bladder mucosa) suture at intervals of 4 mm with absorbable suture material.
- At the end of the operation, the integrity of the fistula closure is checked by filling the bladder with blue solution. The vaginal wound edges are then treated with single button sutures.

In postoperative care of the patients, ensuring unobstructed urine flow is of crucial importance. If the urine cannot flow freely, this leads to an overstretching of the urinary bladder and a corresponding tension on the wound sutures. In addition, the patients should drink a lot to dilute the urine, which serves to prevent urinary infections. Since the patients are immobilized for the first two weeks after the operation, care should be taken to keep the bed linens dry to prevent the occurrence of moisture-related ulcers (decubitus). Therefore, we formulated the 3 D's of postoperative monitoring in Dori:

- **Dropping** to ensure unobstructed urine flow via a permanent catheter!
- **Drinking** to ensure sufficient fluid intake!
- **Drying** to keep the bed linens dry!

For further deepening of the individual surgical steps, reference is made here to the standard work by Kees Waaldijk: "step-by-step surgery of vesicovaginal fistulas; a full-color atlas" and to our review article (Wacker et al. 2009).

12.6 Prevention

12.6.1 Prevention of Birth Injuries

It is well researched that it is beneficial for the course of birth if the birthing person can move freely. However, the body position adopted does not affect the extent and frequency of birth injuries, with the exception of the lithotomy position (Eason et al. 2000). An upright birth position is associated with fewer episiotomies compared to the supine or lithotomy position, but it is also associated with an increasing number of second-degree perineal tears. The side position and the all-fours position are particularly beneficial for preventing birth injuries (Meyvis et al. 2012).

12.6.2 Prevention of Vesicovaginal Fistulas

As Waaldijk was able to demonstrate, most obstetrically caused fistulas are due to protracted birth processes and as a result of a birth standstill. The presence of a birth standstill of more than 6 hours leads to a significant increase in the frequency of vesicovaginal fistulas (Waaldijk 1994). Therefore, as already described in Chap. 11 (Conducting the birth), it is sensible and necessary to document and monitor the course of the birth, especially in rural Africa, using a partogram (Wacker 1994; Wacker et al. 1998).

Furthermore, it is important to ensure comprehensive care for birthing women in easily accessible and well-functioning obstetric facilities, especially in rural Africa.

Answers to the initial questions
1. C is correct
2. All are correct
3. A, B and C are correct

References

Bräuer ND, Antón J, George PM, Kuntner L, Wacker J (2014) Handling postpartum haemorrhage – obstetrics between tradition and mordernity in post-war Sierra Leone Tropical Doctor. https://doi.org/10.1177/0049475514557579. tdo.sagepub.com

Buppasiri P, Lumbiganon P, Thinkhamrop J, Thinkhamrop B (2014) Antibiotic prophylaxis for third- and fourth degree perineal tear during vaginal birth. Cochrane Database Syst Rev 2014(11) Art. No.: CD005125

Deutsche Gesellschaft für Gynäkologie und Geburtshilfe (DGGG) (2020) Management von Dammrissen III. und IV. Grades nach vaginaler Geburt. S 2k-Leitlinie. http://www.awmf.org/leitlinien/aktuelle-leitlinien.html. Accessed 14 Jan 2022

Eason E, Labreque M, Wells G, Feldmann P (2000) Preventing perineal trauma during childbirth: a systematic review. Obstet Gynecol 95(3):464–471
Fitzgerald MP, Pelvic Floor Disorders Network et al (2007) Risk factors for anal sphincter tear during vaginal delivery. Obstet Gynecol 109(1):29–34
Fleming VE, Hagen S, Niven C (2003) Does perineal suturing make a difference? The SUNS trial. BJOG 110(7):684–689
Frohlich J, Kettle C (2011) Perineal care. BMJ Clin Evid. 1401. https://www.ncbi.nlm.nih.gov/pubmed/25752310. Accessed 22 Jan 2022
Garthus-Niegel S, von Soest T, Vollrath ME, Eberhard-Gran M (2012) The impact of subjective birth experiences on post-traumatic stress symptoms: a longitudinal study. https://www.ncbi.nlm.nih.gov/pubmed/22940723. Accessed 23 Jan 2022
Hancock B (2005) First steps in vesicovaginal Fistula repair. The Royal Society of Medicine Press, London
Hedayati H, Parsons J, Crowther CA (2003) Rectal analgesia for pain from perineal trauma following childbirth. Cochrane Database Syst Rev 2003(3) Art. No.: CD003931
Jiang H, Qian X, Carroli G, Garner P (2017) Selective versus routine use of episiotomy for vaginal birth. Cochrane Database Syst Rev 2:CD000081
Kammerer S (2007) Die vesicovaginale Fistel in der Sahelregion von Burkina Faso. Motivation und Mobilisation der betroffenen Frauen unter Berücksichtigung der lokalen Verhältnisse vor Ort. Eine Analyse des Projektes ‚Fistelklinik Dori'. Inauguraldissertation; Ruprecht-Karls-Universität Heidelberg
Kindberg S, Seehafer P (2022) Geburtsverletzungen – vermeiden, erkennen, versorgen. Elwin Staude-Verlag GmbH, Hannover
Langley V, Thoburn A, Shaw S, Barton A (2006) Second degree tears: to suture or not? A randomized controlled trial. Br J Midwifery 14(9):550–554
Meister MR et al (2016) Predicting obstetric anal sphincter injuries in a modern obstetric population. Am J Obstet Gynecol 215(3):310
Meyvis I, van Rompaey B, Goormans K, Lambers S, Mistiaen W (2012) Maternal positions and other variables: effects on perineal outcomes in 557 births. Birth 39(2):115–120
Ministere de la Santé; Burkina Faso (2012) Programm nationale de lutte contre les fistulas obstétricales
Royal College of Obstetricians and Gynaecologists (RCOG) (2015) The management of third-and fourth-degree perineal tears. Green-top Guideline 29. https://www.rcog.org.uk/guidance/browse-all-guidance/green-top-guidelines/third-and-fourth-degree-perineal-tears-management-green-top-guideline-no-29/. Accessed 21 Mar 2022
Samuelsson E et al (2002) A prospective observational study on tears during vaginal delivery: occurrences and risk factors. Acta obstet Gynecol Scand 81:44–49
SBU (2021) – Diagnostik samt erfarenheter av bemötande och information. Statens beredning för medicinsk och social utvärdering (SBU), Stockholm. SBU-rapport nr 323. ISBN 978-91-88437-67-9
Soerensen MM, Bek KM, Buntzen S, Højberg KE, Laurberg S (2008) Long-term outcome of delayed primary or early secondary reconstruction of the anal sphincter after obstetrical injury. Dis Colon Rectum 51(3):312–317
UNICEF, WHO (1992) Ten steps to successful breastfeeding, step 4. http://tensteps.org. Accessed 16 Mar 2017
Waaldijk K (1994) Step-by-step surgery of vesicovaginal fistulas; a full-colr atlas. Campion Press, Edinburgh
Wacker J (1994) Geburtsverletzungen in Geburtshilfe unter einfachen Bedingungen. Springer, Heidelberg, pp 225–227
Wacker J et al (1998) Introduction of a simplified round partogramm in rural maternity units: Seno province, Burkina Faso. West-Africa Trop Doct 28:146–152

Wacker J, Hailegiorgis A, Barth A, Zanré Y (2009) Vesicovaginale Fisteln – Über den Einsatz von Ärzten in den ländlichen Regionen Afrikas gynäkol prax 33. Hans Marseille, München, pp 679–694
Wacker J, Nikièma P, Kaboré E, Sontie Tiemasse AS, Thieba B, Zanré Y (2020) Häufigkeit und Versorgung von Geburtsverletzungen in Afrika Coloproctology. https://doi.org/10.1007/s00053-020-00458-5
WHO (2022a) ICD-10-PCS. Procedure codes, Section 1 – Obstetrics – 10E Delivery
WHO (2022b) ICD-11 codes. https://icd.who.int/browse11/l-m/en. Accessed 22 Feb 2022

Further Reading

Ahmed S, Tuncalp O (2014) Burden of obstetric fistula: from measurement to action. Lancet Glob Health 3:e243–e244
Wacker J (2007) Die verlorenen und verstoßenen Frauen von Dori. Zusammenhalt von Familien und Zerrüttung von Beziehungen am Beispiel der Frauen mit vesico-vaginaler Fistel (VVF). In: Trotha R-v (eds) Kultur und Gerechtigkeit. Nomos, Baden-Baden

The Treatment of Preeclampsia in Poor and Rich Countries

13

Jürgen Wacker, Laeticia Nwaeburu and Abdoulaye N'Diaye

Contents

Introductory Questions

1. The preeclampsia is a disease in pregnancy that particularly:
   A. affects young pregnant women under 20 years old
   B. affects older pregnant women over 35 years old
   C. often occurs in the first pregnancy
   D. its frequency can be reduced by prophylactic administration of ASA

J. Wacker (✉)
ehemaliger Chefarzt der Frauenklinik Bruchsal, Bruchsal, Germany
e-mail: wacker@menschenfuerfrauen.de

L. Nwaeburu
Klinikum Ingolstadt, Frauenklinik, Ingolstadt, Germany

A. N'Diaye
Frauenklinik, Hopital Saint Camille, Ouagadougou, Burkina Faso

J. Wacker et al. (eds.), *Global Women's Health*,
https://doi.org/10.1007/978-3-662-69700-9_13

2. The preeclampsia is
   A. one of the most common causes of maternal mortality worldwide
   B. does not represent an increase in maternal mortality
   C. is detected earlier in rich countries than in poor countries
   D. can only be treated in women's clinics with intensive care units
3. How do the guidelines for the diagnosis and therapy of hypertensive pregnancy diseases differ in poor and rich countries?
   A. Not at all
   B. By the recommended drugs (magnesium, antihypertensive)
   C. By the existing infrastructure in the respective clinics
   D. By the qualification of the existing staff

13.1 Introduction

Worldwide, approximately 300,000 women die from diseases during pregnancy and complications during childbirth. 99% of these deaths occur in developing countries (LDC). In these countries, pregnancy and childbirth complications are the most common cause of death in women of childbearing age, see Chap. 8. Every maternal death is a tragedy, it is a tremendous loss for the family, the community, and society, because in the hands of the woman lies the future of societies and nations of this earth. Therefore, maternal health is a human right and its improvement is one of the United Nations' Millennium Development Goals.

Hypertensive pregnancy diseases are responsible for about 10–15% of maternal mortality depending on the study, however, 90% of these women die in poor countries. The disease mainly affects the young first-time mother or the older first-time mother. The causes of its development are complex and not fully understood, but it is known that both **endogenous and exogenous factors** play a role in the development of this disease. In recent years, an imbalance between angiogenesis and antiangiogenesis has been described as a key factor in the causative chain of preeclampsia.

Overview

Definition of preeclampsia and classification of hypertensive diseases in pregnancy according to the International Society of Hypertension in Pregnancy (ISSHP) cited in (Wacker 2020)

- Gestational hypertension
- Preeclampsia: Hypertension and proteinuria with/without edema
- Severe forms of preeclampsia: HELLP syndrome and eclampsia
- Chronic hypertension

- Superimposed preeclampsia
- Other hypertensive complications
- Other diseases with hypertensive complications; e.g., collagen diseases, hyperthyroidism

13.2 Pathogenesis of Preeclampsia

The twentieth century was, according to Pierre-Yves Robillarda, the "**le siècle des lumières**" for understanding this complex disease. There were important steps for this:

- Discovery of the blood pressure cuff
- The presence of elevated blood pressure values in both pre-eclamptic and eclamptic women
- The description of the risk factors of a preeclampsia
- The understanding that trophoblast implantation in humans is much deeper than in other mammals
- The association of organ manifestation with nonspecific endothelial damage
- The immunological and vascular backgrounds

13.2.1 Endogenous Factors

Today we know that placenta implantation plays a crucial role in the development of the disease. It is suspected that the implantation of the placenta in pre-eclamptic patients is disturbed very early on. The trophoblast invasion in healthy pregnancies leads to the loss of elasticity of the uterine spiral arteries via cell adhesion receptors and a **insensitivity to vasopressive substances** (e.g., to **Angiotensin II**), which in turn leads to an increase in uterine perfusion. In hypertensive pregnancy diseases, this mechanism is disturbed, leading to inadequate blood flow to the placenta. The resulting placental ischemia has both fetal and maternal effects. In placental bed biopsies of pre-eclamptic women, a lack of conversion of the spiral arteries into low-pressure vessels can be detected. In short, preeclampsia is characterized by the lack of pregnancy-related decrease in vascular resistance in the uterine arteries. This results in poor placental blood flow (placental insufficiency), the logical consequence is intrauterine fetal growth restriction. In addition, systemic changes in the Renin-Angiotensin-Aldosterone System (RAAS) are also found (Wacker 1992, 2020).

In addition to these described **endogenous and endocrinological changes** that lead to the clinical full picture of a preeclampsia, there are also **exogenous factors** that either favor the development of preeclampsia or aggravate the course of an existing preeclampsia.

13.2.2 Exogenous Factors

As a doctor in the development service (DED) EH in the Sahel of Dori in the north of Burkina Faso, I observed that the frequency of pregnant women with severe preeclampsia significantly increased towards the end of the dry season! The basis of the women's diet in the Sahel was millet, enriched with sauces of corresponding vegetables or leaves from shrubs and trees depending on the season. Popular, because nutritious and tasty, were the fresh leaves of the Baobab monkey bread tree, which could only be picked during the rainy season, because the Baobab lost its leaves during the dry season. In a prospective study conducted at three different hospitals in Zimbabwe, we were able to show a **correlation between the frequency of preeclampsia and climatic changes (rainy season)** in 1998 (Wacker et al. 1998b). As an explanation, we suggested the influence of heat and humidity on blood vessels and the production of vasoactive substances. Obviously, dry and rainy seasons also change the vegetation of the respective countries and thus also the diet of the people living there (Wacker et al. 1998b). Based on these results and starting from the already known different content of the main foods (millet, maize, Baobab leaves and other food components) in vitamins, we conducted a prospective study in the Antenatal Clinic of the Mpilo Governmental Hospital in Bulawayo, Zimbabwe, in 1997. With the help of the **Erythrocyte Glutathione Reductase Activations Coefficient Test (EGRACT)**, we determined the Riboflavin status in pregnant women of the Antenatal Clinic. There were statistically significant differences in the Riboflavin status between pregnant women with a normal course of pregnancy and pregnant women who developed preeclampsia later in pregnancy (Wacker et al. 2000). The reduced and **insufficient concentrations of Riboflavin-dependent cofactors** Flavin Adenine Dinucleotide **(FAD)** and Flavin Adenine Mononucleotide **(FAM)** found in this study could explain the changes known in the pathophysiology of preeclampsia such as mitochondrial dysfunction, increased oxidative Stress and disturbances in the release of NO (Wacker et al. 2000).

It is generally known from history that famine leads to a dramatic increase in preeclampsia among malnourished pregnant women, as was observed during the Spanish Civil War in Madrid and during the Second World War in Leningrad, which was besieged by German troops. Based on publications by Chapell and Seed (1999) and Raijmakers and Dechend (2004) and the increasingly reported importance of oxidative stress in the pathophysiology of preeclampsia, we conducted a prospective double-blind study (Placebo vs. Riboflavin 15 mg) (group size each 815 pregnant women) in eight different Primary Health Care (PHC) facilities in Ouagadougou (Burkina Faso) from May 2004 to June 2005. In this study, there were no significant differences in the frequency of preeclampsia. In a further study in Venezuela, we added Vitamin C to Vitamin B_2 (Riboflavin) and found a significant difference in the severity of preeclampsia with milder courses in the group with vitamin supplementation (Elsen et al. 2012). Compared to the pregnant women studied in the study conducted in Burkina Faso, the BMI of the pregnant women studied in Venezuela was higher and the nutritional status of the women was better than in Burkina Faso! This could be explained by the fact that hunger and malnutrition are more decisive in the development of preeclampsia than the mere substitution of supplied vitamins!

13.3 Diagnosis

A preeclampsia can be very dangerous for the mother and the child, therefore the correct and timely diagnosis is absolutely necessary. The main symptoms of this disease

A preeclampsia exists with any (even pre-existing) elevated blood pressure >140/90 mm Hg in pregnancy with at least one newly occurred organ manifestation:

Renal

- Proteinuria > 300 mg/d/l
- Protein/Creatinine > 30 mg/mmol
- Serum Creatinine > 0.90 mg/dl (79.6 μmol/l)
- Oliguria < 80 ml/4 h

Hepatic

- Upper abdominal pain
- Increase in transaminases (twice above the reference values)

Neurological abnormalities

- Headaches
- Visual disturbances, visual impairments up to blindness
- Hyperreflexia, clonus
- Convulsions (Eclampsia)
- Stroke

Pulmonary

- Respiratory insufficiency
- Pleural effusion
- Pulmonary edema

Preeclampsia-specific systems

- Changes in angiogenic factors (e.g. sFlt-1/PIGF)

During the development of preeclampsia research, some test procedures were already described in the 1980s and 1990s of the last century to predict or rule out preeclampsia before the appearance of clinical symptoms (Roll Over Test, Angiotensin II i.V. Test etc.) (Wacker et al. 1992).

Currently, the determination of the quotient from sFlt-1/PIGF from the peripheral blood of the pregnant woman is used for early and precise determination of the occurrence of a preeclampsia:

The quotient sFlt-1/PIGF (sFlt= soluble fms-like tyrosine kinase 1, PIGF = placental growth factor) can be used as early markers for the prediction of a preeclampsia, as the pathophysiology of the development of this disease leads to an increase in this quotient before the clinical manifestation. In a prospective randomized clinical study, **Zeisler et al.** (2016) demonstrated the effective benefit of this biomarker.

In summary, it can be stated that the use of the sFLT-1/PIGF quotient significantly improves the correct diagnosis without affecting the decision for hospital admission.

13.4 Management of Preeclampsia

The initial assessment of patients with hypertensive pregnancy diseases should be carried out by trained professionals (NICE guideline, 2019 p. NICE guideline). The following Fig. 13.1 shows the individual components of management in preeclampsia.

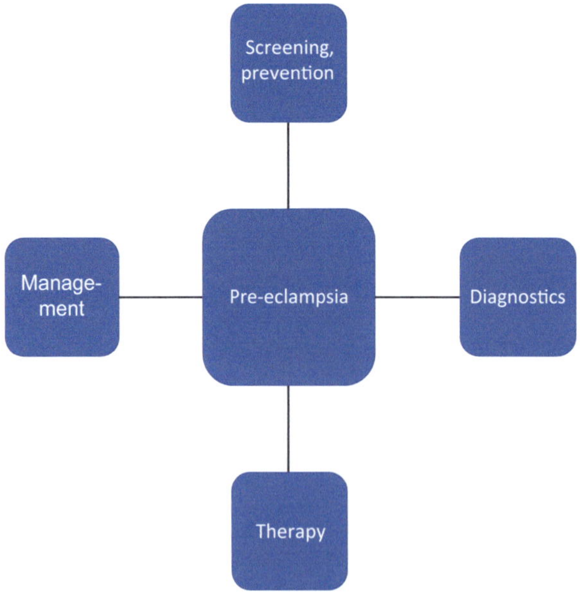

Fig. 13.1 Overview of the management of preeclampsia

Hypertensive pregnancy disorders are among the most common risk factors associated with intensive care admission in obstetrics. Despite the enormous advances in the research of the cause and diagnosis of preeclampsia, the only causal therapy remains the delivery of the child and removal of the placenta.

Primary goals of disease management are

- Pregnancy prolongation, to reduce the fetal risks associated with prematurity, indicated between the 24th and 34th week of gestation
- Reducing maternal risk due to preeclampsia-related complications

A balance must be found between maternal and fetal benefit.

For this, one should distinguish between the management of mild, moderate, and severe preeclampsia.

Outpatient care of the pregnant woman is possible in the absence of prodromes of preeclampsia and blood pressure values below 160/100 mm Hg.

During outpatient check-ups, blood pressure, body weight, protein excretion in the urine, and the general well-being of the pregnant woman must be closely monitored.

Admission to an obstetric department is necessary in the presence of the following findings:

- Blood pressure increase >160/100 mmHg
- Rapid weight gain (more than 1 kg/week, facial edema) due to fluid retention
- Pathological sFlt-1/PIGF ratio >85 or >110
- Clinical manifestation or prodromal symptoms such as unclear upper abdominal pain, headaches, visual disturbances, etc.
- Indications of a fetal threat (decreasing fetal movements, conspicuous CTG, pathological Doppler examination, intrauterine growth retardation (IUGR) and oligohydramnios)
- Lack of compliance for outpatient care

Obstetric management after admission to the clinic:

- Clarification and exclusion of an acute maternal and fetal emergency
- Continuous blood pressure measurement
- Ultrasound examination of the child, fetal weight! Doppler
- Continuous CTG examination mandatory at the start of intravenous antihypertensive treatment
- Control of reflexes
- Laboratory values and protein excretion in the urine (rapid test and 24-hour urine)
- Exclusion of the presence of a HELLP syndrome

The HELLP syndrome is a severe form of preeclampsia.

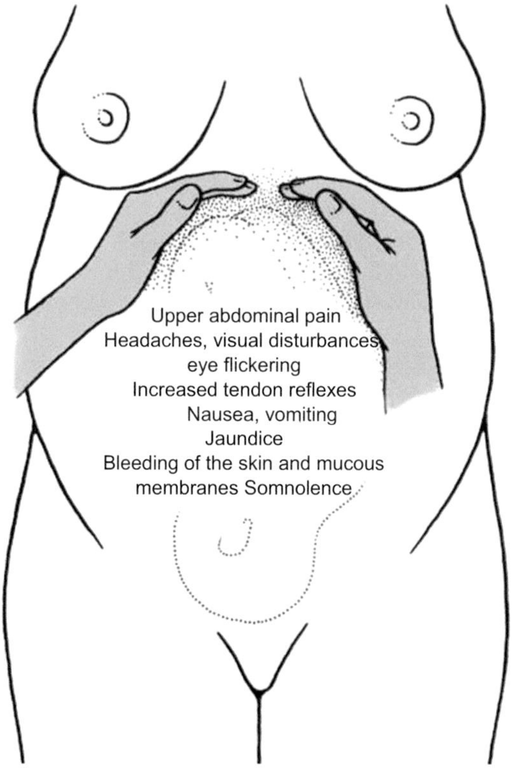

Fig. 13.2 Clinical symptoms in HELLP syndrome. (From: Wacker 2020)

Figure 13.2 shows the clinical symptoms in the presence of a HELLP syndrome.

The HELLP syndrome must be differentially diagnosed from the following diseases:

- Acute fatty liver of pregnancy (Acute Fatty Liver of Pregnancy/AFL)
- Appendicitis
- Hyperemesis gravidarum
- Idiopathic thrombocytopenia
- Urolithiasis
- Gallstone disease
- Duodenal ulcer/Gastroenteritis
- Systemic lupus erythematosus
- Hemolytic-uremic syndrome
- Hepatitis
- Thrombotic thrombocytopenic purpura

To confirm the diagnosis of HELLP syndrome, the following laboratory parameters, shown in Fig. 13.3, must be determined.

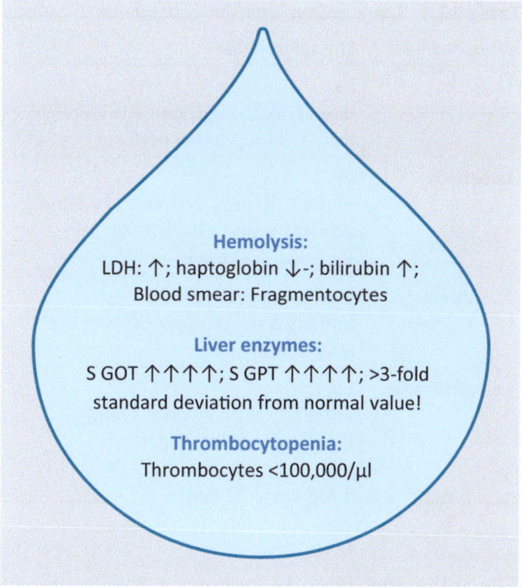

Fig. 13.3 Laboratory changes in HELLP syndrome. (From: Wacker 2020)

Once the diagnosis of HELLP syndrome is confirmed, a timely delivery must be performed.

13.5 Therapy

The goals of treating preeclampsia are to avoid maternal complications due to hypertension, coagulation disorders, and an eclamptic seizure, as well as to avoid child complications and the consequences of prematurity. For lowering high blood pressure, the rule is:

▶ **Not too fast and not too far!** This means for clinical practice: **In order not to endanger the child's blood supply: Do not lower blood pressure more than 10% of the systolic initial value per hour and not below 140 mmHg!**

Example

Procedure for hypertensive crisis/eclampsia during pregnancy and childbirth:

Urapidil i.v.; initially inject 6.25 mg slowly over 2 min.
Then 3–24 mg/h with NaCl perfusor
Magnesium sulfate i.v.: Initially 4–6 g in 50 ml in 15–20 min as a short infusion
Maintenance dose 1–2 g/h ◀

Table 13.1 Drug antihypertensive acute therapy: Substances and dosage

Drug	Dosage scheme	Note
Urapidil	i.v. initially 6.25 mg i.v. slowly (2 min) then 3–24 mg/h (via perfusor)	Better tolerability and controllability
Labetalol	i.v. initially 50 mg i.v. slowly (1–3 min), possibly repeat after 30 min. Perfusor: 120 mg/h	Austria, Switzerland
Nifedipine	p.o. initially 5 mg p.o., possibly repeat after 20 min	- less controllability
Dihydralazine	i.v. initially 5 mg i.v. (over 2 min) then 2–20 mg/h (via perfusor) or 5 mg every 20 min	Onset of action after 3–5 min, sometimes only after 20 min, especially with bolus administration (and then often overshooting)

The following Table 13.1 shows the recommendations for severe hypertension in pregnancy.

13.5.1 Global Women's Health: Same Guidelines for Different Circumstances Require Different Procedures in Clinical Practice

As described in Chap. 19, the guidelines for the treatment of hypertensive diseases in pregnancy are similar between Burkina Faso, Germany, Cameroon, and Switzerland. Doctors and midwives in these countries know what to do to optimally help patients with preeclampsia, but have different financial resources and therefore different equipment in their clinics. Intensive care units are far away and financially unaffordable for most patients in poor countries. Despite this situation, which is a consequence of the poverty in many African countries, there are encouraging approaches:

In many countries of our world, there are no referring specialists and trained midwives who can admit the sick pregnant women to a clinic. Often, pregnant women in the poorest countries turn to village midwives (Traditional Birth Attendants, TBAs), who have only been briefly trained and often cannot read or write. Even under these conditions of poverty, it is important to admit pregnant women with hypertensive diseases to the nearest maternity clinic in time. In a study conducted in the Sahel of Burkina Faso, we were able to demonstrate that it is possible to have blood pressure measurement as part of prenatal care carried out by traditional village midwives. As part of a multi-day training in Dori, the village midwives were introduced to auscultation and the handling of a blood pressure cuff. Using a sphygmanometer marked with red arrows, the village midwives learned to distinguish between normal and pathological blood pressure values. Each of the referring village midwives of the CHR Dori received a blood pressure monitor at the end of the training for use in their respective village. It was shown that at the end of the study, the number of admitted pregnant women with preeclampsia could be increased to four times the number before the study was conducted (Wacker et al. 1998).

13.6 Treatment in Poor and Rich Countries Fundamentally Differs (Laeticia Nwaeburu)

While management in rich countries is characterized by speed, prevention, and better outcomes, it is a disaster in poor countries, much dependent on the availability of money and proximity to a hospital with doctors. The preeclampsia not only poses a risk during pregnancy but also years later, as the consequences of a past preeclampsia are not to be neglected, as shown in this meta-analysis. Data from more than 3 million women show that women who had preeclampsia have an increased risk of cardiovascular diseases, with almost a fourfold increased risk of arterial hypertension 14 years after a past preeclampsia, a twofold increased risk of coronary heart disease and a 1.8-fold increased risk of stroke each after 12 and 10 years after the preeclampsia.

While the indication for antihypertensive treatment of patients with severe hypertension is the same in the guidelines from Germany and Cameroon, different antihypertensives are available to doctors in the two countries. A discrepancy between scientific knowledge and clinical implementation is noticeable. Considering that the large multicenter study comparing the tolerability between dihydralazine and urapidil was already published in 2006 (Wacker et al. 2006), but urapidil was only recognized as the first choice for severe hypertension in the new guideline of 2019, a discrepancy between scientific knowledge and clinical implementation is also recognized! In the first case, this discrepancy is due to the still existing poverty of the population in Cameroon (Fomulu 2013), whereas in Germany the delayed implementation of scientific findings into clinical practice must be explained by other factors.

Answers to the initial questions

1. All answers are correct
2. A, B, C are correct
3. C is correct

References

Chapell L, Seed P (1999) Effect of antioxydants on the occurence of preeclampsia in women at increased risk: a randomised trial. Lancet 354:810–816
Elsen C, Rivas-Echeverria C, Wacker J et al (2012) Vitamin E, A and B^2 as possible risk factors for preeclampsia – under consideration of the PROPER study ('Prevention of preeclampsia by high-dose riboflavin supplementation'). Geburtsh Frauenheilk 72:846–852
Raijmakers MT, Dechend R (2004) Oxydative stress and preeclampsia: rationale for antioxydant clinical trials. Hypertension 44:374–380
Wacker J (2020) Präeklampsie und hypertensive Schwangerschaftserkrankungen; HELLP-Syndrom. In: Wacker J, Sillem M, Bastert G, Beckmann MW (eds) Therapiehandbuch Gynäkologie und Geburtshilfe. Springer, Heidelberg, pp 115–146
Wacker J, Mistry NJ, Bauer H, Vecsei P, Bastert G (1992) Mineralocorticoids and mineralocorticoid receptors in mononuclear leucocytes in patients with pregnancy induced hypertension. J Clin Endocrin Metabolism 74:910–913
Wacker J, Schulz M, Frühauf J, Chiworra FM, Solomayer E, Bastert G (1998b) Seasonal change in the incidence of preeclampsia in Zimbabwe. Acta Obstet Gynecol Scand 77:712–716
Wacker J, Frühauf J, Schulz M, Chiworra FM, Volz J, Becker K (2000) Riboflavin deficieny and preeclampsia. Obstet Gyncol 96:38–44
Wacker J, Wagner B, Briese V, Schauf B, Heilmann L, Bartz C, Hopp H (2006) Antihypertensive therapy in patients with pre-eclampsia: a prospective randomised multicentre study comparing dihydralazine with urapidil. Eur J Obstet Gynecol Reprod Biol 127:152–157
Zeisler H, Liurba E, Chantraine F et al (2016) Prededtive value of the sFlt-1/PIGF Ratio in women with suspected preeclampsia. N Engl J Med 374(1):13–22.N e

Furhter reading

August P (2009) Management of hypertension in pregnancy. www.uptodate.com. Accessed 2010
AWMF (1999) Leitlinie zur Diagnostik und Therapie hypertensiver Schwangerschaftserkrankungen 2019
Duley L, Meher S, Abalos E (2006) Management of preeclampsia. BMJ 332:463–468
Formulu, FJ (2007) Mortalité maternelle à hôpital Générale deYaoundé: Etude retrospective sur 5 années (2002–2006). Health Sciences and Disease. Medizinische Fakultät der Universität Yaoundé (Kamerun)
Heilmann L, Rath W, Wacker J (1998) Diagnostik, Therapie und geburtshilfliches Vorgehen bei schweren hypertensiven Schwangerschaftserkrankungen. Frauenarzt 39:1706–1716
Hoestermann C, Ogbaselassie G, Wacker J, Bastert G (1996) Maternal mortality in the main referral hospital in The Gambia. West Africa. Trop Med Int Health 1:710–717
Maggee LA, Cham C, Waterman EJ, Ohlsson A, Dadelszen P (2003) Hydralazine for treatment of severe hypertension in pregnancy: meta-analysis. BMJ 327:955–965
Magpie Trial Collaborative Group (2002) Do women with pre-eclampsia, and their babies, benefit from magnesium sulphate? The Magpie trial: a randomized placebo-controlled trial. Lancet 359:1877–1890
Neugebauer J, Zanré Y, Wacker J (2006) Riboflavin supplementation and preeclampsia. Int J Gynecol Obstet 93:136–137
Robillard PY, Dekker G, Chaouat G, Bouteiller P, Scioscia M, Hulsey TC (2018) Preeclampsia and the 20th century: ‚Le siècle les Lumières'. Pregnancy Hypertens 13:107–109
Schulz M, Wacker J, Bastert G (2002) Glutathione levels and antoxidative status in pre-eclampsia. Int J Gynecol Obstet 78:157–158
Sibai (1998) Treatment of hypertension in pregnancy. N Engl J Med 335:257–265
Wacker J, Lewicka S, Haack D, Bastert G (1993) Hypertension in pregnancy. J Steroid Biochem Moec Biol 45:65–68

Wacker J, Müller J, Unkels R, Grischke EM, Bastert G (1994) Antihypertensive Therapie bei Schwangerschaftsinduzierter Hypertonie (SIH) mit Urapidil. Zbl Gynäkol 116:271–273

Wacker J, Unkels R, Dehne C (1998a) Training birth attendants in the detection of preeclampsia/eclampsia. Int J Gynecol Obstet 62:287–288

Wacker J, Werner P, Walter-Sack I, Bastert G (1998c) Treatment of hypertension in patients with preeclampsia: a prospective parallel-group study comparing dihydralazine with Urapidil. Nephrol Dial Transplant 13:318–325

Wacker J, Schild R, Hormuth V (2005) Präeklampsie und Evidence based Medicine (EbM). Geburtshilfe Frauenheilkd 65:530–533

Wacker J, Tackenberg M, Pöschl J, Merle U, Morath C, Rath W (2021) Vorzeitige Plazentalösung und HELLP-Syndrom in Zeiten von Corona – Cave stuporem coronae. Geburtsh Frauenheilk 81:45–45

Weinstein L (1985) Preeclampsia/eclampsia with hemolysis, elevated liver enzymes and thrombocytopenia. Obstet Gynecol 66:657

The Performance of Caesarean Section in Poor and Rich Countries (Misgav-Ladach-Sectio, "the Gentle Caesarean Section")

14

Michael Stark, Jürgen Wacker and Judith Lindert

Contents

M. Stark
c/o Regus (NESA), Unter den Linden, Berlin, Germany
e-mail: mstark@nesacademy.org

J. Wacker (✉)
ehemaliger Chefarzt der Frauenklinik Bruchsal, Bruchsal, Germany
e-mail: wacker@menschenfuerfrauen.de

J. Lindert
Klinik für Kinderchirurgie der Universität Rostock, Hamburg, Germany
e-mail: judithlindert@globalsurgery-germany.de

J. Wacker et al. (eds.), *Global Women's Health*,
https://doi.org/10.1007/978-3-662-69700-9_14

Introductory Questions

1. The name Misgav Ladach refers to:
   A. First author of the method
   B. The name of a clinic in Jerusalem
   C. The first patient
   D. The first child delivered by this method
2. What two advantages of this method are named by most authors?
   A. Less blood loss
   B. Longer operation duration
   C. Shorter operation duration
   D. Necessity of higher analgesic administration
3. Child development in caesarean section
   A. is always easier than with a vaginal birth
   B. should be performed in premature births with standing amniotic sac.
   C. to be performed with a deep head stuck in the pelvis through a reverse breech development
   D. requires good training and constant practice

14.1 Introduction

Every surgical procedure consists of hundreds of movements. Each has an origin and its history, each serves a specific purpose and should have a specific execution path.

It is surprising that to this day there is no standardized method of caesarean section that is justified by the methods of evidence-based medicine. Moreover, even in the respective maternity clinics **in poor and rich countries**, different variations of caesarean section are performed.

Today, alternative endoscopic or robot-assisted interventions exist for most abdominal operations. **In this respect, the caesarean section will be the only indicated laparotomy in the future as well.**

The result of our considerations for optimizing the individual steps of the operation is the so-called Misgav-Ladach section method. The Misgav-Ladach method has since proven to be a surgical procedure that achieves much better results with few, simple, optimized steps than the traditional methods used for decades.

14.2 Surgical Technique

This chapter mainly deals with the surgical technique of the caesarean section and not with the routine use of anticoagulants, antibiotics etc.

The **positioning of the birthing woman in a Trendelenburg position** facilitates access to the lower abdominal cavity and makes the use of abdominal cloths unnecessary, as the small intestine loops fall backwards. The use of abdominal cloths causes adhesions (Down et al. 1980). Amniotic fluid, which remains in the abdominal cavity, acts bacteriostatically (Larsen and Davis 1984; Larsen and Galask 1975). If abdominal cloths are used, the amniotic fluid is absorbed by them and its protection is lost.

The Trendelenburg position influences the spread of regional anesthesia (Setayesh et al. 2001). Air embolism, even if it does not clinically appear, is more common in caesarean sections than one might think (>50%), and a deep Trendelenburg position can therefore cause damage (Lowenwirt et al. 1994). These factors must be taken into account when positioning the patient, and if there is suspicion of embolism, an immediate reverse Trendelenburg position should be established and the abdominal cavity filled with physiological saline solution. Since most caesarean sections are performed under regional anesthesia, the comfort of the patient and the anesthetist's assessment of the steepness of the position should also be considered.

The legs of the birthing woman should lie parallel. If these are abducted, tension is created on the fascia, which makes closure difficult.

It is extremely important that the fascia is tension-free when sewing. For this, the legs of the birthing woman must not be abducted.

14.2.1 Type of Abdominal Incision

Since the first described cesarean section by **Ferdinand Kehrer** on 25.09.1881 in Meckesheim near Heidelberg (North Baden, Rhein-Neckar district), where both mother and child survived, abdominal incisions in cesarean sections have traditionally been performed with a longitudinal cut. Since uterotomies were performed with a longitudinal cut in these years, this was a logical and optimal approach.

In 1897, **Johannes Pfannenstiel** described a transverse cut as an alternative to the then usual longitudinal cut, which brings aesthetic advantages (Pfannenstiel 1897). Here, the power of tradition becomes apparent. For many years, the Pfannenstiel cut was used without ever conducting comparative studies. Only 74 years later, Mowat and Bonnar compared longitudinal cuts with Pfannenstiel transverse cuts in cesarean sections. Some expected advantages of the transverse cut were indeed confirmed (Mowat and Bonnar 1971).

In 1972, **Joel-Cohen** described an alternative transverse cut, in which the opening of the fascia occurs over the linea arcuata. The comparison of the cesarean section adapted Joel-Cohen cut with the Pfannenstiel cut showed that febrile morbidity and the consumption of painkillers are significantly lower (Stark and Finkel 1994). Since the conversion of the uterotomy from longitudinal to transverse cuts by **John Martin Munro-Kerr** in the year 1924 (Hewitt 1961), uterotomies are performed worldwide in this form. The combination of the Munro-Kerr and the modified Joel-Cohen cuts provides an optimal access route to the lower uterine segment.

14.2.2 Performing the Abdominal Incision

A superficial cut, exclusively through the cutis, is performed within a physiological transverse line of the skin at a height of 3 cm below an imaginary line that connects the two anterior superior iliac spines. To achieve an accurate cross-section within a skin line, the cut should be precisely planned from the outset and the skin marked accordingly. The marking allows the (right-handed) surgeon to stretch the intended starting point to the left and guide the cut towards the right marking, without causing an asymmetrical cut.

The **following illustration shows the incision in the Misgav-Ladach cesarean section method** (Fig. 14.1):

In the middle of the cut, where no significant bleeding can occur, the opening is deepened by a cross-section to the fascia. In the fascia, a transverse opening of 4–5 mm is created, through which one can see the fibers of the rectus abdominis muscles.

A straight scissors with rounded edges is applied on both sides of the fascia with an opening of 2–3 mm, with one of the scissor blades above and one below the fascia. The scissors are pushed laterally to the left until the length of the planned opening is reached, then similarly pushed to the right along the course of

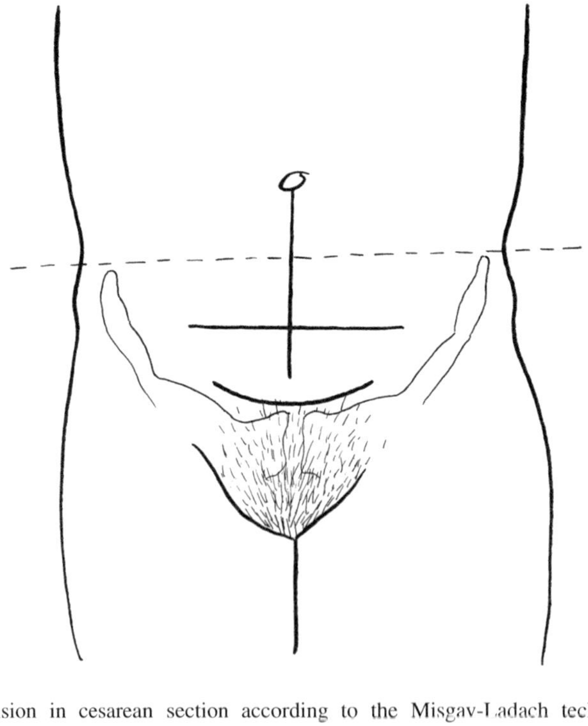

Fig. 14.1 Incision in cesarean section according to the Misgav-Ladach technique. (From: Wacker 2020)

the fascia, so as not to injure it. This opens the fascia under the blood vessels and the adipose tissue.

The opening in the fascia is pulled up and down in the middle of the cut using the two index fingers, allowing the surgeon and his assistant to each place their two index and middle fingers (of the right hand) below the rectus abdominis muscles. Together, they slowly pull the muscles towards themselves, and with them the adipose tissue and the blood vessels, which have lateral elasticity, as far as desired, until the desired width of the opening is reached. Hemostasis is rarely necessary. With this method, several operations can be performed without a single hemostasis.

If the pulling force is not sufficient, as might be the case with overweight women or a subsequent operation due to adhesions, each surgeon can use four fingers for pulling. In such a case, however, the index finger and the middle finger of the left hand should be placed directly on the index finger and the middle finger of the right hand and a joint pull should be performed. The reason for this is that blood vessels—similar to a string on a musical instrument—have lateral elasticity, but little longitudinal elasticity. Pulling with four fingers side by side tends to separate the fingers of the two hands from each other, which can lead to tension and tearing of the blood vessels.

14.2.3 Opening the Peritoneum

The peritoneum has no blood vessels of its own. Since it envelops the intra-abdominal structures, a blind opening with sharp instruments such as scissors or scalpel could possibly lead to injuries of the small intestine loops.

A small opening is created by repeated stretching of the peritoneum using two index fingers (Stark 2009). If this is pulled up and down, the peritoneum is opened transversely. It is important to perform this step well above the bladder to avoid damaging it.

14.2.4 Uterotomy

The Scottish doctor John Martin Munro-Kerr (1868–1960) demonstrated the advantages of the **transverse incision in the lower uterine segment over the then traditional longitudinal incision** in 1924.

One advantage of this change is the reduced blood loss. Also, in subsequent pregnancies, fewer ruptures occur, as the fibers are positioned transversely during the development of the lower segment. This transverse opening thus runs relatively physiologically along the fibers and is therefore less traumatic. The longitudinal incision is rarely used today due to the risks of ruptures in subsequent pregnancies (Borso 1957). However, there are situations where some obstetricians prefer a longitudinal incision in the lower segment, such as in prematurity or multiple pregnancies (Neeser et al. 1988).

The question of whether the bladder should be pushed down is still open. Even though there are short-term advantages when the uterus is opened above the bladder fold (Hohlagschwandtner et al. 2001), the long-term comparison still requires further prospective studies. We prefer to open the uterus as low as possible, as there are fewer muscle fibers and more connective tissue (6.4% muscle tissue in the lower uterine segment versus 68.8% in the corpus uteri). This causes less damage to the myometrium.

Both the length of the abdominal incision and the width of the opening of the lower segment must be planned according to the weight estimate and the position of the child. In the case of breech presentation, for example, one should plan generously in order to be able to perform the birth non-traumatically.

14.2.5 Placental Detachment

After the development of the child, the placenta can be detached manually or by gentle traction of the umbilical cord with pressure from above.

According to a Cochrane Database Review, manual detachment of the placenta causes more bleeding and a higher incidence of endometritis (Wilkinson and Enkin 2000). This is certainly true in cases where premature rupture of membranes has already occurred (Lasley et al. 1997).

14.2.6 Suturing the Uterotomy

The uterus can be sutured with exteriorization (Exteriosation) of the uterus or within the body. Both methods have their supporters.

The advantages of exteriorization during suturing include the ability to suture faster (Darj and Nordström 1999; Hershey and Quilligan 1978; Wahab et al. 1999), and the ability to manually contract the uterus and thereby reduce blood loss. Other advantages include a better view of the intestinal loops and the necessary inspection of the ovaries.

14.3 Suturing Technique

There are several variants for suturing the uterus: a two-layer suture, where one layer is continuous and the other is sutured with individual button sutures, or those where the corners are sutured separately beforehand and then two-layer continuous or individual button sutures are used.

As early as the 1970s, Csucs et al. were able to demonstrate that single-layer suturing of the uterus forms anatomically better scars (Csucs et al. 1972). Advocates of single-layer suturing were also Jelsemaet et al. (1993). Even though there are claims that single-layer suturing can cause more ruptures in subsequent pregnancies (Bujold et al. 2002), there are numerous case examples that single-layer suturing has no disadvantages (Hudić et al. 2010).

In 2016, Bennich et al. were able to show that a two-layer suture has no influence on the thickness of the uterine wall.

The preference for single-layer suturing is based on the physiological fact that a rigorous involution of the uterus takes place immediately after birth. The suture material only serves for hemostasis in the first hours. Later, the myometrium loses volume, and the suture material lies freely around the contracted tissue. The more suture material is used, the more foreign body reactions occur, which in turn leads to an increased need for pain medication. Even though several prospective studies need to be conducted in this regard, for us the optimal way of suturing is a single-layer, continuous, and overcast suture.

Individual sutures cause more tissue reactions due to the larger number of knots, weakening the scar. The larger the needle, the fewer steps are needed to achieve hemostasis. We use an 80 mm round needle with a 90 cm long thread. The larger the needle, the less suture material is needed. Less inserted suture material also means a lower foreign body reaction.

After sewing, blood and amniotic fluid are in the peritoneal cavity. Clots can be manually removed, as no abdominal towels should be used. Liquid blood is absorbed by the peritoneum or through the lymphatic pathways. The amniotic fluid acts bacteriostatically at higher temperatures (Larsen and Davis 1984). Nevertheless, in case of suspicion of amnionitis, the abdominal cavity should be rinsed with a physiological saline solution.

14.3.1 Closing the Peritoneum or Better Leaving the Peritoneum Open

Surgeons of all disciplines have taken for granted that every anatomical layer should be returned to its original position. This task was facilitated by the introduction of anesthesia in 1846 by Morton, allowing surgeons to operate without the suffering pressure caused by their patients' pain.

The Peritoneum cannot be sewn by joining its edges. If you sew the peritoneum, bridges of blood vessels form over its edges, which become foci for adhesions.

As Ellis (1980) has proven, the coelom cells form a new peritoneum within a few days.

In 1983, we began to leave the parietal peritoneum open and since 1984 the visceral peritoneum. In 1991, we were able to demonstrate that significantly fewer adhesions are found in cases of repeated cesarean sections where the peritoneum was left open in the previous operation (Stark 1993).

Closing the peritoneum prolongs the duration of the operation, causes more foreign body reactions and thus more pain and adhesions and should therefore be avoided. This applies to both the parietal and the visceral peritoneum (Royal College of Obstetrics and Gynaecology—RCOG 2002).

Closing the peritoneum prolongs the duration of the operation, causes more foreign body reactions and thus more pain and adhesions and should therefore be avoided (Royal College of Obstetrics and Gynaecology—RCOG2002).

14.3.2 Closure of the Fascia

Above the linea arcuata, the fascia is two-layered on the lateral side. It is significant to include both layers in the suture. We grasp both layers of the fascia on both sides with a Péan clamp each, and 3/4 of the way to the assistant, the cranial and caudal part of the fascia is provided with another Péan clamp each. The first suture is performed below the fascia in such a way that the two layers are sewn from inside to outside and then from outside to inside, so that the knot lies below the fascia. This reduces foreign body reactions and local postoperative sensitivity under the skin.

After the knot, continue sewing, first from inside to outside and then continuously towards the assistant, who holds the two Péan clamps located at the previously mentioned approach point. This ensures that the assistant's hands do not cross with the surgeon's hands. The assistant should not hold the instruments too far apart to avoid tension on the fascia, nor too close together to give the surgeon the opportunity to see into the abdominal cavity and to ensure that no loops or a portion of the omentum are included in the suture. As soon as the suture reaches both clamps, the assistant removes them and holds the last Péan clamp, which holds the two layers together on his side. It is important to also grasp both layers with the needle at its end. The clamp is removed after the knot has been set.

Another advantage of sewing from the surgeon's side towards the assistant is that the surgeon can constantly determine the tension of the suture material with his left hand. Also, the dynamics of his approach are not interrupted.

14.3.3 Skin Closure

There are studies comparing the cosmetic results of various suture methods in traditional cesarean section. In the closure of a Pfannenstiel incision, the intracutaneous skin suture has yielded the best cosmetic results (Lindholt et al. 1994). However, there are no studies comparing different suture methods in the modified Joel-Cohen incision. We believe that the drainage is better the fewer sutures are applied, as this results in fewer hematomas and seromas. Our own version involves closing the skin incision with three sutures, two lateral and one median, which are applied with a very large cutting needle and deep, almost to the fascia. Allis clamps are applied to the cut ends for a few minutes between the sutures to achieve optimal adaptation.

The lateral sutures are removed after 48 hours. After the operation, a skin swelling occurs. The inelastic sutures cannot give way, resulting in pressure and local pain and also permanent skin stripes. All of this can be avoided by removing the lateral sutures; and indeed, we have observed that the pain at the lateral suture sites subsides immediately after the suture removal. The remaining single suture in the middle is removed after five days.

The first presentations and publications of the Misgav-Ladach cesarean section (Stark and Finkel 1994; Stark et al. 1995) met with great resonance, and since then this method has quickly gained worldwide popularity due to its advantages. It has been proven that

- the mobilization of the patient occurs faster (both after uncomplicated operations without and with complications) (Björklund et al. 2000),
- the operation duration (Federici et al. 1997; Li et al. 2001) and the hospital stay (Federici et al. 1997) are shorter,
- the operation can be performed with short-term anesthesia (for example with 2 "hyperbaric" Mepivacain)
- generally less pain medication is needed and
- the overall cost efficiency is more favorable than with other methods (Moreira et al. 2002);
- less and weaker pain (Belci et al. 2015)

Even though the Misgav-Ladach method is currently the most used cesarean section method in some countries, we must continue to critically examine each step of work and be open to new ideas, because insistence on traditions and stagnation is a great danger to the development of surgery.

14.4 Difficult Child Development in Cesarean Section

As described in detail above, the cesarean rate has increased in most Western countries. The rate of secondary cesareans has increased the most. Notably, there is an increase in cesareans performed at a fully dilated cervix. These cesareans can be technically extremely difficult because the child's head often gets stuck in the small pelvis like a champagne cork and is hardly dislocatable towards the uterotomy. Therefore, the development of the child is associated with not to be underestimated dangers for mother and child.

Therefore, this chapter will discuss measures and procedures for a child's head impacted deep in the mother's pelvis.

Based on oral communications from my Burkinabe colleague Dr. Abdoulaye N'Diaye and on the basis of a review article by R. Zimmermann (2015) on this topic, we would like to describe this problem of child development with an impacted child's head:

According to R. Zimmermann, it is similar to the presence of a shoulder dystocia, a nightmare, as the fetal head is stuck like a champagne cork in the small pelvis and cannot be pulled out with any of the usual measures. Zimmermann refers to this condition as 'cephalic dystocia'.

Complications of a cephalic dystocia:

According to Zimmermann, uncontrolled extraction attempts can cause serious damage to both the child and the mother. Known are skull fractures or intracranial hematomas in the child due to too much pressure on the head. But also plexus paresis or fractures of the arm and clavicle are described. Due to the often greatly extended uterotomy development time, the children are depressed and acidotic.

According to R. Zimmermann, the following procedure is recommended:

Preparation

If, despite a fully dilated cervix, the control center for a vaginal-operative delivery is too high and the indication for a cesarean section is given, the procedure should be started with increased urgency (maximum 20–40 minutes). Of great importance is the palpable or sonographic exact determination of the attitude, especially the position of the fetal back. It is recommended to reduce the contractions until the start of the operation with a ß-mimetic tocolysis i.v. The patient is positioned on the operating table with about 40° spread legs to allow an assistant access to the vagina if necessary.

Start of Operation

In a caesarean section during the expulsion phase, the lower uterine segment is often strongly stretched. When entering at the usual place, one often encounters the vagina, which has been strongly displaced cranially, instead of the uterus. Therefore, R. Zimmermann recommends making the Pfannenstiel skin incision about 2 cm further cranially than usual. The uterotomy is also performed about 4 cm higher than usual. This procedure provides more space for the development of the child and prevents the opening of the vagina.

Procedure for Dorsoposterior Presentation

R. Zimmermann describes in a review article in 2015 the development of the child from a reversed breech position. This procedure goes back to the Indian doctor and is also practiced by doctors working in Africa (oral communication from Abdoulaye N'Diaye; Berhan and Berhan 2014). In this procedure, the two fetal arms are first gently released and brought in front of the mother's abdominal wall. This avoids a later, necessary, more difficult arm release. After the arm release, the fetal feet are located and released. Initially, only one foot can often be released. Cranial traction of the upper half of the uterotomy by the assistant can be helpful in tight conditions. In very difficult space conditions, according to R. Zimmermann, a widening of the uterotomy—T-shaped or arc-shaped is rarely necessary. As a third step, the fetal buttocks and then the fetal trunk are extracted by certain and continuous traction on both thighs. In the last step, the child is grasped with the Bracht maneuver and the head is rotated from the straight to the transverse position with a twisting motion. With pressure from the outside by the assistant, the head slides effortlessly through the uterotomy.

The following illustration from the article by R. Zimmermann from 2015 shows this procedure of the development of the child from a reversed breech position in four steps (Fig. 14.2):

In many clinics, the child's head wedged into the maternal pelvis is pushed up from the vagina with the hand or with the help of two fingers. This method, described as the push-and-pull method, positions the patient primarily in the lithotomy position. Landesman and Graber described this procedure in 1984. Since pushing up with fingers exerts great pressure on the child's head, with the risk of skull fractures and brain hemorrhages, R. Zimmermann has suggested the use of a 60 mm Silc Cup silicone vacuum from Medela/Menox as an alternative to hand/fingers. Originally, this device was made to be attached to the fetal head with a vacuum, but in this case, it is used as a pushing, not a pulling instrument. With the silicone cap, the pressure is much better distributed on the skull cap when pushing

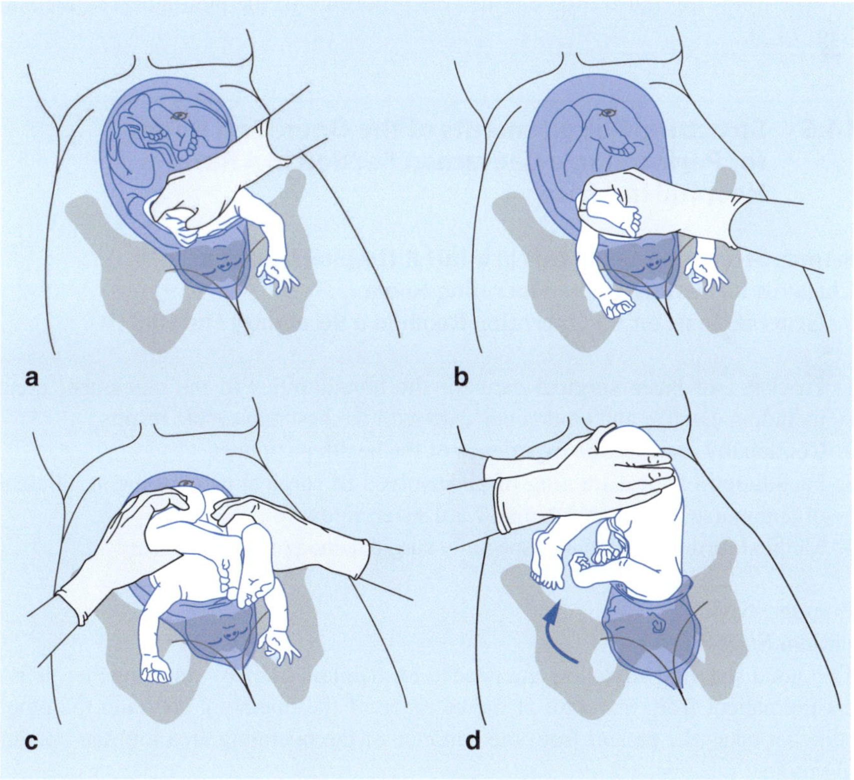

Fig. 14.2 Development of the child from a reversed breech position. (From: Zimmermann 2015)

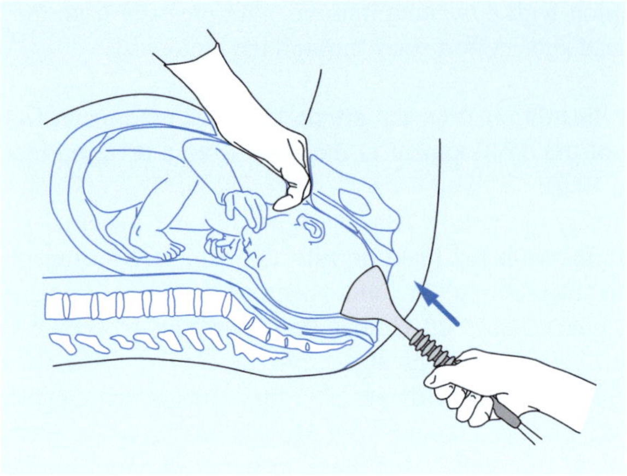

Fig. 14.3 Pull-Push Method. (From: Zimmermann 2015)

up. The following illustration clarifies the procedure of the pull-and-push method (Fig. 14.3).

14.5 Structural Requirements of the Operating Room for Performing a Caesarean Section in a Rural Hospital in Africa

Setting, Structures, Standards in a Rural Hospital in Africa
Checklist for Setting Up an Operating Room
General Goals for an Operating Room in a Secondary Hospital

1. Provision of basic surgical care for the communities in the catchment area, including elective and emergency care with the best achievable results.
2. Continually increase the experience of the health personnel
3. Facilitation of local training of all involved in surgical care (surgeon, clinical officer, nurse, nurse, anesthetist, ward sister, midwife)
4. Medical further education, especially surgical and perioperative care

Preoperative
Patient Stretcher(s)
Two good standard stretchers are needed to maintain asepsis. One stretcher delivers the patient from the ward at the entrance of the operating area and the other stretcher takes the patient from the entrance of the operating area into the operating room.

The carrier should have at least the following properties:

- Have stands for infusion bottles with intravenous fluids
- Be adjustable
- High flexibility
- Buy from a supplier who guarantees a low resource area

Some of the best brands are: Stryker, Hill-Rom, Avante

Perioperative
Operating table
This is the center of the entire surgical process, as it connects the patient and the surgeon, and there is a good selection of operating tables that offer the following:

- "Comfort" for surgeons
- Patient comfort
- "Comfort" for anesthetists
- Adjustability
- Material easy to clean
- Durability and maintenance
- Affordability

Usable brands include: Skytron, Steris, Stryker

Patient monitors
At this point, the patient's vital functions (blood pressure, oxygen saturation, pulse rate, respiratory rate, and temperature) and other perimeters must be constantly monitored throughout the surgical procedure to ensure a safe operation.

Another monitor is needed for the postoperative observation period, especially for difficult or long procedures.

Appropriate brand specifications include: Phillips, Aurora, Mindray.

Operating lights (40,000–160,000LUX)
These provide the lighting needed for the surgical procedure. They can either be fixed (ceiling), procedure light, or standing portable or/and spotlight. These properties should be considered when selecting the right lights:

- Color temperature
- Depth
- Shadow dilution
- Lamp duration and availability of replacement lamps in Sierra Leone
- Voltage stability

Some surgical spotlights would be required for certain procedures and also as a backup in case of a power outage, e.g. USB Charging useful, Life-Box

Oxygen concentrators
These are needed to provide the appropriate amount of gas, as the anesthesia machine is not usable.

Diamedica is one of the brands used in most African countries due to its functionality for cost-effective source environment settings.

Suction machines
These can range from portable to non-portable machines and their main purpose is to drain unwanted fluid from the operating area as well as for anesthesia, for which two machines are needed.

Appropriate brand specifications include: De Vibiss, Allied, Medline

Medicine cabinets
These are needed to store and access medications that allow the doctor and anesthetists to prescribe them.

Surgical instruments
Depending on performance orientation in Bellwether procedures: Sectio, laparotomy, and treatment of open fractures

Others
The following smaller devices are also crucial for the operating room:

- Mayo stands
- Hand tables
- Patient stirrups
- Infusion stands
- Surgical instruments and storage containers
- Roof for half the area to dry, to allow drying of surgical drapes

Postoperative
An autoclave, which is essential for the sterilization process, is needed.

Answers to the Introductory Questions

1. B
2. A, C,
3. B, C, D

References

Berhan Y, Berhan A (2014) A meta-analysis of reverse breech extraction to deliver a deeply impacted head during cesarean delivery. Int J Gynecol Obstet 124:99–105

Björklund K, Kimaro M, Urassa E, Lindmark G (2000) Introduction of the Misgav-Ladach caesarean section at an African tertiary centre: a randomised controlled trial. Br J Obstet Gynecol 107(2):209–216

Borso A (1957) Dehiscence of hysterotomy wounds after cesarean section performed with longitudinal incision of the lower segment. Minerva Ginecol 15; 9(17):742–747

Bujold E, Bujold C, Hamilton EF, Harel F, Gauthier RJ (2002) The impact of a single-layer or double-layer closure on uterine rupture. Am J Obstet Gynecol 186(6):1326–1330

Csucs L, Kott I, Solt I (1972) Mono-layer sutures of uterine incision in cesarean section based on clinical experience and animal experiments. Zentralbl Gynäkol 26; 94(34):1121–1126

Darj E, Nordström ML (1999) The Misgav-Ladach method for cesarean section compared to the Pfannenstiel method. Acta Obstet Gynecol Scand 78:37–41

Down RH, Whitehead R, Watts JM (1980) Why do surgical packs cause peritoneal adhesions? Aust N Z J Surg 50(1):83–85

Ellis H (1980) Internaloverhealing: the problem of intraperitoneal adhesions. World J Surg 4:303–306

Federici D, Lacelli B, Muggiasca L, Agarossi A, Cipolla L, Conti M (1997) Cesarean section using the MisgavLadach method. Int J Gynecol Obstet 57(3):273–279

Hershey DW, Quilligan EJ (1978) Extraabdominal uterine exteriorization at cesarean section. Obstet Gynecol 52(2):189–192

Hewitt J (1961) J.M. Munro Kerr. J Obstet Gynaecol Br Emp 68:510–514

Hohlagschwandtner M, Ruecklinger E, Husslein P, Joura EA (2001) Is the formation of a bladder flap at caesarean necessary? A randomized trial. Obstet Gynecol 98(6):1089–1092

Hudić I, Fatusić Z, Kamerić L, Misić M, Serak I, Latifagić A (2010) Vaginal delivery after Misgav-Ladachcesarean section – is the risk of uterine rupture acceptable? J Matern Fetal Neonatal Med 23(10):1156–1159

Larsen B, Davis B (1984) Enhancement of the antibacterial property of amniotic fluid by hyperthermia. Obstet Gynecol 63(3):425–429

Larsen B, Galask RP (1975) Host resistance to intraamniotic infection. Obstet Gynecol Surv 30(10):675–691

Lasley DS, Eblen A, Yancey MK, Duff P (1997) The effect of placental removal method on the incidence of postcesarean infections. Am J Obstet Gynecol 176(6):1250–1254

Li M, Zou L, Zhu J (2001) Study on modification of the MisgavLadach method for cesarean section. J Tongji Med Univ 21(1):75–77

Lindholt JS, Moller-Christensen T, Steele RE (1994) The cosmetic outcome of the scar formation after cesarean section: percutaneous or intracutaneous suture? Acta Obstet Gynecol Scand 73(10):832–835

Moreira P, Moreau JC, Faye ME et al (2002) Comparison of two cesarean techniques: classic versus MisgavLadachcesarean. J Gynecol Obstet Reprod 31(6):572–576

Mowat J, Bonnar J (1971) Abdominal wound dehiscence after caesarean section. Br Med J 2(756):256–257

Neeser E, Niehues U, Hirsch HA (1988) Maternal morbidity following cesarean section. Comparison of isthmo-corpus longitudinal section and isthmian transverse section in premature labor. Geburtshilfe Frauenheilkd 48(1):8–12

Pfannenstiel J (1897) Über die Vorteile des suprasymphysären Faszienquerschnitts für die gynäkologischen Koliotomien, zugleich ein Beitrag zu der Indikationsstellung der Operationswege. Samml Klein Vortr Gynäkol:68–98. (KlinVortr NF Gynäk 1900; 97: 268)

Royal College of Obstetrics and Gynaecology – RCOG (2002) Peritoneal closure guideline no. 15, July
Setayesh AR, Kholdebarin AR, Moghadam MS, Setayesh HR (2001) The Trendelenburg position increases the spread and accelerates the onset of epidural anesthesia for Cesarean section. Can J Anaesth 48(9):890–893
Stark M (1993) Clinical evidence that suturing the peritoneum after laparotomy is unnecessary for healing. World J Surg 17(3):419
Stark M (2009) In the era of 'non-closure of the peritoneum', how to open it? (Not every simple method is optimal, but every optimal method is simple). Acta Obstet Gynecol Scand 88(1):119
Stark M, Finkel AR (1994) Comparison between the Joel-Cohen and Pfannestiel incision in caesarean sections. Eur J Obstet Gynaecol Reprod Biol 53:121–122
Stark M, Chavkin Y, Kupfersztain C, Guedj P, Finkel AR (1995) Evaluation of combinations of procedures in cesarean section. Int J Gynaecol Obstet 48(3):273–276
Wahab MA, Karantzis P, Eccersley PS, Russell IF, Thompson JW (1999) A randomised, controlled study of uterine exteriorisation and repair at caesarean section. Br J Obstet Gynaecol 106(9):913–916
Wilkinson C, Enkin MW (2000) Manual removal of placenta at caesarean section. Cochrane Database Syst Rev 2:CD000130
Zimmermann R (2015) Schwierige Kindesentwicklung bei der Sectio. Der Gynäkologe, pp 599–610

Further Reading

Alamia V, Meyer BA (1999) The development of a scoring system, obstetric parameter that predict successful vaginal delivery after caesarean birth. Obstet Gynecol 93(Suppl):49
Ansaloni L, Brundisini R, Morino G, Kiura A (2001) Prospective, randomized, comparative study of MisgavLadach versus traditional cesarean section at Nazareth Hospital, Kenya. World J Surg 25(9):1164–1172
Belci D, Di Renzo GC, Stark M, Đurić J, Zoričić D, Belci M, Peteh LL (2015) Better outcome regarding the intensity of pain, presence of neuropathic and chronic pain and the level of satisfaction about cosmetic appearance of the scar (Morbidity and chronic pain following different techniques of caesarean section: a comparative study). J Obstet Gynaecol 35(5):442–446
Bennich G, Rudnicki M, Wilken-Jensen C, Lousen T, Lassen PD, Wøjdemann K (2016) Impact of adding a second layer to a single unlocked closure of a Cesarean uterine incision: randomized controlled trial. Ultrasound Obstet Gynecol 47(4):417–422. https://doi.org/10.1002/uog.15792
Bundesgeschäftsstelle für Oualitätssicherung – BQS (2008) Qualitätsreport. http://www.bqs-institut.de/
Deutsche Gesellschaft für Gynäkologie und Geburtshilfe – DGGG (2006) Stellungsnahme zur Frage der erlaubten Zeit zwischen der Indikationsstellung und Sectio (E-E-Zeit) bei einer Notlage. http://www.google.de/search?q=Stellungsnahme+zur+Frage+der+erlaubten+Zeit+zwischen+der+Indikationsstellung+und+Sectio+%28E-E-Zeit%29+bei+einer+Notlage&channel=linkdoctor
Dodd JM, Crother CA, Huertas E, Guise JM, Dell H (2009) Planned elective repeat caesarean section versus planned vaginal birth for women with a previous caesarean birth. Cochrane Database Syst Rev 4:CD004224
Dudenhausen JW (2009) Indikationen zur abdominalen Schnittentbindung. In: Stark M (eds) Der Kaiserschnitt. Urban & Fischer, München/Jena, pp 80–84
Flamm BL, Goings JR, Liu Y, Wolde-Tsadik G (1994) Elective repeat caesarean delivery versus trial of labor: a prospective multicenter study. Obstet Gynecol 83:927–934

Hauth JC, Owen J, Davis RO (1992) Transverse uterine incision closure: one versus two layers. Am J Obstet Gynecol 167:1108–1111
Husslein P, Wertaschnigg D (2002) Elective cesarean section – delivery mode of the future or social misconception? Therapie Umsch 59(12):660–666
Jelsema RD, Wittingen JA, Vander Kolk KJ (1993) Continuous, nonlocking, single-layer repair of the low transverse uterine incision. J Reprod Med 38(5):393–396
Landesman R, Graber EA (1984) Abdominovaginal delivery: modification of the cesarean section operation to facilitate delivery of the impacted head. Am J Obstet Gynecol 148:707–710
Landon MB, Hauth JC, Leveno KJ et al (2004) Maternal and perinatal outcome associated with a trial of labor after prior cesarean delivery. N Engl J Med 25:2581–2589
Lowenwirt IP, Chi DS, Handwerker SM (1994) Nonfatal venous air embolism during cesarean section: a case report and review of the literature. Obstet Gynecol Surv 49(1):72–76
McMahon MJ, Luther ER, Bowes WA, Olsham AF (1996) Comparison of a trial of labor with an elective second caesarean section. N Engl J Med 335:689–695
Meininger D, Byhahn C, Kessler P et al (2003) Intrathecal fentanyl, sufentanil, or placebo combined with hyperbaric mepivacaine 2% for parturients undergoing elective cesarean delivery. Anesth Analg 96(3):852–858
Mozurkewich EL, Hutton EL (2000) Elective repeat cesarean delivery versus trial of labour: a meta-analysis of the literature from 1989 to 1999. Am J Obstet Gynecol 183(5):1187–1197
Notzon FC, Cnattingius BP et al (1994) Cesarean section delivery in the 1980s: international comparison by indication. Am J Obstet Gynecol 170:495–504
Odent M (2009) Wie steht es um die Zukunft einer durch Kaiserschnitt entbundenen Zivilisation. In: Der Kaiserschnitt von Michale Stark. Urban & Fischer, München/Jena, pp 396–411
Paterson CM, Saunders NJ (1991) Mode of delivery after one caesarean section: audit of current practice in a health region. Br Med J 303:818–821
Phelan JP, Ahn MO, Diaz F et al (1989) Twice a cesareansection, always a cesarean? Obstet Gynecol 73:161–165
Rageth C, Juzzi C, Grossenbacher H (1999) Delivery after previous caesarean: a risk evaluation. Obstet Gynecol 93:332–337
Rumler-Detzel P (2006) Wunsch-Sectio – aus juristischer Sicht. Gesundheits Recht 5:241–244
Schlund GH (2008) Kommentar zur juristischen Problematik einer Wunschsectio. Gynäkol Praxis 32:237–238
Stark M (1994) Technique of caesarean section: MisgavLadach method. In: Popkin DR, Peddle LJ (eds) Women's health today. Perspectives on current research and clinical practice. Proceedings of the XIV. World congress of gynaecology and obstetrics, Montreal. Parthenon/New York, pp 81–85
Wacker J (2009) Re-Sectio. In: Stark M (eds) Der Kaiserschnitt. Urban & Fischer, München/Jena, pp 177–187
Wacker J (2010) Kaiserschnitt vs. Natürliche Geburt. Geburtsh Frauenheilkd 70:840–843
Wacker J, Baldé MD, Bastert (2005) Obstetrics unplugged, 2nd edn. Printhouse Heidelberg – Verlag Regionalkultur, Ubstadt-Weiher
Wacker J, Sillem M, Bastert G, Beckmann MW (2020) Therapiehandbuch Gynäkologie und Geburtshilfe, 3rd edn. Springer, Heidelberg
Weinstein D, Benshushan A, Tano V, Zilberstein R, Rojanski N (1996) Predictive score for vaginal birth after cesarean section. Am J Obstet Gynecol 174:192–198
Wolff F (2008) Aktuelles zur Wunschsectio. Juristische Konsequenzen. Gynäkol Praxis 32:231–244
Zimmermann R (2012) Handbuch Geburtshilfe. Eigenverlag, Zürich
jtgga.2016.16131. eCollection 2016.

Effects of Modern Obstetrics on Human Development Using the Example of Premature Termination of Pregnancy

15

Michel Odent, Michael Stark and Jürgen Wacker

Contents

Introductory Questions

1. What role could the increase in melatonin levels play in the late phase before birth?
   A. Component of birth preparation
   B. Synergy between melatonin and the inhibitory neurotransmitter GABA
   C. Possible interaction with oxytocin

M. Odent
London, UK

M. Stark
c/o Regus (NESA), Berlin, Germany
e-mail: mstark@nesacademy.org

J. Wacker (✉)
ehemaliger Chefarzt der Frauenklinik Bruchsal, Bruchsal, Germany
e-mail: wacker@menschenfuerfrauen.de

J. Wacker et al. (eds.), *Global Women's Health*,
https://doi.org/10.1007/978-3-662-69700-9_15

2. What we can learn from African mothers:
   A. Most intimate form of bonding by mothers who carry their infants wrapped in a cloth on their backs
   B. Adoption of other, more successful birthing positions than lying on the back
   C. Long-lasting memory of the course of birth
3. What was the disaster of the introduction of powdered milk as baby food instead of natural breastfeeding by a Swiss company in the 1970s and how was this problem resolved?
   A. Diarrhea in infants
   B. Dehydration of infants
   C. Malnutrition of infants
   D. African midwives and doctors were supported by development workers to jointly and sustainably advocate for a renaissance of natural breastfeeding.

15.1 Introduction

In his book "The Caesarean Section", in which Michael Stark, along with several co-authors, some of whom are internationally known obstetricians, extensively discusses the topics surrounding delivery by caesarean section, particularly the Misgav-Ladach method he developed, there is a sentence by the Heidelberg philosopher Karl Jaspers above the foreword by Joachim W. Dudenhausen:

> No one has the truth, we are all seeking it!

Michel Odent describes in Chapter 27 of Michael Stark's book 'The Caesarean Section' under the heading 'What is the future of a civilization born by caesarean section' possible effects of the mode of delivery on the emotional and psychological development of humans (Michel Odent 2009). The author of this chapter, the French doctor and obstetrician Michael Odent, became internationally known as a representative of the "Gentle Birth" developed by Frédérick Leboyer. In 1987, he founded the Primal Health Research Centre in London, which researches the influence of prenatal experiences on health. In a section of his chapter titled "From the non-human to the human mammal", Odent describes the observations of Eugene Marais on Kaffir antelopes in South Africa and the studies of Krehbiel and Poindron on ewes, in which the ewes were given chloroform or epidural anesthesia during birth, and afterwards did not care for their own lambs (Marais 1937; Krehbiel et al. 1987). For Odent, ethologists like Konrad Lorenz and Harlow were and are true pioneers who had come to the tacit agreement that the mother-child relationship represents the prototype of love. Under the section "The Responsibility of the Pioneers", Odent writes (2009): "Since the famous Einstein letter to President Roosevelt in October 1939, warnings about human-induced existential risks have been voiced by those who, as pioneers of scientific or technical progress, were at the root of the danger." Furthermore, Michel Odent (2009) writes in specific reference to Michael Stark's book: "Today it is our duty, as representatives of the community of obstetricians, to focus in this book initiated and edited by Michael Stark on the threats that have not yet been perceived by scientifically and medically versed philosophers. The fact that Michael Stark asked the author Michel Odent to write a chapter on the future of a civilization that has come into the world by caesarean section—a topic that greatly concerns the editor—is in itself a warning".

In the early phase of our book project "Global Women's Health" and after a longer conversation with Michael Stark in December 2021, similar questions arose for me, as a doctor, author and former development aid worker:

- What happens when we simply export our Western medicine, which is literally reflected in the guidelines of our medical societies, to other countries and continents?
- What do we know about the experiences of other cultures in dealing with birth, health, illness and death?
- What possibilities are there for scientific and human exchange on an equal footing between poor and rich countries?
- How can we succeed in aligning our medical knowledge with the nature and workings of nature?

Michel Odent has spent his life intensively dealing with the medicine of people from other cultures and especially with their handling of birth. When I subsequently asked Michel Odent in December 2021 if he would like to contribute to the success of our book project, he immediately agreed and sent me the following contribution:

15.2 Effects of Shortening the Duration of Pregnancy Through Induction of Labor on Human Development. About the Physiological Significance of the Late Phase of Pregnancy

In the context of modern obstetrics, it is becoming increasingly common to shorten the duration of pregnancy through interventions such as induction of labor or caesarean section before birth. According to English statistics for the period 2020–2021, for example, the rate of labor inductions was 34.4% and the rate of caesarean sections before the onset of labor and the start of birth was 18.3% (NHS Digital Maternity Statistics 2022). For this reason, we summarize the conclusions of current studies that suggest that the importance of the short phase of "physiological birth preparation" is underestimated (Odent 2019).

A Spanish-Dutch team has shown that there is a gradual reduction in the volume of gray matter during late pregnancy (Hoekzema et al. 2016). The observed reductions are not randomly distributed throughout the brain, but are located in areas of the cerebral cortex that play a key role in sociability. It seems that the need for privacy already increases in late pregnancy before labor begins.

The increase in melatonin levels in the phase before birth could also be seen as a component of birth preparation. We must keep in mind the synergy between melatonin, the inhibitory neurotransmitter GABA (Kivela 1991; Nakamura et al. 2001) and oxytocin (Sharkey et al. 2009).

The peak production of ALLO (allopregnanolone) by the placenta in the days before birth also becomes an important chapter of physiological birth preparation. ALLO is a positive modulator of GABA (Children's National Health System 2018).

Such findings and results of research are of utmost importance in a time when the concept of neocortical inhibition becomes a key to understanding human nature in general and physiological processes such as the sense of smell (Endevelt-Shapira et al. 2014) and birth (Odent 1987) in particular.

After thousands of years of cultural conditioning related to socialized births, we have the consistent conclusions of documents about ethnic groups that have maintained their Paleolithic lifestyle into the twentieth century: women have isolated themselves for birth (Everett 2008; Eaton et al. 1988; Shostak 1990; Schiefenhovel 1978). Interestingly, in these documents, infant and toddler death is portrayed as a major issue, while maternal and perinatal deaths are hardly mentioned (one case in the report by Daniel Everett, who lived like a Pirahã/Pirrara in the Amazon jungle for more than twenty years). There are several explanations for the comparatively safe birth in the Paleolithic era. First, there were the effects of a hundred-thousand-year natural selection, so that a woman's ability to pass on her genes was linked to her ability to give birth. We must also consider that the first pregnancy usually occurred shortly after puberty. In addition, women protected themselves from negative cultural interventions in the perinatal period by satisfying their need for privacy.

The first prerequisite to question millennia-old traditions and cultural imprints is to start from the useful question, which is not: "Why are human births difficult?" It is: "Why are human births occasionally easy and quick, regardless of individual morphological peculiarities?" If the starting point is the useful question, the focus is not on mechanical considerations, which have probably been overestimated so far, but on the reduced neocortical control, as the solution that evolution has found to make human births possible and potentially easy. Even in the twenty-first century, there are still people who are aware of this solution. They know that women after an easy and quick birth usually cannot remember details, apart from the effects of some sensory perceptions—especially the sense of smell. Their behavior would have been unacceptable in other situations for a civilized woman (e.g., screaming or cursing). They were in unexpected, bizarre, and primitive body postures. The neocortical control was obviously reduced.

On the day when the concept of neocortical inhibition is considered a key to understanding human birth, we will be on our way to accepting that a birthing woman must first feel protected from stimuli such as language, light, and all situations that increase attention. We will be able to ask ourselves how and to what extent it is still possible to desocialize human births. One will be interested in the phase of physiological birth preparation.

The investigation of human birth within the framework of brain physiology will provide reasons to preserve published information from being forgotten, which despite its great scientific value and probable practical implications has remained almost undiscovered. An example: According to a Swedish study, the risk of developing prostate cancer in old age is lower the longer a boy has spent in the womb (Ekbom et al. 2000). The authors examined a large cohort of men born in Stockholm between 1889 and 1941. In the cohort, a total of 834 cases of prostate cancer were identified between 1958 and 1994. The study included 1880 control persons. The reasons why this study has remained unnoticed are obvious in the current phase of the history of information technology. First, it was published in a reputable, but highly specialized scientific journal that is not read by most health care practitioners. And even if the published article had reached the practitioners, it is very likely that most readers would not have gone beyond the title: experts in prostate cancer are not interested in the length of fetal life, while obstetricians and midwives are not conditioned to think long-term and are not interested in the risk that a newborn boy might one day develop prostate cancer.

The study of the phase of "physiological birth preparation" should be a way to identify future topics. We recently learned that the particles of Vernix caseosa, which detach from the skin of the fetus and float in the amniotic fluid, are swallowed by the fetus and are involved in the development of the intestinal flora. The new focus is on their extraordinary richness in saturated branched-chain fatty acids. We remind that molecules of branched-chain fatty acids are characterized by the presence of one or two methyl groups (CH3) on the carbon chain. There is renewed interest in Vernix caseosa since we learned that humans are not the only mammals whose skin is covered with Vernix: marine mammals such as sea lions and seals develop a human-like Vernix. There are indications for comparative studies of human intestinal flora and the intestinal flora of some marine mammal species. The importance of branched-chain fatty acids has been underestimated so far. Only one work is mentioned in which their antitumor activity in human breast cancer cells is described, with the focus on their effect on fatty acid biosynthesis (**Sawitree Wongtangtintharn** 2004).

In the age of over-specialization, it is urgently necessary to develop new ways of classifying scientific data in order to facilitate the finding of secured knowledge with practical implications.

In the meantime, it would be a dangerous goal to reduce the number of obstetric interventions (Odent 2004a). The priority is to investigate physiological processes, including the phase before the onset of labor.

15.3 Rethinking Traditions

In a time when the perinatal period is considered critical for the development of the ability to love, an overview of those documented rituals and beliefs whose effects disrupt the physiological processes is a first step to understand the current turning point in the history of our species. It reveals the extent of what has been a cross-cultural phenomenon for millennia.

Today, female genital mutilation is mainly observed in Africa and among individual immigration populations in Europe (Momoh et al. 2001; Wacker and Zerm 2020). According to a WHO study, genital mutilations are estimated to result in one to two perinatal deaths per 100 births, the risk increases in the case of extensive techniques (Banks et al. 2006). In Nigeria, the "Gishiri cut" often follows genital mutilation during childbirth. This operation is performed by a traditional birth attendant on women with prolonged labor. The birth attendant uses a knife to make a soft tissue cut with the aim of enlarging the birth canal. The Gishiri cut is a major risk for the occurrence of genital fistulas (Ampofo et al. 1990).

According to Michel Odent, the birth guidance by a midwife leads to a mixing of the cultural milieu with the physiological process. One of the basic needs of a human infant during birth is privacy, which must be protected. The need for protection was originally satisfied by the proximity of the mother of the birthing woman or another familial mother figure of the community. This was the origin of the midwife. At a certain stage in history, the midwife seems to have tended to strengthen her role, take more influence, and become an active "coach".

Betsy Lozoff showed in her study of 186 non-industrialized societies that less than 2% of women in such societies routinely give birth alone and in only another 2% is this allowed to women at all (Lozoff 1983). In 62% of the 71 societies, birth attendants actively try to influence the birth: by manual manipulation, massaging or stretching the cervix, even by throwing themselves on the stomach or, as reported by Brigitte Jordan in documenting the practices of the Maya people in Yucatan, simply by explaining the birth process (Jordan 1983). In some cultures, birth attendants guided the laboring women by telling them how to breathe. Sheila Kitzinger reported, for example, that in Jamaica women are instructed to breathe superficially in the late opening phase because it is believed that the fetus could slip into the maternal chest (Kitzinger and MacCormak 1982).

15.4 Lost Evolutionary Advantages

Among the doctors and midwives who performed their "development service" in different African countries in the 1980s, many were inspired by the reports of the **ethologists** and the ideas of Sheila Kitzinger and Brigitte Jordan. They longed for exoticism and found extremes. They were confronted with the consequences of poverty, which brought about diseases with extreme manifestations and obstetric emergencies of unprecedented scale. From romantics, they became realists, carried by the humility to serve, and comforted by the hope of being able to help.

Michel Odent wrote about this in 2009 under the heading "Lost Evolutionary Advantages":

'The widespread distribution of the described traditional beliefs and rituals suggests that, despite their disadvantages, they had an evolutionary advantage until now. Indeed, the disadvantages of clinging to traditional rituals are enormous: There are still hundreds of thousands of maternal deaths per year due to bleeding, and a postpartum hemorrhage is almost always the result of inadequate intervention. While some of those who confuse science with technology proclaim that "the end of science" has already been reached (Horgan 2003), our hope is indeed more than ever carried by the scientific search for truth.'

15.5 Encouraging Experiences and Perspectives for the Future

There are also encouraging examples of mutual "learning" in development cooperation. After the disaster of introducing powdered milk as baby food instead of natural breastfeeding by a Swiss company in the 1970s, African midwives and doctors, supported by German development workers, managed to promote and enforce the renaissance of breastfeeding sustainably!

We learned the most intimate form of bonding from African mothers when we saw the mothers carrying their infants wrapped in a cloth on their backs.

We learned from African mothers that there are other, more successful birthing positions than lying on the back!

We were surprised by African mothers how intensely they experience their birth process, and remember it even after years (Wacker et al. 1989; Wacker 2010)!

We have learned that we can better understand human destinies if we respect nature and its laws.

Today we need a real science, not to challenge nature, but to question deeply rooted beliefs, to understand the truth in nature. According to Odent, this is a necessary step to rediscover—with the help of a physiological perspective—the basic needs of the birthing woman and her newborn.

Answers to the Initial Questions

1. Correct: A, B, C
2. Correct: A, B, C
3. Correct: A, B, C, D

References

Ampofo EK, Omotora BA, Otu T, Uchebo G (1990) Risk factors of vesico-vaginal fistulae in Maiduguri, Nigeria: a case control study. Trop Doct 20:138–139
Banks E, Meirik O, Farley T et al (2006) WHO study group on female genital mutilation and obstetric outcome: WHO collaboration prospective study in six african countries. Lancet 367:1835–1841
Children's National Health System (2018) Placental ALLO levels rise during pregnancy and peak as fetuses approach full term. www.sciencedaily.com/releases/2018/05/180505091803.htm
Eaton SB, Shostak M, Konner M (1988) The paleolithic prescription. Harper and Row, New York
Ekbom A et al (2000) Duration of gestation and prostate cancer risk in offspring. Cancer Epidemiol Biomarkers Prev 9(2):221–223
Endevelt-Shapira Y, Shushan S, Roth Y, Sobel N (2014) Disinhibition of olfaction: human olfactory performance improves following low levels of alcohol. Behav Brain Res 272:66–74. https://doi.org/10.1016/j.bbr.2014.06.024. Epub 2014 Jun 25
Everett D (2008) Don't sleep, there are snakes. Profile Books
Hoekzema E et al (2016) Pregnancy leads to long-lasting changes in human brain structure. Nat Neurosci. https://doi.org/10.1038/nn.4458
Horgan J (2003) Rational mysticism: disspatches from the border between science and spirituality. Houghon Mifflin, Boston
Jordan B (1983) Birth in four cultures. Eden Press, Montreal
Kitzinger S, MacCormak CP (1982) The social context of birth: some comparisons between childbirth in Jamaica and Britain. In: MacCormak CP (eds) Ethnography of fertility and birth. Academic Press, New York, pp 181–203
Kivela A (1991) Serum melatonin during human pregnancy. Acta Endocrinol 124(3):233–237
Krehbiel D, Poindron P, Lévy F et al (1987) Peridural anesthesia disturbs maternal behavior in primiparous and multiparous parturient ewes. Physiol Behav 40:463–472
Lozoff B (1983) Birth and 'bonding' in non-industrial societies. Dev Med Child Neurol 25:595–600
Marais EN (1937) The soul of the white ant. Metuen, London
Momoh C, Ladhani S, Lochrie DP, Rymer J (2001) Female genital mutilation: analysis of the first twelve months of a southern London specialist clinic. BJOG 108:186–191
Nakamura Y et al (2001) Changes of serum melatonin level and its relationship to feto-placental unit during pregnancy. J Pineal Res 30(1):29–33
NHS-Statistiken (2022). https://digital.nhs.uk/data-and-information/publications/statistical/nhs-maternity-statistics/2020-21#
Odent M (1987) The fetus ejection reflex. Birth 14:104–105
Odent M (2004a) Making sense of rising caesarean section rates: Die Senkung der Kaiserschnittraten sollte nicht das Hauptziel sein. BMJ 329. https://doi.org/10.1136/bmj.329.7476.1240-b. (Published 18 November 2004) Cite this as: BMJ 2004;329:1240.3
Odent M (2004b) Im Einklang mit der Natur – Neue Ansätze der sanften. Geburt Mabuse/Walter, Düsseldorf
Odent M (2009) Wie steht es um die Zukunft einer durch Kaiserschnitt entbundenen Zivilisation. In: Stark M (eds) der Kaiserschnitt. Urban & Fischer/Elsevier, pp 396–411
Odent M (2019) Die menschliche Geburtsvorbereitung. In: The future of Homo. World Scientific, Hackensack
Schiefenhovel W (1978) Childbirth among the Eipos, New Guinea. Film presented at the Congress of Ethnomedicine. Gottingen
Sharkey JT, Puttaramu R, Word RA, Olcese J (2009) Melatonin synergizes with oxytocin to enhance contractility of human myometrial smooth muscle cells. J Clin Endocrinol Metab 94(2):421–427. https://doi.org/10.1210/jc.2008-1723. Epub 2008 Nov 11
Shostak M (1990) Nisa. Earthscan, London

Wacker J, Zerm C (2020) Über die Bedeutung von FGM bei schwangeren Migrantinnen. Geburth Frauenheilk 80:31–34

Wacker J, Ouedraogo G, Maier K et al (1989) Introduction of a labour chart in a regional hospital in Burkina Faso; effects on caesarean section rate and maternal mortality. Trop Med Parasitol 40:505

Wacker J (2010) Kaiserschnitt vs. Natürliche Geburt. Geburtshilfe Frauenheilkd 70:840−843

Wongtangtintharn S, Oku H, Iwasaki H, Toda T (2004) Effect of branched-chain fatty acids on fatty acid biosymyhesis of human brain cancer cells. J Nutr Science Vitaminol Tokyo 50(2):137–143

Malignant Diseases of Women Worldwide

16

Antje Henke, Jürgen Wacker, Abdoulaye N'Diaye and Eva J. Kantelhardt

Contents

A. Henke (✉)
Global & Planetary Health AG, Institut für Medizinische Epidemiologie, Biometrie und Informatik, Proflizentrum Gesundheitswissenschaften, Medizinische Fakultät der Martin-Luther-Universität Halle-Wittenberg, Halle, Germany
e-mail: Antje.henke@uk-halle.de

J. Wacker
ehemaliger Chefarzt der Frauenklinik Bruchsal, Bruchsal, Germany
e-mail: wacker@menschenfuerfrauen.de

A. N'Diaye
Frauenklinik, Hopital Saint Camille, Ouagadougou, Burkina Faso

E. J. Kantelhardt
Global & Planetary Health AG; Klinik und Poliklinik für Gynäkologie, Medizinische Fakultät der Martin-Luther-Universität Halle-Wittenberg, Universitätsklinikum Halle (Saale), Halle (Saale), Germanye-mail: eva.kantelhardt@uk-halle.de

J. Wacker et al. (eds.), *Global Women's Health*,
https://doi.org/10.1007/978-3-662-69700-9_16

Three questions worth considering will be posed at this point. You will find the answers at the end of this chapter.

Introductory Questions

1. The following diseases are the most common worldwide:
   A. Infectious diseases
   B. HIV, Malaria, and Tuberculosis
   C. Cancer
   D. Inflammatory bowel diseases
2. On which continent is the highest disease-specific mortality for malignant diseases in % of the population found?
   A. Asia
   B. Africa
   C. America
   D. Europe
   E. Australia
3. What is the main reason for the increase in cancer worldwide?
   A. Modern lifestyle
   B. Better diagnostics
   C. Aging population
   D. Increase in smoking

16.1 Introduction

According to the International Agency for Research on Cancer of the World Health Organization (IARC/WHO), cancer is one of the most common causes of death worldwide and claimed more than 10 million victims alone in 2020 (International Agency for Research on Cancer 2021). With a projected growth rate of 64% between 2020 and 2040, cancer will increasingly burden global public health—especially women in countries with limited resources—in the coming years. More people now die from malignant tumors than from infectious diseases (such as HIV, malaria, and tuberculosis) worldwide. The greatest challenge is the introduction and quality assurance of comprehensive and interdisciplinary oncological care that covers all levels of health systems. This can only happen through international cooperation, education, and knowledge transfer.

The IARC collects cancer registry data internationally and tries to make forecasts on this basis. Thus, the IARC determined a number of 19.1 million new cases worldwide for 2020; 10 million were men and 9.22 million were women (International Agency for Research on Cancer 2021).

The IARC is committed to collecting cancer data as accurately as possible worldwide. This can only be achieved in the long term with the support of countries and their governments, which introduce, promote, and ultimately provide data from population-based cancer registries in their respective countries. The data collections of the population-based cancer registries that report to the IARC are checked according to standardized quality criteria in terms of completeness and countability. Especially in low- to middle-income countries (LMICs), high-quality data is lacking, as this requires cancer registries with well-trained documenters who work on the basis of oncology centers with sufficient staff, diagnostic possibilities, and functioning documentation. In many Sub-Saharan African countries, cancer registries are only gradually being introduced; of the 49 countries, 25 have valid registry data from a total of 35 cancer registries. These are connected in the Network of African Cancer Registries (AFCRN, www.afcrn.org) and report their data to the IARC (Ferlay et al. 2018).

The cancers with the most deaths worldwide include lung, colorectal, stomach, liver, and breast cancer. One in five men and one in six women will develop cancer in their lifetime, and in one in eight men and one in eleven women, malignant tumors are the cause of death (Bray et al. 2018). Experts predict a massive increase in malignant diseases due to a growing and aging population, risk factors such as smoking, obesity, lack of exercise, and poor nutrition: By 2040, the incidence is expected to double compared to today. In many countries, despite the possibility of prevention, there is still a high burden of oncogenic infections e.g., by the Human Papillomavirus (HPV), Hepatitis B and C viruses, malaria, and HIV infections (Bray et al. 2018; Morhason-Bello et al. 2013). In women, malignant tumors often occur in the breast (breast carcinomas) and on the cervix (cervical carcinomas). Breast carcinomas are the most commonly diagnosed malignant disease in women (24.2%) and the most common cause of cancer-related death.

> "Every year, more than 2 million women worldwide are diagnosed with breast or cervical cancer, but a woman's place of residence, socioeconomic status, and life circumstances largely determine whether she develops one of these cancers and ultimately survives. There are proven and cost-effective treatment options for these two common cancers, but for so many women, access to them is unattainable. These inequalities highlight the urgent need for sustainable investments in low- and middle-income countries." (Ginsburg et al. 2017).

In Sub-Saharan Africa (SSA), the five-year survival rate for breast cancer is less than 40% compared to over 94% in Europe. Cervical carcinoma ranks fourth in incidence (accounting for 6.6% of all cancers) and mortality (accounting for 7.5%) among cancers in women worldwide (Bray et al. 2018). While the incidence of cervical carcinomas is significantly declining in high-income countries (HIC), it remains the leading cause of cancer deaths in LMICs, accounting for a quarter of all cancer diagnoses. Women-specific cancers are often overlooked in national health policy in these countries (Stefan 2015).

Due to the enormous unequal burden of women-specific cancers worldwide, the World Health Organization (WHO) has declared breast and cervical carcinomas, along with cancers in children, a global health problem. The implementation of WHO cancer strategies is intended to help combat these diseases comprehensively. The three pillars of the "Global Breast Cancer Initiative" launched by the WHO in 2020 are (Anderson et al. 2021):

1. Education and intensified early detection
2. Timely diagnosis
3. Comprehensive disease management and easy access to therapy

The WHO program for the elimination of cervical carcinoma has the following goals: to vaccinate 90% of girls by the age of 15; to screen 70% of women between the ages of 35 and 45 at least once with an adequate method and to adequately treat 90% of women with an invasive or pre-invasive lesion. To implement this, education strategies, HPV vaccination campaigns, and screening programs, strengthening pathology for timely diagnosis and referral for multidisciplinary treatment are proposed. In addition, a multidisciplinary approach is required to combat cancer in general, which must include prevention, access to treatment options, and palliative care. International cooperation is needed to address the substantive, practical, and financial challenges.

16.2 Epidemiology of Malignant Diseases in Women

16.2.1 Epidemiology of Cervical Carcinoma

In contrast to other female-specific cancers such as endometrial and ovarian carcinoma, younger women often also suffer from cervical carcinoma (HPV vaccination guideline 2022). Worldwide, 570,000 new cases of cervical carcinoma are diagnosed annually, and about 311,000 women die from cervical carcinoma (Arbyn et al. 2020). Globally, the highest incidence rates are found in SSA, as well as in South and Central Asia and South America (Bray et al. 2018). The lowest incidence rates are in Western Asia, North America, and Australia/New Zealand (Bray et al. 2018).

The rates of annual new cases vary geographically: They range from 75/100,000 women in Eswatini, followed by 73/100,000 in Malawi (World Cancer Research Fund) to lower rates such as 4/100,000 in Germany or 5/100,000 in Israel (Robert Koch Institute 2017; Fisher et al. 2016). Overall, 84% of new cases and 87 to 90% of deaths occur in LMICs. In Europe in 2018, cervical carcinoma was only in seventh place with 3.8% of newly diagnosed malignant diseases (Say et al. 2014). Women in SSA lose more years of life to cervical carcinoma than to any other type of cancer. Often, it affects them at a stage in life when they are crucial for the social and economic stability of their families (Denny and Anorlu 2012).

The reason for the decline in the incidence rate in HICs is the success story of early detection programs: In many HICs, Papanicolaou smears (Pap smears) were introduced nationwide in the 1960s and 1970s, which detect pre-invasive lesions. After the important role of human papillomaviruses in the development of cervical carcinoma was recognized in the 1990s, Gardasil, the first vaccine against

HPV, was approved in the European Union in 2006 (Smith et al. 2015). Nowadays, HPV-DNA tests enable more efficient prevention programs.

In SSA, access to these prevention measures is often difficult. About 60 to 75% of the affected women live in rural areas; especially for these women, long travel distances, inadequate supply structures, and ignorance about cervical carcinomas pose major obstacles (Denny and Anorlu 2012; Henke et al. 2021). In addition, there are cultural and socio-economic barriers that hinder comprehensive cancer prevention (Denny and Anorlu 2012; Busolo and Woodgate 2015).

In Asia, the largest and most populous continent with its 48 countries, most of which are classified as LMICs, cervical carcinoma is the third most common type of cancer. Central and South America (CSA), with over 600 million inhabitants, also bear a large cancer burden. According to GLOBOCAN 2020 data, there were over 59,000 new cases of invasive cervical carcinoma and over 31,500 deaths annually, making the disease the first or second most common cancer in many countries in the region (The Global Cancer Observatory 2021). Recent forecasts suggest that the number of cases will almost double in the next 15 years if no further measures are taken. These numbers are high compared to Europe, where care has made progress in recent decades, leading to a significant decrease in incidence and significantly better survival, especially in early stages.

16.2.2 Epidemiology of Breast Cancer

The most common cancer worldwide is breast cancer with 2.1 million cases annually. While the care of breast cancer patients in HICs has made massive progress and a five-year survival rate of 94% has been achieved in Europe, there are drastic differences globally.

In almost all LMICs, breast cancer is the most common cancer—albeit with a lower overall population-based age-adjusted frequency than in HICs. Nevertheless, the population-based age-adjusted survival probability, for example in SSA, is only about half as high as in Europe or North America after five years (22.2 versus 13 per 100,000 women in Africa compared to Europe) (Adeloye et al. 2018; Joko-Fru et al. 2020a). Due to unequal access to early detection measures, women often have a higher cancer stage at initial diagnosis and thus significantly worse survival probabilities (Black and Richmond 2019; Kantelhardt et al. 2014).

The improvement in survival rates in high-income countries is attributed to early detection through screening and effective treatment. A report by the IARC has shown that mammography screening in women aged 50 to 69 reduces breast cancer mortality by 25% (Black and Richmond 2019).

Unfortunately, population-based mammography screening programs are not feasible in most LMICs due to the young population structure and are not possible for the older population due to lack of resources and capacities.

The main reasons for the low survival rates for both cervical cancer and breast cancer are difficult access to medical facilities and the associated late presentation with malignant tumors in the hospital; poor nutrition and comorbidities, such as anemia, malaria, and HIV infection; long waiting times for diagnosis and therapy and financial obstacles, which make the completion and even the start of treatment difficult (Morhason-Bello et al. 2013; Joko-Fru et al. 2021). In addition, the number of cancer centers in LMICs is often limited and the care of cancer patients is usually only possible in urban centers, which are sometimes many hours away from the women's place of residence. Little is known about women in rural areas who develop cancer—many also have no access to medical care over a long course of illness (Ayele et al. 2021).

16.2.3 Epidemiology of Other Gynecological Cancers in Women

Ovarian cancer ranks 4th or 5th in new cases in women in LMICs. Prevention or early detection is not possible, surgical and systemic therapy must be carried out at centers (Piszczan et al. 2019). In countries with a higher prevalence of HIV, there is also a slightly larger number of women with vulvar or vaginal cancers compared to countries with lower HIV prevalence. These are often not immediately recognized, but diagnosed in higher stages and thus also show low survival probabilities (Kroeber et al. 2018). In this context, the training of gynecologic oncologists through international cooperation plays a significant role in treating the often young affected women due to the population structure.

16.3 Risk Factors for Malignant Diseases in Women

Cervical carcinoma, and to some extent vulvar carcinoma, is causally linked to the persistence of high-risk HPV (especially type 16 and 18). It most commonly occurs in women between the ages of 40 and 49. Worldwide, the HPV prevalence in women is estimated to be between 2 and 44%, and for Europe between 8 and 15% (Baseman and Koutsky 2005). Other sexually transmitted infections, such as herpes simplex viruses or Chlamydia trachomatis, which can trigger chronic inflammation, promote the occurrence of cervical and vulvar carcinomas (Hawes and Kiviat 2002). In addition, infectious diseases such as HIV, as well as malnutrition, increase the likelihood of developing cervical carcinoma. Certain behaviors such as smoking also increase the risk. Worldwide, women with low socioeconomic status have a higher risk of developing cervical and vulvar carcinoma. They often experience societal disadvantage compared to men, especially in terms of access to health services. In addition, poor hygiene conditions are an important cofactor. Sociocultural factors that increase the risk of HPV infection are particularly prevalent in some SSA countries; these include early marriage and many births. In addition, the risk of contracting HPV doubles in polygamy and changing partnerships. Feelings of shame regarding health care and a dominant decision-making right of the man over health issues in the family can be further factors that hinder cancer prevention.

As risk factors for breast cancer, genetic predisposition, a high density of breast gland tissue, hormonal (postmenopausal women are more frequently affected) and reproductive factors (fewer children, less breastfeeding time) as well as obesity, lack of exercise, smoking and increased alcohol consumption are considered (World Health Organization (WHO) 2020). These risk factors for breast cancer are increasingly common in LMICs due to lifestyle changes and changes in reproductive factors. Thus, an average annual increase in new case rates of up to 8% can be seen in SSA alone (Joko-Fru et al. 2020b).

16.4 Women's Motivations for Cancer Prevention

The factors that motivate women worldwide for cancer prevention are diverse. Ensuring "good" health, fear of the consequences of cervical cancer, and the desire to maintain a good relationship with health personnel are among the main motivations for screening (Bukirwa et al. 2015).

In so-called "shame cultures", the shamefulness of a possible disease, the discomfort with the examination procedure, and the discomfort of exposing the intimate area—in addition to other barriers (access to the health system, health costs, transport routes, ignorance about the disease)—are the most common reasons for not participating in cancer prevention (Busolo and Woodgate 2015; Henke et al. 2021). Another obstacle to cancer prevention is the fear of being diagnosed as HIV-positive, as this is associated with high stigma in many countries. In addition, there is often a lack of encouragement for screening from peers and relatives. Furthermore, women sometimes receive insufficient information from primary care providers about referral procedures and they are afraid during the waiting times between the screening and the receipt of the results (Momberg et al. 2017). Other important limitations mentioned in studies in LMICs include lack of health literacy, disrespectful treatment by health care workers, rejection by the husband, social influence, lack of knowledge about screening, and religious influence. Women's behavior in accessing cancer prevention is highly influenced by knowledge/awareness and attitude. Overall, there is little knowledge about malignant diseases in women and among health care providers, sometimes even across different education levels (Henke et al. 2021).

In addition to the efforts of health professionals, community health workers can play an important role. Community Health Workers (CHWs) are key to mobilizing and educating the community against diseases, as they enjoy trust in the respective population and have extensive experience. In many countries, cancer awareness campaigns are already being conducted (building on experiences e.g. with HIV)—for example, information is disseminated via radio and television and health professionals and CHWs are specifically trained in cancer prevention (Mensah et al. 2020).

▶ In addition to the infrastructural deficiencies at the primary and secondary levels of health systems and the inadequately trained personnel, low awareness of cancer, negative health beliefs, lack of time, and low health literacy (Health Literacy) are mentioned at the individual level as barriers to participating in cancer prevention. Fear of cancer diagnosis, stigmatization, and little knowledge about screening methods are further obstacles to prevention. An HPV test with a self-collection kit can lead to significantly higher acceptance (Gizaw et al. 2019).

16.5 Prevention Strategies and Precautions for Cervical Cancer

The WHO classifies cervical cancer as a global health problem. The WHO guidelines on HPV vaccinations, screening programs, treatment options, and palliative care are intended to help member countries achieve their goals in combating cervical cancer. In HICs, it is recommended to perform cervical cancer screening using a Pap smear or HPV DNA testing. If findings are suspicious, a colposcopy is performed or HPV screening and cytology must be repeated at a later date.

Therefore, visual inspection of the cervix with acetic acid (VIA) and Lugol's solution has proven to be a cost-effective alternative, which is learned and performed by various trained health service providers in training. This can demonstrably reduce the incidence of preinvasive lesions and cervical cancer. In LMICs that have national cancer plans, this method is often recommended as a "see and treat" method and is used by public health services and international aid organizations. With the use of simple resources (such as acetic acid and a cryotherapy device), precancerous lesions can be detected and treated immediately. In addition, local health workers can be trained in VIA screening during these operations. However, the VIA method is highly dependent on the examiner, so the WHO now recommends laboratory-based precision testing of HPV DNA when resources are sufficient. Due to the higher requirements of this method for infrastructure and trained personnel, there is still no nationwide implementation in SSA (Gizaw et al. 2020). In this context, telemedicine, telepathology, and smartphone-enhanced training are becoming increasingly important.

The HPV vaccination has also found its way into national cancer prevention guidelines in some LMICs. To support national vaccination campaigns, the WHO launched HPV vaccination programs for countries in SSA in 2011, which are supported by the public-private Global Alliance for Vaccines and Immunization (GAVI-Alliance) (GAVI. The Vaccine Alliance 2013). According to the WHO, as of March 2017, vaccines for 11-year-old girls had been included in the national vaccination programs in 71 countries (37%), and in 11 countries (6%) also for 11-year-old boys—so more than 200 million doses were administered worldwide!

16.6 Cancer treatment for Women in low to middle Income Countries

The first contact with the health system in LMICs usually takes place at the basic health station (at village/community level). The staff in these facilities have basic medical knowledge. The limited number of large medical facilities, difficult access routes and poor communication between health facilities favor late diagnoses and long waiting times between diagnosis and the start of therapy. An additional challenge in SSA is the belief in traditional medicine. Thus, up to 80% of the population first contact traditional healers before seeking help in the public health system, thereby delaying the time of diagnosis and the start of therapy.

The lack of pathologists is also a major obstacle to ensuring a cancer diagnosis; most African countries have between none and only 4 pathologists per million inhabitants, while this number in Europe and the USA is 50 (Ross 2008; Wilson et al. 2019). The staging is often limited to clinical examination due to the lack of diagnostic imaging.

In many LMICs, there are hardly any opportunities to perform radiation therapy. In almost half of the countries in SSA, there are no radiation therapy facilities. Where such facilities are available, there is usually one device available for several million people (as in Madagascar, Nigeria, Sudan, Kenya, Senegal, Zimbabwe and Cameroon). Adequate surgical options as part of the treatment of breast and cervical cancers are often lacking. Another problem arises as almost all oncological centers are located in cities, and therapy there, especially for the rural population, is often associated with high costs and long travel distances. The current significant lack of oncological-surgical and especially gynecological-oncological trained professionals will increasingly contribute to the bottleneck of care in the future (Griesel et al. 2021).

In LMICs, it can be observed in gynecological-oncological diseases that women often present with advanced stages at initial diagnosis and often only have limited access to comprehensive therapy. The resulting poor survival chances are associated with great suffering for the affected women and their families, as well as significant economic damage to society. The prevention measures established in HICs are only partially transferable to LMICs due to sometimes high material and personnel costs. However, the stringent implementation of adapted and cost-efficient care strategies would already lead to significantly better survival.

Answers to the initial questions:

1. With 19.3 million new cases and 10 million cancer deaths worldwide in 2020, cancer diseases have overtaken infectious diseases. In total, it is estimated for both sexes that half of all cancer cases and 58.3% of cancer deaths in 2020 will occur in Asia, where 59.5% of the world's population live. Europe accounts for 22.8% of all cancer cases and 19.6% of cancer deaths, although it only affects 9.7% of the world's population, followed by North and South America with 20.9% of the incidence and 14.2% of the mortality worldwide (Arbyn et al. 2020).
2. The proportion of cancer deaths in Asia (58.3%) and in Africa (7.2%) is higher compared to Europe, America or Australia, which is due to the different distribution of cancer types and the higher mortality rates in these regions (Arbyn et al. 2020)
3. A, B and C are correct.

References

Adeloye D, Sowunmi OY, Jacobs W, David RA, Adeosun AA, Amuta AO et al (2018) Estimating the incidence of breast cancer in Africa: a systematic review and meta-analysis. J Glob Health 8(1):10419. https://doi.org/10.7189/jogh.08.010419

Anderson BO, Ilbawi AM, Fidarova E, Weiderpass E, Stevens L, Abdel-Wahab M, Mikkelsen B (2021) The Global Breast Cancer Initiative: a strategic collaboration to strengthen health care for non-communicable diseases. Lancet Oncol 22(5):578–581. https://doi.org/10.1016/S1470-2045(21)00071-1

Arbyn M, Weiderpass E, Bruni L, de Sanjosé S, Saraiya M, Ferlay J, Bray F (2020) Estimates of incidence and mortality of cervical cancer in 2018: a worldwide analysis. Lancet Glob Health 8(2):e191–e203. https://doi.org/10.1016/S2214-109X(19)30482-6

Ayele W, Addissie A, Wienke A, Unverzagt S, Jemal A, Taylor L, Kantelhardt EJ (2021) Breast awareness, self-reported abnormalities, and breast cancer in rural Ethiopia: a survey of 7,573 women and predictions of the National Burden. Oncologist 26(6):e1009–e1017. https://doi.org/10.1002/onco.13737

Baseman JG, Koutsky LA (2005) The epidemiology of human papillomavirus infections. J Clin Virol 32(Suppl 1):S16–S24. https://doi.org/10.1016/j.jcv.2004.12.008

Black E, Richmond R (2019) Improving early detection of breast cancer in sub-Saharan Africa: why mammography may not be the way forward. Glob Health 15(1):3. https://doi.org/10.1186/s12992-018-0446-6

Bray F, Ferlay J, Soerjomataram I, Siegel RL, Torre LA, Jemal A (2018) Global Cancer Statistics 2018: GLOBOCAN estimates of incidence and mortality worldwide for 36 cancers in 185 countries. CA Cancer J Clin 68(6):394–424. https://doi.org/10.3322/caac.21492

Bukirwa A, Mutyoba JN, Mukasa BN, Karamagi Y, Odiit M, Kawuma E, Wanyenze RK (2015) Motivations and barriers to cervical cancer screening among HIV infected women in HIV care: a qualitative study. BMC Womens Health 15:82. https://doi.org/10.1186/s12905-015-0243-9

Busolo DS, Woodgate RL (2015) Cancer prevention in Africa: a review of the literature. Glob Health Promot 22(2):31–39. https://doi.org/10.1177/1757975914537094

Denny L, Anorlu R (2012) Cervical cancer in Africa. Cancer Epidemiol Biomarkers Prev 21(9):1434–1438. https://doi.org/10.1158/1055-9965.EPI-12-0334

Ferlay J et al (2018) Cancer today (powered by GLOBOCAN 2018). IARC CancerBase No. 15. http://publications.iarc.fr/577. Zugegriffen: 23. März 2022

Fisher M, Schejter E, Solt I, Renart G (2016) Cervical cancer in Israel 2016: facts, insights and thoughts for the future. Harefuah 155(9):563–566

GAVI. The vaccine alliance (2013) Tanzania, UR. Country Fact Sheet. https://www.gavi.org/programmes-impact/country-hub/africa/tanzania-ur. Zugegriffen: 15. Apr. 2022

Ginsburg O, Bray F, Coleman MP, Vanderpuye V, Eniu A, Kotha SR et al (2017) The global burden of women's cancers: a grand challenge in global health. The Lancet 389(10071):847–860. https://doi.org/10.1016/S0140-6736(16)31392-7

Gizaw M, Teka B, Ruddies F, Abebe T, Kaufmann AM, Worku A et al (2019) Uptake of cervical cancer screening in Ethiopia by self-sampling HPV DNA compared to visual inspection with acetic acid: a cluster randomized trial. Cancer Prev Res (Phila) 12(9):609–616. https://doi.org/10.1158/1940-6207.CAPR-19-0156

Gizaw M, Teka B, Ruddies F, Kassahun K, Worku D, Worku A et al (2020) Reasons for not attending cervical cancer screening and associated factors in rural Ethiopia. Cancer Prev Res (Phila) 13(7):593–600. https://doi.org/10.1158/1940-6207.CAPR-19-0485

Griesel M, Seraphin TP, Mezger NC, Hämmerl L, Feuchtner J, Joko-Fru WY et al (2021) Cervical cancer in sub-Saharan Africa: a multinational population-based cohort study on patterns and guideline adherence of care. Oncologist. https://doi.org/10.1002/onco.13718

Hawes SE, Kiviat NB (2002) Are genital infections and inflammation cofactors in the pathogenesis of invasive cervical cancer? J Natl Cancer Inst 94(21):1592–1593. https://doi.org/10.1093/jnci/94.21.1592

Henke A, Kluge U, Borde T, Mchome B, Serventi F, Henke O (2021) Tanzanian women's knowledge about cervical cancer and HPV and their prevalence of positive VIA cervical screening results. Data from a prevention and awareness campaign in Northern Tanzania, 2017–2019. Glob Health Action 14(1):1852780. https://doi.org/10.1080/16549716.2020.1852780

HPV-Impfleitlinie (2022) Leitlinie zur HPV Impfung. https://www.hpv-impfleitlinie.de/leitlinie_02.html. Zugegriffen: 4. Apr. 2022

International Agency for Research on Cancer (2021) Globocan 202. Cancer Today. https://gco.iarc.fr/today/data/factsheets/populations/900-world-fact-sheets.pdf. Zugegriffen: 18. März 2022

Joko-Fru WY, Miranda-Filho A, Soerjomataram I, Egue M, Akele-Akpo M-T, N'da G et al (2020a) Breast cancer survival in sub-Saharan Africa by age, stage at diagnosis and human development index: A population-based registry study. Int J Cancer 146(5):1208–1218. https://doi.org/10.1002/ijc.32406

Joko-Fru WY, Jedy-Agba E, Korir A, Ogunbiyi O, Dzamalala CP, Chokunonga E et al (2020b) The evolving epidemic of breast cancer in sub-Saharan Africa: results from the African Cancer Registry Network. Int J Cancer 147(8):2131–2141. https://doi.org/10.1002/ijc.33014

Joko-Fru WY, Griesel M, Mezger NCS, Hämmerl L, Seraphin TP, Feuchtner J et al (2021) Breast cancer diagnostics, therapy, and outcomes in sub-Saharan Africa: a population-based registry study. J Natl Compr Canc Netw 1–11. https://doi.org/10.6004/jnccn.2021.7011

Kantelhardt EJ, Zerche P, Mathewos A, Trocchi P, Addissie A, Aynalem A et al (2014) Breast cancer survival in Ethiopia: a cohort study of 1,070 women. Int J Cancer 135(3):702–709. https://doi.org/10.1002/ijc.28691

Kroeber ES, Mathewos A, Wondemagegnehu T, Aynalem A, Gemechu T, Piszczan S et al (2018) Vulvar cancer in Ethiopia: a cohort study on the characteristics and survival of 86 patients. Medicine 97(9):e0041. https://doi.org/10.1097/MD.0000000000010041

Mensah K, Assoumou N, Duchesne V, Pourette D, DeBeaudrap P, Dumont A (2020) Acceptability of HPV screening among HIV-infected women attending an HIV-dedicated clinic in Abidjan, Côte d'Ivoire. BMC Womens Health 20(1):155. https://doi.org/10.1186/s12905-020-01021-6

Momberg M, Botha MH, van der Merwe FH, Moodley J (2017) Women's experiences with cervical cancer screening in a colposcopy referral clinic in Cape Town, South Africa: a qualitative analysis. BMJ Open 7(2):e013914. https://doi.org/10.1136/bmjopen-2016-013914

Morhason-Bello IO, Odedina F, Rebbeck TR, Harford J, Dangou J-M, Denny L, Adewole IF (2013) Challenges and opportunities in cancer control in Africa: a perspective from the African Organisation for Research and Training in cancer. Lancet Oncol 14(4):e142–e151. https://doi.org/10.1016/s1470-2045(12)70482-5
Piszczan S, Desalegn D, Petros H, Gurmu M, Kroeber ES, Addissie A et al (2019) Clinical characteristics and survival of patients with Malignant Ovarian tumors in Addis Ababa, Ethiopia. Oncologist 24(6):e303–e311. https://doi.org/10.1634/theoncologist.2018-0869
Robert Koch Institut (2017) Cervical cancer. Ed. v. Robert Koch Institut. Robert Koch Institut. https://www.krebsdaten.de/Krebs/EN/Content/Cancer_sites/Cervical_cancer/cervical_cancer_node.html. Zugegriffen: 28. März 2022
Ross E (2008) Traditional healing in South Africa: ethical implications for social work. Soc Work Health Care 46(2):15–33. https://doi.org/10.1300/j010v46n02_02
Say L, Chou D, Gemmill A, Tunçalp Ö, Moller A-B, Daniels J et al (2014) Global causes of maternal death: a WHO systematic analysis. Lancet Glob Health 2(6):e323–e333. https://doi.org/10.1016/S2214-109X(14)70227-X
Smith LM, Strumpf EC, Kaufman JS, Lofters A, Schwandt M, Lévesque LE (2015) The early benefits of human papillomavirus vaccination on cervical dysplasia and anogenital warts. Pediatrics 135(5):e1131–e1140. https://doi.org/10.1542/peds.2014-2961
Stefan DC (2015) Cancer care in Africa: an overview of resources. J Glob Oncol 1(1):30–36. https://doi.org/10.1200/JGO.2015.000406
The Global Cancer Observatory (2021) Latin America and the Caribbean, fact sheet. https://gco.iarc.fr/today. Zugegriffen: 4. Apr. 2022
Wilson ML, Atun R, DeStigter K, Flanigan J, Fleming KA, Horton S et al (2019) The Lancet commission on diagnostics: advancing equitable access to diagnostics. The Lancet 393(10185):2018–2020. https://doi.org/10.1016/s0140-6736(19)31052-9
World Health Organization (WHO) (2020) Breast cancer. Factsheet

The Treatment of Breast Cancer in Poor and Rich Countries

17

Maria Eleni Hatzipanagiotou, Abdoulaye N'Diaye, Leonie Ströbele and Jürgen Wacker

Contents

M. E. Hatzipanagiotou (✉)
Departement of Gynecology and Obstetrics, University Medical Centre Regensburg, Regensburg, Germany

A. N'Diaye
Département de gynécologie, Hôpital Saint Camille de Ouagadougou, Centre de Santé Saint Camille, Ouagadougou, Burkina Faso

L. Ströbele
Klinik für Frauenheilkunde und Geburtshilfe, UKGM Standort Gießen, Gießen, Germany

J. Wacker
ehemaliger Chefarzt der Frauenklinik Bruchsal, Bruchsal, Germany
e-mail: wacker@menschenfuerfrauen.de

J. Wacker et al. (eds.), *Global Women's Health*,
https://doi.org/10.1007/978-3-662-69700-9_17

Introductory Questions (multiple answers are possible)

1. Breast cancer is a disease that particularly
   A. can affectyoung women
   B. shows a familial clustering
   C. often occurs in women in postmenopause
   D. is the most common malignancy in women in wealthy countries
2. Breast cancer
   A. is curable in 70% of cases in wealthy countries
   B. is often diagnosed late in poor countries
   C. can be detected early in mammography
   D. can only be treated in breast centers
3. How do the guidelines for the diagnosis and therapy of breast cancer differ in poor and wealthy countries?
   A. Not at all
   B. By the application of the following drugs: Trastuzumab, Pertuzumab and Anthracyclines/Taxanes
   C. By the existing infrastructure in the respective clinics
   D. By the qualification of the existing staff

17.1 Global Epidemiology

Breast cancer is the most common cancer in women worldwide (Gelband et al. 2015). In 2020, 2.3 million women were diagnosed with breast cancer worldwide and there were 685,000 deaths (World Health Organization n.d.-a). However, there are considerable global differences, with a higher incidence in "high-income countries" (HICs, 92 per 100,000 in North America) than in "low- and middle-income countries" (LMICs, 27 per 100,000 in Central Africa and East Asia) (Torre et al. 2016; Ginsburg et al. 2017). The incidence of breast cancer is steadily increasing in almost all countries of the world, while mortality rates in HICs continue to decline (Sung et al. 2021). Particularly in Sub-Saharan Africa (SSA), breast cancer incidences have increased very rapidly in recent decades. Between the mid-1990s and mid-2010s, incidence rates in Malawi (Blantyre), Nigeria (Ibadan), and the Seychelles increased by >5% per year, and in South Africa (Eastern Cape) and Zimbabwe (Harare) by 3 to 4% per year. The age-standardized relative 5-year survival in 12 African countries south of the Sahara was 66% for cases diagnosed between 2008 and 2015, in stark contrast to 85 to 90% for cases diagnosed between 2010 and 2014 in HICs (Gelband et al. 2015).

17.2 Reasons and Risk Factors for the Development of Breast Cancer

Risk factors for the development of breast cancer can be divided into non-modifiable, modifiable, and genetic risk factors. Non-modifiable factors include female sex, age, early menarche, and late menopause (Winters et al. 2017). In HICs, most breast cancers are diagnosed at the age of 60–70 years, while the average age at diagnosis in LMICs is between 40–50 years (Winters et al. 2017). High income and high educational status are associated with better breast cancer-specific survival compared to women with low income and poor education (Winters et al. 2017). Modifiable risk factors include obesity, physical inactivity, and alcohol consumption (Danaei et al. 2005). A young maternal age at the birth of the first child, multiparity, and long breastfeeding periods (>12 months) are protective for the development of breast cancer (Winters et al. 2017; Britt et al. 2007). Approximately 10% of breast cancer cases are genetically determined (Shiovitz and Korde 2015). Pathological mutations in known risk genes lead to a cumulative risk of developing breast cancer by the age of 80 of 72% (BRCA1) and 69% (BRCA2) respectively (Kuchenbaecker et al. 2017). Regarding the genetic changes in women with breast cancer in LMICs, there is a significant lack of data, mainly due to limited molecular biological diagnostic possibilities (Sagna et al. 2019; Biancolella et al. 2021).

17.3 Prevention and Screening

For the reduction of mortality and morbidity from breast cancer, screening and early detection are essential. In Germany, women over 30 years of age should have a clinical breast examination once a year (Albert and Co/Fallenberg and Co n.d.). In addition, mammography screening is recommended for the age group 50–69 years at two-year intervals. It is controversial whether the breast cancer screening methods applicable to HICs can be used with the same effectiveness in LMICs, not least because of economic aspects (Mishra et al. 2021; Mandal and Basu 2018). It should also be considered that with a growing number of screened women, medical follow-up care must be ensured. Moreover, the population in LMICs is often significantly younger, and therefore the use of mammography is questionable, as mammography can produce false findings, especially in young women with consequently denser breast tissue (Panieri 2012). Women with breast cancer in LMICs often present in late stages (Jemal et al. 2011), which significantly limits the prognosis. Reasons for late consultations include low awareness and lack of knowledge about breast cancer, mythical explanations, and mistrust in the health system (Gyedu et al. 2018). Other reasons for late consultations are poor accessibility of health facilities, high costs for diagnosis and therapy, poor knowledge among medical staff, and a lack of health insurance (Akuoko et al. 2017; Kantelhardt et al. 2015; Gadgil et al. 2015). Due to the gradual process of breast cancer, which is usually painless at the beginning, many women wait too long before consulting a health facility. A point of attack conducive to prevention, especially in LMICs, is the creation of awareness ("awareness creation"). This includes the implementation of training programs for health sector workers. The goal is to educate the civilian population about risk factors (see above), recognizing symptoms, and the importance of having symptoms checked in a timely manner. Self-help groups for survivors and cooperation with community groups can play a central role in information dissemination and inform women about symptoms and treatment options for breast cancer (Breast Cancer Initiative 2.5 n.d.-a).

17.4 Stages of Breast Cancer and Histological Classification

Clarity and precision about the extent of cancer are essential for prognosis, therapy, and staging (O'Sullivan et al. 2017). The pTNM status (local-regional tumor spread, local-regional lymph node involvement, distant metastasis) according to the current TNM classification (Brierley et al. 2016) serves this purpose. Based on this, the international classification into UICC stages 0 to IV according to UICC (see Table 17.1) (DKFZ n.d.) is carried out.

Table 17.1 UICC stages Breast cancer

UICC Stage 0	In-situ carcinoma without affected lymph nodes and without metastases (Tis N0 M0)
UICC Stage I A	Maximum 2 cm tumor without lymph node involvement or distant metastases (T1 N0 M0)
UICC Stage I B	No or maximum 2 cm tumor with micrometastases in the lymph nodes, but without distant metastases (T0/T1 N1mi M0)
UICC Stage II A	No or maximum 2 cm tumor with few affected lymph nodes, but without distant metastases (T0/1 N1 M0), or larger, but maximum 5 cm tumor without lymph node involvement or distant metastases (T2 N0 M0)
UICC Stage II B	Larger, but maximum 5 cm tumor with few affected lymph nodes, but without distant metastases (T2 N1 M0), or tumor larger than 5 cm, but without lymph node involvement or distant metastases (T3 N0 M0)
UICC Stage III A	No or maximum 5 cm tumor with medium spread lymph node involvement, but without distant metastases (T0–T2 N2 M0), or tumor larger than 5 cm, with affected lymph nodes, but without distant metastases (T3 N1/N2 M0)
UICC Stage III B	Tumor of any size with extension to chest wall or skin, regardless of lymph node involvement, but without distant metastases (T4 with N0, N1 or N2, M0)
UICC Stage III C	Extensive lymph node involvement regardless of tumor size, but no distant metastases (any T, N3, M0)
UICC Stage IV	Distant metastases present, regardless of tumor size and lymph node involvement (any T, any N, M1)

Table 17.2 The most important molecular subtypes of breast cancer

Luminal A	ER- and/or PgR-positive and HER2-negative and Ki-67 low
Luminal B	HER2-negative: ER- and/or PgR-positive and HER2-negative and Ki-67 high
	HER2-positive: ER- and/or PgR-positive and HER2-positive and Ki-67 high or low
HER2-positive	ER- and PgR-negative and HER2-positive
triple-negative	ER-, PgR- and HER2-negative

The axillary lymph node status is considered the strongest prognostic factor for recurrence-free and overall survival in breast cancer. In newly diagnosed breast cancer from UICC Stage II onwards, staging (lung, liver, skeleton) should be performed (Department of Health n.d.). Here, a tomography of the thorax/abdomen and a bone scintigraphy are performed in HICs.

Pathomorphological assessments are the most important basis for decision-making for surgical, radiation therapy, and especially for systemic therapy of breast cancer (Hammond et al. 2010; Wolff et al. 2013). Breast cancers are differentiated based on an immunohistochemical algorithm, (Cheang et al. 2009; Hugh et al. 2009; Prat et al. 2013), which forms the basis for further therapy (Table 17.2).

17.5 Diagnostic

If a woman shows symptoms and complaints, a clinical examination, imaging techniques such as mammography, ultrasound examination, possibly MRI, and biopsy for diagnosis are recommended (Guidelines Program Oncology n.d.). In case of unclear or suspicious breast findings, an invasive clarification is carried out by means of punch or vacuum biopsy, which capture the pretherapeutic necessary tumor biological factors for therapy planning (tumor type, grading, hormone receptor status, HER2, Ki-67).

The method of choice for the detection of hormone receptors is immunohistochemistry. The testing of the HER2 receptor is technically more complex, but extremely important for therapy planning (Breast Cancer Initiative 2.5 n.d.-b). For histological clarification of suspicious lymph nodes, the punch biopsy should be used.

Situation of Pathology in LMICs: A recently published Lancet series highlighted the state of pathology and laboratory medicine in low-income countries (Horton et al. 2018; Sayed et al. 2018; Wilson et al. 2018). The main problems that affect the quality of pathology can be summarized in lack of equipment, inefficient organization, and insufficiently qualified personnel. The majority of laboratories do not meet the required standards (ISO n.d.). The current number of staff cannot possibly meet the needs of a growing population. Many pathological examinations are often not feasible or exceed financial resources. As a result, certain examinations are shifted abroad by patients who can pay (Ziegenhorn et al. 2020), which can lead to dependencies and can stagnate the development of domestic pathology services.

A "Pathology Package" developed by Fleming et al. could be used by political decision-makers in LMICs to bring structure and quality to local pathology services. The package is divided into four levels, from level 1, related to primary health care, to level 4, which concerns the level of care of university hospitals. Crucial to the "Pathology Package" is that the laboratories of the various levels should work together as an organization. It enables the efficient referral of patients, the joint use and purchase of laboratory material, the exchange of personnel and knowledge, the provision of training and further education, as well as research opportunities. Especially with regard to the provision of an affordable immunohistochemical (IHC) technique, the implementation of the package could pave the way through the support of partner laboratories (Fleming et al. 2017). As another useful tool, the Breast Health Initiative 2.5 has developed a strategy plan for the diagnosis of breast cancer in LMICs, depending on the level of resources (Breast Cancer Initiative 2.5 n.d.-b). The different resource levels are divided into basic, limited, enhanced, and maximal (Table 17.3) (Yip et al. 2008).

Table 17.3 Strategy plan for the diagnosis of breast cancer for LMICs. (Modified after (Breast Cancer Initiative 2.5 n.d.-b))

Resource level	Basic	Limited	Enhanced	Maximal
Clinical	History Physical examination Clinical breast examination Preservation of tissue samples for further diagnostics	Ultrasound-guided fine needle aspiration of sonographically suspicious axillary lymph nodes Sentinel lymph node biopsy	Mammography or ultrasound-guided biopsies SLN biopsy with radiotracer	
Imaging and laboratory tests		Breast ultrasound Chest X-ray, bone scintigraphy Liver ultrasound Complete blood count	Mammography CT Cardiological examination	PET, breast MRI, BRCA 1 and 2 testing Second opinion mammography
Pathology	Diagnosis depending on breast tumor with suitable technique Pathology report Hormone receptor status TNM status	ER hormone receptor status by immunohistochemistry Resection margin, DCIS Lymphovascular invasion LK status	Measurement of HER-2 overexpression or gene amplification PR hormone receptor status by immunohistochemistry	Immunohistochemical staining of LK for cytokeratin to detect micrometastases Second opinion pathology Creating gene profiles

For SSA, the National Cancer Comprehensive Network has developed guidelines for prevention, diagnosis, and therapy (NCCN n.d.). In addition, the WHO Regional Office for Africa (WHO-AFRO) has launched a process to improve laboratory quality on the way to accreditation (Stepwise Laboratory Quality Improvement Process Towards Accreditation, SLIPTA) (Datema et al. 2020). Furthermore, population-based cancer registries, which contain patient, pathology, therapy, and outcome data, can provide indications of improvements in care and survival over time.

17.6 Management of Surgical and Medicinal Therapy of the Primary Disease

17.6.1 Surgical Therapy

After correct breast, axilla, and possibly spread diagnostics, including the histological processing of the preoperatively taken punches, individual therapy planning is carried out. Surgical therapy is one of several steps in the treatment of early breast cancer. Here, the complete removal of the tumor with free resection margins (R0) as a prerequisite for a low local recurrence risk is in the foreground (Oncology Guidelines Program L 2021). Breast-conserving therapy (BCT) with subsequent radiation of the affected breast is equivalent in terms of survival to mastectomy alone (Oncology Guidelines Program L 2021; Fisher et al. 2002). In the case of clinically and sonographically inconspicuous axillary lymph nodes, sentinel lymph node biopsy is performed. Axillary dissection is performed in the case of axillary lymph node involvement, either as primary surgical therapy or after neoadjuvant chemotherapy (Working Group for Gynecological Oncology n.d.).

The type of surgical intervention must be adapted to the available expertise and existing resources. In the most resource-poor environments, modified radical mastectomy including axillary dissection is the standard surgical treatment, as no radiotherapy is available and there are no possibilities for pathological evaluation of the resection margins or marking of sentinel lymph nodes. Even at the basic care level, significant investment in the quality of surgical care is often required. The more resources are available, the more likely BCT, which requires adjuvant radiation of the affected breast, or a sentinel biopsy are considered as possible options (Breast Cancer Initiative 2.5 n.d.-a).

17.6.2 Adjuvant Endocrine Therapy

After determining the steroid hormone receptors on the surgical specimen, adjuvant endocrine therapy with aromatase inhibitors (AI) or tamoxifen or as part of studies with CDK4/6 inhibitors is performed in endocrine-sensitive carcinomas. The standard duration is 5–10 years.

For systemic adjuvant therapy, tamoxifen offers one of the most cost-effective options. The costs for AI can be significantly higher. Tamoxifen is listed by the WHO as an essential drug, was widely available, patent-free, and has an estimated average price of 0.09 USD per tablet. In regions with very low resources, pathological testing is limited to confirming breast cancer. In some areas, health services prescribe tamoxifen for all patients with breast cancer without prior determination of hormone receptors. This should be critically viewed, as women with hormone receptor-negative tumors do not benefit from endocrine therapy and are still exposed to unwanted side effects and costs. In HICs, the percentage of hormone receptor-positive breast cancers is about 60–75%, and that of triple-negative breast cancers is about 15–20% of breast cancer diseases. The rate of triple-negative breast cancers in LMICs is up to 40–55%. This different prevalence underscores the importance of correct pathological diagnosis. CDK4/6 inhibitors are generally not affordable for patients in LMICs. In addition, these drugs require therapy monitoring by specialized professionals with regular consultation, which further complicates the use of these drugs. Health systems and professionals at all resource levels must determine which drugs are suitable for their patient groups and what available resources are available to enable therapies (Breast Cancer Initiative 2.5 n.d.-c).

Backgrounds for Misdirection in Drug Supply
The uninterrupted, sustainable, and unrestricted worldwide availability of essential drugs is, especially in a multi-year cancer therapy like breast cancer, essential for the chances of cure. The fact that this is unfortunately not always the case is shown by the example of Tamoxifen, which since January 2022 can no longer be fully supplied by several manufacturers/distributors. The exact reasons for the supply shortage are not yet fully clarified. Possibly individual stockpiling during the lockdowns of the COVID-19 pandemic is one of the causes. Last but not least, economic reasons also play a major role in drug production, which is highlighted in this section. Tamoxifen is a very cost-effective drug and therefore not profitable for pharmaceutical companies. The fact that profit thinking should be abandoned in the worldwide sustainable drug supply requires a rethink (German Board and College of Obstetrics and Gynecology n.d.).

17.6.3 Chemotherapy and Targeted Anti-HER2 Therapy

In cases of clear indication for chemotherapy, neoadjuvant therapy should be preferred. In HR+/HER2 carcinomas with "high risk", an anthracycline-containing chemotherapy is performed followed by adjuvant endocrine therapy (see above). For triple-negative carcinomas, the addition of carboplatin is recommended due to improved response rates (Schneeweiss et al. 2019). In Her2-positive carcinomas, a sequential anthracycline-based or anthracycline-free chemotherapy is performed with simultaneous administration of targeted anti-HER2 therapy (Piccart et al. 2021; Schneeweiss et al. 2013). The introduction of the monoclonal anti-HER2 antibody Trastuzumab was one of the most important steps in breast cancer therapy in recent years, yet this drug is not available in most resource-poor environments. Since targeted substances are very expensive, the introduction of biosimilars is the only way to make these substances widely available in LMICs. If a targeted anti-HER2 therapy is available in a region, the infrastructure for testing the HER2 receptor must also be available. In LMICs, where advanced disease is often present at the time of initial diagnosis of breast cancer and the rate of hormone receptor-negative breast cancers is high, the benefit of chemotherapy can be significant. If chemotherapy is started—in rural areas sometimes also made possible by financial support from an entire village—the dropout rates before completion of therapy are high. Studies in LMICs can lead to the establishment of evidence-based medicine in these environments using and optimizing existing resources (Breast Cancer Initiative 2.5 n.d.-d).

Seven chemotherapy substances (carboplatin, cyclophosphamide, doxorubicin, docetaxel, fluorouracil, methotrexate, paclitaxel), which are used for the treatment of breast cancer, are included in the WHO list of essential medicines of 2021 (World Health Organization n.d.-b).

The safe and effective application of cytostatics should be carried out by specially trained personnel. However, in LMICs, the application is often carried out by general practitioners, surgeons, or radiation therapists, so specialized oncological training for non-oncological personnel should take place and protocols and standardized procedures adapted to the respective environment should be established.

17.6.4 Radiotherapy

After BCT adjuvant radiation of the affected breast is obligatory (Haviland et al. 2013). After mastectomy, radiation of the chest wall should be performed in cases of >3 affected lymph nodes, in T3/T4 tumors, and in young patients with a high risk of recurrence. Radiation of the axilla should be performed in cases of clear clinical involvement or positive sentinel status and incomplete or non-performed axillary dissection (Working Group for Gynecological Oncology n.d.).

In LMICs, due to the often already locally advanced breast cancer diseases, the proportion of women who would benefit from radiotherapy is particularly large, but the gap between demand and available supply is growing. The estimated deficit is 7000 radiotherapy devices worldwide. In 29 out of 52 African countries, there is no radiation unit. 85% of the world's population live in LMICs, but less than 35% of the world's radiotherapy facilities are located in these countries. Even in resource-poor environments, it should be a political goal to offer radiotherapy in a cost-effective manner and make it accessible to patients. In addition, trained personnel and sufficient equipment (e.g., simulator, planning computer system, tools for dosimetry) are prerequisites for implementation. The high investment costs can be minimized through modern financing approaches and joint efforts with international institutions, partnerships with NGOs, and public-private organizations to enable treatment for breast cancer patients.

Findings from the Lancet Oncology Commission have shown that investment in radiotherapy not only enables the treatment of a large number of cancer patients but also reduces mortality and brings positive economic benefits (Breast Cancer Initiative 2.5 n.d.-e).

17.7 Recurrence and Metastasized Breast Cancer

When diagnosing a locoregional recurrence, correct staging (tomography of the thorax/abdomen, bone scintigraphy) must be performed, as distant metastases can be detected in about 20% of these cases.

If it is an intramammary recurrence after breast-conserving therapy, mastectomy is performed. In the case of a chest wall recurrence without distant metastases, tumor excision is performed. The goal of surgical therapy is R0 resection. Systemic therapy is carried out analogously to the primary disease depending on the present histological subtype and taking into account previous therapies.

If metastasis is detected in the imaging, it is a palliative situation. The therapy goals now primarily include improving quality of life through symptom control, extending progression-free survival, and increasingly overall survival. Systemic therapy approaches are in the foreground, the planning of therapy should take place after histological evaluation of a metastasis. Metastasis mainly occurs in the lungs, liver, bones, and lymph nodes.

In HICs, due to the multitude of available substances, long-term courses are to be expected in most patients even in the situation of incurable disease. In the case of osseous metastases, osteoprotective therapy is carried out in addition to tumor-specific therapy to reduce skeletal complications and bone pain (Working Group for Gynecological Oncology n.d.). CDK4/6 inhibitors are now standard in HICs in the first-line treatment of metastatic hormone receptor-positive breast cancer (Gao et al. 2020). In the case of Her2-neu-positive breast cancer, various targeted substances, such as Trastuzumab or Pertuzumab, are used in the metastatic situation. In the case of triple-negative breast cancer, checkpoint inhibitors have now found their way into first-line therapy in addition to the classic chemotherapies. Research is also continuously being carried out on new substances, such as Sacituzumab Govitecan, which are used in HICs. For this therapy, for example, annual therapy costs of approximately 260,000 EUR or 310,000 USD are incurred. This corresponds to around 7650 € per dose (DGHO German Society for Hematology and Medical Oncology e. V. 2021/2022). These costs are mentioned here as an example, the therapy costs for other newer drugs are at a comparable level (Information from the Drug Commission of the German Medical Association n.d.), with the benefit of extending survival by usually a few months. In contrast, the availability of tumor-specific substances in LMICs is significantly limited. Available drugs in LMICs are mainly endocrine therapies with Tamoxifen and Aromatase inhibitors, as well as Fulvestrant, even in the case of metastases. Trastuzumab has been available as a biosimilar since 2018, but the excellent prognosis improvement through targeted anti-HER2 therapies is largely limited to HICs. In LMICs, only a few patients benefit from the great advances that have been made in the areas of metastatic breast cancer in recent years. In addition to tumor-specific therapy, symptom relief, psychosocial support, spiritual aspects, and adequate pain therapy play an important role. At least access to pain medication and the management of psychosocial suffering should be considered a priority in any health system for ethical reasons. These areas should also be realized in regions with very low resources, involving the family and the village community.

17.8 Treatment of Breast Cancer in West Africa (Using Burkina Faso as an Example)

In Burkina Faso, there is no established guideline for breast cancer, but there is a strategic plan for the fight against cancer in general. Initiatives and plans exist from associations for the fight against breast cancer, which are led by medical oncologists. According to the WHO in 2016, breast cancer accounts for 12.3% of the most common types of cancer in Burkina Faso and is second only to cervical cancer. According to a recent study in Burkina Faso, Leonie Stroebele et al. (2018) observed an increase in breast cancer (Stroebele et al. 2018). 60% of the budget for medical expenses is needed for cancer diseases.

The prevention in the country is mainly based on raising awareness to reduce or eliminate risk factors and communication for social behavior change, especially for self-examination of the breasts. In Burkina Faso, mammography screening is recommended every 2 years from the age of 40. If abnormalities are found, a biopsy should be taken. The findings are available within 2 to 3 weeks.

Political objectives are the promotion of breast cancer prevention through:

- Educational measures with the community for self-examination of the breasts
- Systematic screening for breast tumors in health services
- Improvement of access to mammography from the age of 40
- Early treatment of breast tumors
- Management of breast cancer through surgery, chemotherapy, and radiation therapy

The differences in the treatment of breast cancer between the major cities and the provinces in the country are glaring:

- Oncologists and surgical gynecologic oncologists are only available in the two major cities of Ouagadougou and Bobo Dioulasso.
- Although many regional hospitals have mammography units for screening and diagnosis, most are out of operation due to staff shortages. The same applies to histological examination possibilities. Even in the two largest cities, the corresponding equipment is only available in the high-demand major clinics and hospitals. Many specialists work in private clinics rather than public hospitals due to better earning opportunities.

- The country's only radiation therapy center is located in Ouagadougou (since 2021).
- The average cost of breast cancer treatment is between 2 and 3 million CFA francs (approx. 3330 to 5000 USD). In 2020, the gross domestic product per capita in Burkina Faso was around 831 USD (Gross Domestic Product (GDP) 2026).
- There are often difficulties in accessing cytostatics.
- General health insurance is still in its infancy, most patients are not insured and have to fully cover the cost of care.

All these elements contribute to the delay in the diagnosis and treatment of breast cancer in Burkina Faso and result in most breast cancer cases in the country being discovered late. However, intensified awareness and education are showing a slow trend towards earlier diagnosis. Only since the beginning of 2021 have the three essential pillars for the treatment of breast cancer in terms of surgery, chemotherapy, and radiation therapy been available in Burkina Faso, at least theoretically allowing a curative treatment approach.

17.9 Outlook

Currently, the goals for the diagnosis and therapy of breast cancer are very different globally. This is due to the subjective therapy wish of each woman, which can be met in HICs through very expensive drugs. In contrast, the objective global inequality and unequal distribution of resources, which leads to the significant differences in breast cancer-specific survival. It remains open which goals should be set globally for breast cancer to achieve global justice.

Answers to the Initial Questions

1. All are correct
2. A, B and C are correct
3. C and D are correct

References

Akuoko CP, Armah E, Sarpong T et al (2017) Barriers to early presentation and diagnosis of breast cancer among African women living in sub-Saharan Africa. PloS One 12:e0171024. https://doi.org/10.1371/journal.pone.0171024

Albert und Co/Fallenberg und Co (o. J.) Diagnostik und Therapie früher und fortgeschrittener Mammakarzinome. Früherkennung und Diagnostik. https://www.ago-online.de/fileadmin/ago-online/downloads/_leitlinien/kommission_mamma/2021/Einzeldateien/2021D_03_Frueherkennung_und_Diagnostik_MASTER_final_20210302.pdf. Zugegriffen: 25. Jan. 2022

Arbeitsgemeinschaft für Gynäkologische Onkologie (o. J.) Empfehlungen gynäkologische Onkologie Kommission Mamma. https://www.ago-online.de/leitlinien-empfehlungen/leitlinien-empfehlungen/kommission-mamma. Zugegriffen: 25. Jan. 2022

Biancolella M, Ouédraogo NLM, Zongo N et al (2021) Breast cancer in West Africa. Molecular analysis of BRCA genes in early-onset breast cancer patients in Burkina Faso. Hum Genomics 15:65. https://doi.org/10.1186/s40246-021-00365-w

Breast Cancer Initiative 2.5 (o. J.-a) Treatment: locoregional therapy: Surgery for breast cancer. https://www.fredhutch.org/content/dam/www/research/divisions/public-health-sciences/epidemiology/bci-25/KSPDF/KS%20Treatment%20Surgery%20030617.pdf. Zugegriffen: 7. Febr. 2022

Breast Cancer Initiative 2.5 (o. J.-b) Diagnosis. Biopsy, pathology and subtypes. https://www.fredhutch.org/content/dam/www/research/divisions/public-health-sciences/epidemiology/bci-25/KSPDF/KS%20Diagnosis%20Biopsy%20030617.pdf. Zugegriffen: 7. Febr. 2022

Breast Cancer Initiative 2.5 (o. J.-c) Systemic therapy: hormonal therapy and targeted agents. https://www.fredhutch.org/content/dam/www/research/divisions/public-health-sciences/epidemiology/bci-25/KSPDF/KS%20Treatment%20Hormonal%20030617.pdf. Zugegriffen: 7. Febr. 2022

Breast Cancer Initiative 2.5 (o. J.-d) Systemic therapy: chemotherapy for breast cancer. https://www.fredhutch.org/content/dam/www/research/divisions/public-health-sciences/epidemiology/bci-25/KSPDF/KS%20Treatment%20Chemo%20030617.pdf. Zugegriffen: 7. Febr. 2022

Breast Cancer Initiative 2.5 (o. J.-e) Locoregional therapy: radiation therapy for breast cancer. https://www.fredhutch.org/content/dam/www/research/divisions/public-health-sciences/epidemiology/bci-25/KSPDF/KS%20Treatment%20Radiation%20030617.pdf. Zugegriffen: 7. Febr. 2022

Brierley J, Gospodarowicz MK, Wittekind CH (2016) TNM classification of malignant tumours, 8. ed. Wiley, Chichester/West Sussex

Britt K, Ashworth A, Smalley M (2007) Pregnancy and the risk of breast cancer. Endocr Relat Cancer 14:907–933. https://doi.org/10.1677/ERC-07-0137

Bruttoinlandsprodukt (BIP) pro Kopf in Burkina Faso bis 2026. https://de.statista.com/statistik/daten/studie/399057/umfrage/bruttoinlandsprodukt-bip-pro-kopf-in-burkina-faso/. Zugegriffen: 25. Jan. 2022

Cheang MCU, Chia SK, Voduc D et al (2009) Ki67 index, HER2 status, and prognosis of patients with luminal B breast cancer. J Natl Cancer Inst 101:736–750. https://doi.org/10.1093/jnci/djp082

Danaei G, Vander Hoorn S, Lopez AD et al (2005) Causes of cancer in the world. Comparative risk assessment of nine behavioural and environmental risk factors. Lancet 366:1784–1793. https://doi.org/10.1016/S0140-6736(05)67725-2

Datema TAM, Oskam L, Broerse JEW et al (2020) Review of the stepwise laboratory quality improvement process towards accreditation (SLIPTA) version 2:2015. Afr J Lab Med 9:1068. https://doi.org/10.4102/ajlm.v9i1.1068

Department of Health (o. J.) Diagnosis, staging and treatment of patients with breast cancer. Diagnosis, staging and treatment of patients with breast cancer. National Clinical Guideline No. 7; Stand: 14.02.2022

DGHO Deutsche Gesellschaft für Hämatologie und Medizinische Onkologie e. V. NUB Antrag 2021/2022 Sacituzumab Govitecan. https://www.dgho.de/arbeitskreise/a-g/drg-gesundheitsoekonomie/nub-2022/22-124-sacituzumab-govitecan-nub-anfrage-dgho-stand-2021-09-30-final.pdf. Zugegriffen: 7. März 2022

DKFZ (o. J.) Brustkrebs: Klassifikation und Stadieneinteilung. Einteilung nach UICC: In welchem Stadium befindet sich der Brustkrebs? https://www.krebsinformationsdienst.de/tumorarten/brustkrebs/stadieneinteilung.php. Zugegriffen: 14. Febr. 2022

Fisher B, Anderson S, Bryant J et al (2002) Twenty-year follow-up of a randomized trial comparing total mastectomy, lumpectomy, and lumpectomy plus irradiation for the treatment of invasive breast cancer. N Engl J Med 347:1233–1241. https://doi.org/10.1056/NEJMoa022152

Fleming KA, Naidoo M, Wilson M et al (2017) An essential pathology package for low- and middle-income countries. Am J Clin Pathol 147:15–32. https://doi.org/10.1093/AJCP/AQW143

Gadgil A, Sauvaget C, Roy N et al (2015) Breast cancer awareness among middle class urban women – a community-based study from Mumbai, India. Asian Pac J Cancer Prev 16:6249–6254. https://doi.org/10.7314/apjcp.2015.16.15.6249

Gao JJ, Cheng J, Bloomquist E et al (2020) CDK4/6 inhibitor treatment for patients with hormone receptor-positive, HER2-negative, advanced or metastatic breast cancer. A US food and drug administration pooled analysis. Lancet Oncol 21:250–260. https://doi.org/10.1016/S1470-2045(19)30804-6

Gelband H, Jha P, Sankaranarayanan R, Horton S (Hrsg) (2015) Cancer. Disease control priorities, vol 3, 3. ed. Washington, DC. https://doi.org/10.1596/978-1-4648-0349-9

German Board and College of Obstetrics and Gynecology (o. J.) Verknappung des Brustkrebsmedikaments Tamoxifen. https://www.dggg.de/fileadmin/data/Stellungnahmen/DGGG/2022/Empfehlungen_zum_Lieferengpass_Tamoxifen_09.02.2022_01.pdf. Zugegriffen: 9. März 2022

Ginsburg O, Bray F, Coleman MP et al (2017) The global burden of women's cancers. A grand challenge in global health. Lancet 389:847–860. https://doi.org/10.1016/S0140-6736(16)31392-7

Gyedu A, Gaskill CE, Boakye G et al (2018) Differences in perception of breast cancer among Muslim and Christian women in Ghana. J Glob Oncol 4:1–9. https://doi.org/10.1200/JGO.2017.009910

Hammond MEH, Hayes DF, Dowsett M et al (2010) American Society of Clinical Oncology/College Of American Pathologists guideline recommendations for immunohistochemical testing of estrogen and progesterone receptors in breast cancer. J Clin Oncol 28:2784–2795. https://doi.org/10.1200/JCO.2009.25.6529

Haviland JS, Owen JR, Dewar JA et al (2013) The UK standardisation of breast radiotherapy (START) trials of radiotherapy hypofractionation for treatment of early breast cancer. 10-year follow-up results of two randomised controlled trials. Lancet Oncol 14:1086–1094. https://doi.org/10.1016/S1470-2045(13)70386-3

Horton S, Sullivan R, Flanigan J et al (2018) Delivering modern, high-quality, affordable pathology and laboratory medicine to low-income and middle-income countries. A call to action. Lancet 391:1953–1964. https://doi.org/10.1016/S0140-6736(18)30460-4

Hugh J, Hanson J, Cheang MCU et al (2009) Breast cancer subtypes and response to docetaxel in node-positive breast cancer. Use of an immunohistochemical definition in the BCIRG 001 trial. J Clin Oncol 27:1168–1176. https://doi.org/10.1200/JCO.2008.18.1024

Information der Arzneimittelkommission der deutschen Ärzteschaft (o. J.) Keytruda® (Pembrolizumab). https://www.akdae.de/Arzneimitteltherapie/NA/Archiv-SN/201505-Keytruda.pdf. Zugegriffen: 15. Apr. 2022

ISO (o. J.) International Organization for Standardization. Medical laboratories – Requirements for quality and competence. https://www.iso.org/obp/ui/#iso:std:iso:15189:ed-3:v2:en. Zugegriffen: 6. Febr. 2022

Jemal A, Bray F, Center MM et al (2011) Global cancer statistics. CA Cancer J Clin 61:69–90. https://doi.org/10.3322/caac.20107

Kantelhardt EJ, Muluken G, Sefonias G et al (2015) A review on breast cancer care in Africa. Breast Care (Basel) 10:364–370. https://doi.org/10.1159/000443156

Kuchenbaecker KB, Hopper JL, Barnes DR et al (2017) Risks of breast, ovarian, and contralateral breast cancer for BRCA1 and BRCA2 mutation carriers. JAMA 317:2402–2416. https://doi.org/10.1001/jama.2017.7112

Leitlinienprogramm Onkologie (o. J.) S3-Leitlinie Früherkennung, Diagnose, Therapie und Nachsorge des Mammakarzinoms. https://www.awmf.org/uploads/tx_szleitlinien/032-045OLl_S3_Mammakarzinom_2021-07.pdf. Zugegriffen: 13. Febr. 2022

Leitlinienprogramm Onkologie L Hrsg (2021) Interdisziplinäre S3-Leitlinie für die Diagnostik, Therapie und Nachsorge des Mammakarzinoms. Langversion 4.4 – Juni 2021 AWMF-Registernummer: 032-045OL

Mandal R, Basu P (2018) Krebsvorsorge und Früherkennung in Ländern mit niedrigem und mittlerem Einkommen. Aktuelles Szenario und Zukunftsperspektiven. Bundesgesundheitsblatt Gesundheitsforschung Gesundheitsschutz 61:1505–1512. https://doi.org/10.1007/s00103-018-2833-9

Mishra GA, Pimple SA, Mittra I et al (2021) Screening for breast cancer. Cost-effective solutions for low- & middle-income countries. Indian J Med Res. https://doi.org/10.4103/ijmr.IJMR_2635_20

NCCN (o. J.) NCCN harmonized guidelines™ for sub-Saharan Africa. Guidelines for treatment of cancer by type. https://www.nccn.org/global/what-we-do/harmonized-guidelines. Zugegriffen: 7. Febr. 2022

O'Sullivan B, Brierley J, Byrd D et al (2017) The TNM classification of malignant tumours—towards common understanding and reasonable expectations. Lancet Oncol 18:849–851. https://doi.org/10.1016/S1470-2045(17)30438-2

Panieri E (2012) Breast cancer screening in developing countries. Best Pract Res Clin Obstet Gynaecol 26:283–290. https://doi.org/10.1016/j.bpobgyn.2011.11.007

Piccart M, Procter M, Fumagalli D et al (2021) Adjuvant pertuzumab and trastuzumab in early HER2-positive breast cancer in the APHINITY trial. 6 years' follow-up. J Clin Oncol 39:1448–1457. https://doi.org/10.1200/JCO.20.01204

Prat A, Cheang MCU, Martín M et al (2013) Prognostic significance of progesterone receptor-positive tumor cells within immunohistochemically defined luminal A breast cancer. J Clin Oncol 31:203–209. https://doi.org/10.1200/JCO.2012.43.4134

Sagna T, Bonora E, Ouedraogo MNL et al (2019) Identification of BRCA1/2 p.Ser1613Gly, p.Pro871Leu, p.Lys1183Arg, p.Glu1038Gly, p.Ser1140Gly, p.Ala2466Val, p.His2440Arg variants in women under 45 years old with breast nodules suspected of having breast cancer in Burkina Faso. Biomol Concepts 10:120–127. https://doi.org/10.1515/bmc-2019-0015

Sayed S, Cherniak W, Lawler M et al (2018) Improving pathology and laboratory medicine in low-income and middle-income countries. Roadmap to solutions. Lancet 391:1939–1952. https://doi.org/10.1016/S0140-6736(18)30459-8

Schneeweiss A, Chia S, Hickish T et al (2013) Pertuzumab plus trastuzumab in combination with standard neoadjuvant anthracycline-containing and anthracycline-free chemotherapy regimens in patients with HER2-positive early breast cancer. A randomized phase II cardiac safety study (TRYPHAENA). Ann Oncol 24:2278–2284. https://doi.org/10.1093/annonc/mdt182

Schneeweiss A, Denkert C, Fasching PA et al (2019) Diagnosis and therapy of triple-negative breast cancer (TNBC) – Recommendations for daily routine practice. Geburtshilfe Frauenheilkd 79:605–617. https://doi.org/10.1055/a-0887-0285

Shiovitz S, Korde LA (2015) Genetics of breast cancer. A topic in evolution. Ann Oncol 26:1291–1299. https://doi.org/10.1093/annonc/mdv022

Stroebele L, Kantelhardt EJ, Francoise MT, Sarigda M, Wacker J, Grosse-Frie K (2018) Prevalence of breast-related symptoms, health care seeking behaviour and diagnostic needs among women in Burkina Faso. BMC Public Health 18:447

Sung H, Ferlay J, Siegel RL et al (2021) Global Cancer Statistics 2020. GLOBOCAN estimates of incidence and mortality worldwide for 36 cancers in 185 countries. CA Cancer J Clin 71:209–249. https://doi.org/10.3322/caac.21660

Torre LA, Siegel RL, Ward EM et al (2016) Global cancer incidence and mortality rates and trends – an Update. Cancer Epidemiol Biomarkers Prev 25:16–27. https://doi.org/10.1158/1055-9965.EPI-15-0578

Wilson ML, Fleming KA, Kuti MA et al (2018) Access to pathology and laboratory medicine services. A crucial gap. Lancet 391:1927–1938. https://doi.org/10.1016/S0140-6736(18)30458-6

Winters S, Martin C, Murphy D et al (2017) Breast cancer epidemiology, prevention, and screening. Prog Mol Biol Transl Sci 151:1–32. https://doi.org/10.1016/bs.pmbts.2017.07.002

Wolff AC, Hammond MEH, Hicks DG et al (2013) Recommendations for human epidermal growth factor receptor 2 testing in breast cancer. American Society of Clinical Oncology/College of American Pathologists clinical practice guideline update. J Clin Oncol 31:3997–4013. https://doi.org/10.1200/JCO.2013.50.9984

World Health Organization (o. J.-a) Fact sheet breast cancer https://www.who.int/news-room/fact-sheets/detail/breast-cancer. Zugegriffen: 8. Febr. 2022

World Health Organization (o. J.-b) WHO model lists of essential medicines. https://list.essentialmeds.org/?indication=79. Zugegriffen: 15. Febr. 2022

Yip C-H, Smith RA, Anderson BO et al (2008) Guideline implementation for breast healthcare in low- and middle-income countries. Early detection resource allocation. Cancer 113:2244–2256. https://doi.org/10.1002/cncr.23842

Ziegenhorn H-V, Frie KG, Ekanem I-O et al (2020) Breast cancer pathology services in sub-Saharan Africa. A survey within population-based cancer registries. BMC Health Serv Res 20:912. https://doi.org/10.1186/s12913-020-05752-y

The Role of Palliative Medicine in Poor and Rich Countries

18

Jürgen Wacker

Contents

Stein Husebo and Gebhard Mathis quote Ludwig Wittgenstein in the Ethics chapter of their standard work on palliative medicine as follows (Husebo and Mathis 2017):

> "The most important aspects of things for us are hidden by their simplicity and everydayness—one cannot notice it because one always has it in front of one's eyes. The actual foundations of his research do not even occur to man."

Like all human action, the work of the doctor is also subject to ethical evaluations. Every person, every doctor must deal with the following questions:

J. Wacker (✉)
ehemaliger Chefarzt der Frauenklinik Bruchsal, Bruchsal, Germany
e-mail: wacker@menschenfuerfrauen.de

J. Wacker et al. (eds.), *Global Women's Health*,
https://doi.org/10.1007/978-3-662-69700-9_18

Introductory questions

1. When does life begin? Is there life before birth?
2. When may we end a therapy? Are we allowed to disappoint the hopes of the patients?
3. Is palliative help to live with the disease an alternative to any form of euthanasia?
4. Must life-threatening complications always be treated?
5. What does the ethical principle of Albert Schweitzer mean for modern, global medicine: "**I am life that wants to live, in the midst of life that wants to live!**"

18.1 Case study from Burkina Faso

From **Burkina Faso I know the fate of a mother of two children, about 40 years old,** whom we call Aissatou Yameogo, but who had a different name. She was a diligent and universally popular clinic employee who one day, in the early 1990s, complained of increasing fatigue and exhaustion, which was unusual for her, a life-affirming and always active woman. When fever, cough, and an ever-increasing weight loss occurred, Aissatou consulted a doctor in a larger hospital in Burkina Faso, who diagnosed pneumonia. Aissatou noticed a swelling of the lymph nodes and several warts and nodules in the thigh area. After another blood test, the doctor made the **diagnosis AIDS** and recommended the drugs Abacavir and Lamivudine, which the patient could not afford at that time. Since the pneumonia was a severe form of pneumonia, a Pneumocystis jiroveci pneumonia (PcP), Aissatou needed Pentamidine, another expensive drug, as the previously used drugs Cotrimoxazole and Prednisolone were not enough!

Aissatou was moved to the "isolation ward", the AIDS ward of a large hospital in the capital Ouagadougou. After a brief improvement, high fever occurred again, and the coughing fits made Aissatou's weakened body tremble. In the presence of a friendly colleague and her two children, Aissatou died from the effects of AIDS and the subsequent pneumonia (Wacker 2011).

18.1.1 Reflections from the Case Study

Regarding HIV/AIDS, reference is made here to the detailed description by Camilla Rothe in Chap. 10 (Pandemics) of this book. We must acknowledge that to date, 36 million people have died from the effects of HIV/AIDS. Both women and men are affected by this disease.

It is known that HIV-positive and AIDS patients, like Aissatou in our case study, are threatened by a variety of bacterial, parasitic, viral, mycobacterial, and mycotic pathogens, as well as various tumor diseases. The pathogen of the present pneumonia, Pneumocyatis jiroveci, is ubiquitously distributed. With few exceptions, only immunosuppressed patients suffer from this form of pneumonia. The **symptom triad** of Pneumocystis jiroveci pneumonia consists of: **fever**, non-productive cough, and progressive exertional dyspnea. Like most patients, Aissatou also reported increasing fatigue and lack of physical resilience before this triad developed. Obviously, at the time of diagnosis, it was already an advanced finding, as the typical interstitial infiltrates had spread throughout the lung. In the present case, treatment was started with a high dose of trimethoprim/sulfamethoxazole (20 mg trimethoprim/kg body weight/day). Since this therapy did not improve the condition, treatment was continued with intravenous pentamidine (4 mg/kg body weight/day). During the further course of the hospital stay, the patient died from the consequences of the underlying disease AIDS. However, it was not entirely clear in retrospect whether side effects of the intravenous pentamidine treatment, such as hypoglycemia, renal insufficiency, or arrhythmia, may have contributed to the patient's agonizing death.

As already noted above, Aissatou noticed a swelling of the lymph nodes and several warts and nodules in the thigh area. Histologically, the presence of a **Kaposi's sarcoma was confirmed!** Kaposi's sarcoma is, next to non-Hodgkin's lymphomas, the most common malignant neoplasm in HIV-infected individuals. According to Jan van Lunzen, Kaposi's sarcoma as a social stigma not only represents a significant emotional burden for patients. Large, confluent tumor masses with subsequent lymphedema, but also gastrointestinal or pulmonary involvement can pose major physical problems for patients. Although Kaposi's sarcoma can occur at any stage of HIV infection, unlike many other AIDS-defining diseases, according to van Lunzen and Albrecht, the immune defect in affected patients is usually pronounced. Predilection sites of Kaposi's sarcoma are the entire skin surface with emphasis on the lower extremities and the orogenital mucous membranes, but also the lungs, gastrointestinal tract, and, much less frequently, the CNS. Basically, any organ can be affected. Initially, cutaneous Kaposi's sarcoma lesions appear as small, reddish-brown or livid, often elliptical spots. These lie parallel to the skin's cleavage lines and can gradually, but also in bursts, increase in size and color intensity. Aissatou died before the nodules of Kaposi's sarcoma could disfigure her body and face. She remained in the memory of her children and friends as the pretty friend and kind mother she had always been at heart.

As a development aid worker in the Sahel of Burkina Faso, I was repeatedly impressed by the relatives' concern for the well-being of their sick family members. This concern was evident in the patient waiting outside the door leading to the operating room, in the joyful anticipation of the newly delivered mother in the maternity ward, and in the caring concern for the soon-to-be-dying family member. I didn't need to give these faithful and caring families any instructions, they seemed to do everything available to them as a matter of course. They massaged the legs of the "freshly operated" as if they wanted to perform a practical thrombosis prophylaxis, they held the patients' hands as if they wanted to treat themselves, and they fanned the dying with palm fans to facilitate their breathing. In the simple building of our isolation ward in CHR Dori, I experienced impressive "Traditional Palliative Medicine" at the highest human level, I could only watch, admire, and learn!

Even when I myself was a patient with an attack of malaria tropica in Dori, unable to get up from exhaustion and high fever, increasingly overwhelmed by the feeling of having to die soon, I came to enjoy this traditional African palliative medicine in addition to the injection of Quinimax (quinine). I was treated, touched, and my hot forehead was moistened with precious, cold water. "Is death this gentle?", I wondered.

18.2 Development of the Hospice Movement and Palliative Medicine

Cicely Saunders and Elisabeth Kübler-Ross are considered the founders of the modern hospice movement and palliative medicine!

In her insightful article "A Life Journey in the Field of Therapy," Cicely Saunders vividly describes the development of modern, drug therapy. "When I worked as a ward nurse at St. Thomas's Hospital in 1941, we had a very limited selection of drugs at the time, which eventually included sulfonamides, but no other antibiotics and only a few other agents (Saunders 1996)." After her training in social work in Oxford, Cicely Saunders worked as a medical social worker at St. Thomas Hospital in London from 1947–1957. In addition, she volunteered at St. Luke's Hospital in London once or twice a week from 1948. This hospital was one of the few that specialized in terminally ill patients. At that time, it provided 48 beds for people severely ill with cancer. "In St. Luke's," cannabis and cocaine were omitted. Also, the morphine dose was adjusted to the needs of the patients (Saunders 1996). From 1951 to 1957, Saunders studied medicine and worked again at St. Thomas's Hospital. "At that time, revolutionary new drugs appeared that could better treat symptoms. When I started working at St. Joseph's Hospice in October 1958, the first phenothiazines, antidepressants, benzodiazepines, synthetic steroids, and non-steroidal anti-inflammatory drugs were all in use" (Saunders 1996).

In addition to her clinical work at St. Joseph's Hospital, Saunders was involved in research in the field of pain management and palliative care. In 1960, Cicely Saunders formulated the first policy papers for the establishment of a hospice. On July 14, 1967, St. Christopher's Hospice in London was opened with a research department. In 1969, Saunders set up an outpatient hospice service.

Cicely Saunders died on July 14, 2005, at the age of 87, exactly 38 years after the opening of her hospice.

Her commitment to the hospice movement and palliative medicine is unforgettable, and her quotes and advice are still valid for today's practice of palliative medicine:

> "Hospice work and palliative care encompass everything that is related to the mind—the entire scientific claim, experimenting, researching, and studying. But all this must always be connected with a friendship of the heart—with individual and personal care and relationship." (Cicely Saunders 2009)

> "It's not about adding more days to life, but adding more life to days."

18.3 Principles and Goals of Palliative Medicine

What is the goal of a medicine that can no longer defeat diseases, but can still help people?

1. Physical proximity
2. The doctor as a student
3. Answers to questions
4. Treatment of complaints
5. The doctor as part of the family

18.3.1 Physical Proximity

It is considered "old school" when the chief physician greets about 40 patients during a chief physician's visit by handshake. Of course, different hygiene rules apply in times of a pandemic, but even a corona pandemic will eventually be over! What then speaks against greeting patients by handshake, disinfecting the hands, and exchanging some important words? Hygiene and humanity do not exclude each other, but condition each other! In regular clinical operations, we do not have the time to devote as much time to each patient as she needs or thinks she needs. Our task is to recognize which patients need more conversation, more attention.

18.3.2 The Doctor as a Student

Elisabeth Kübler-Ross pointed out very early in her 1966 essay "The dying patient as teacher" that we, as caregivers and doctors, can learn a lot from our teachers, the patients. It seems as if the dying have a clearer view of the truly important things in life, or they are not so easily distracted by superficialities! Or do the dying dare to tell the truth to one's face, even at the risk of hurting the other person? Often, the dying have a sense for when they will die. We, as caregivers and doctors, theoretically know the four life phases in palliative medicine:

Rehabilitation phase—Pre-terminal phase—Terminal phase—Final phase

The prognosis for the last final phase is: a few hours to one day—"the last hours".

Ingeborg Jonen-Thielemann describes in her chapter "Terminal phase" the activity of the dying in the **Final phase** as follows: "State in extremis, person is dying, consciousness not directed towards the outside world. How often we thought bedridden patients, who had withdrawn into themselves, were in this final phase, which often lasted several days and occasionally one or two weeks. It seems as if we, as caregivers and doctors, but also the patients with their relatives, have lost the sense for the approaching death. We must learn again to observe nature and humans and understand that nature and humans influence each other.

18.3.3 Answers to Questions

"Will I still be with my family at Christmas?", several patients asked me during my medical career. As a young doctor, I struggled with whether I should give a corresponding prognosis about the expected lifespan. Over the years, I understood the message contained in the patient's question: "I want to see my family again, whether at Christmas or at Easter. I want to say goodbye to everyone!" Even the dying long for attention, love and tenderness. Most of the questions asked to us aim to maintain these human needs. We must not leave this questioning of the patients for humanity unanswered!

18.3.4 Treating Symptoms

Shortness of Breath (Dyspnea)

- There are various causes that lead to the symptom of shortness of breath: lung diseases, cardiac causes, neuromuscular diseases
- Other causes: anemia, fever, pain, anxiety, rib fractures, ascites, hepatosplenomegaly

In cases of causally untreatable shortness of breath, palliative approach relies on two concepts (Watzke 2017):

- the influence of the emotional-psychological consequences of dyspnea through coping strategies and
- the influence of the perception of dyspnea in the area of receptors in the thoracic wall and brain through opioids.

Opioids have a scientifically proven relieving effect on dyspnea. The mechanism is likely based on the occupation of opioid receptors in the thoracic wall, lung tissue and brain and has nothing to do with an often claimed sedative effect of opioids (Zebraski et al. 2000).

Opioid dosage for shortness of breath (Watzke 2017)

Opioid naive patients:

- Start with oral morphine (or equivalent) 2.5–5 mg
- Wait until the maximum opioid effect is reached
- If the effect is insufficient: repeat the dose or increase the dose by 25–50%
- Determine the daily dose and switch to a long-acting opioid
- Provide 5–15% of the daily dose—hourly if needed—as therapy for breakthrough dyspnea

Patients already on opioids:

- Increase the opioid dose by 25%

Systemic medicinal pain therapy

The WHO guidelines for tumor pain therapy recommend a medicinal, preferably oral pain therapy after careful anamnesis, examination, and determination of the pain diagnosis. These recommendations were confirmed by the Drug Commission of the German Medical Association (WHO 1996). Figure 18.1 shows the WHO step-by-step scheme.

The most important principles of medicinal pain therapy according to the WHO step-by-step scheme are:

- As simple as possible—preferably oral administration of analgesics
- Regular intake according to a fixed schedule, before pain reoccurs
- Individual dosage
- Controlled dose adjustment
- Prophylaxis of side effects through concomitant medication

By consistently applying the 3-step scheme recommended by the WHO for the first time in 1986, a reduction of pain to a tolerable level and thus a significant improvement in quality of life can be achieved in 75–90% of female patients with tumor pain, according to Nauck and Radbruch.

Fever and Infections

The incidence of fever in palliative patients is between 26 and 78%, thus more frequent than dyspnea. Fever can be a subjectively and objectively burdensome

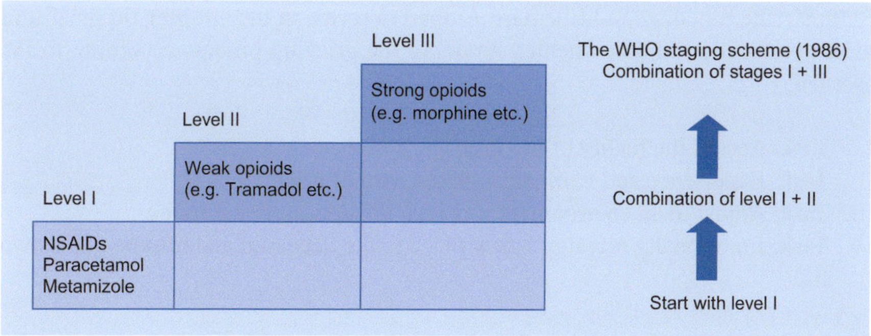

Fig. 18.1 Medicinal pain therapy—The WHO step-by-step scheme. (From: Husebo and Mathis 2017)

symptom. A rise in temperature leads to chills and a drop in temperature to sweating, general weakness, confusion, and dizziness. The following **factors favor the occurrence of infections** in palliative patients:

Impaired cellular immune system, impaired humoral immune system, malnutrition/cachexia, defective skin barriers (decubitus ulcers), ascites/pleural effusions, bedriddenness/immobilization, foreign bodies (bladder catheters, port systems), displacement of normal body flora after antibiotic administration.

In principle, a causal therapy with an antimicrobial drug should be aimed for in the therapeutic decision. In a prospective study on the use of antimicrobial treatment, White et al found that only 21% of palliative patients opted for a recommended antimicrobial treatment. 31% of palliative patients fundamentally rejected an antimicrobial examination. 48% agreed to an antimicrobial treatment only if symptoms caused by the infection should occur. It is important to accept the often clearly expressed wish of palliative patients to forego antimicrobial treatment. It is important to orient oneself to the wishes of the patients, as fever or sweating are perceived very differently as a burden individually.

The following basic measures have proven effective:

- Adequate fluid intake, nursing-physical measures such as cooling of the groin, forearms and lower legs, as well as washings with sage tea.
- Use of Nonsteroidal Anti-inflammatory Drugs such as: Metamizol, Paracetamol and Glucocorticoids to control febrile conditions.
- The neuroleptic **Chlorpromazine** can lower body temperature both in fever and at normal temperature.
- Drug-induced fever and chills can usually be effectively treated with **Pethidine**.
- A subjectively disturbing mild to moderate sweating tendency can be successfully treated with sage extract (Sweatosan N).

18.3.5 The Doctor as Part of the Family

Ruthmareike Smeding and Eberhard Aulbert describe in the **chapter on grief and grief counseling** the task-oriented model of the grieving process according to JW Worden:

I. Task: Accept the reality of the loss
II. Task: Experience and work through the pain of grief
III. Task: Adjust to an environment in which the deceased is missing
IV. Task: Emotionally reassign a new place to the deceased and resume one's own life

Since, according to Smeding and Aulbert, empirical research could not generally confirm the occurrence and sequence of the described phases, and on the other hand, the implementation of these models into practically applicable treatment strategies did not succeed, these stage or phase models were largely abandoned. In their place came models without any sequential or linear conception of the course of grief, which prefer a more component-structured structure of the grieving process (Smeding and Aulbert 2012).

In this community of mourners, the doctor becomes the spiritual counselor, the "pater familias", who mourns and comforts.

18.4 Palliative Care in Nursing Homes or Under Palm Groves (How Elderly, Seriously Ill People Live and Die Worldwide)

In contrast to the high birth rates in poor countries, rich countries have a low birth rate, but a significantly higher proportion of elderly people in the total population. According to the Atlas of Globalization, the proportion of the population over 65 years of age in Germany, Italy, and Japan is more than 21% of the total population, whereas in most African countries significantly less than 5% of the population is older than 65 years (Klingholz 2019)!

The former assumption of the "life-saturated human being, who symptom-free and without life-threatening illness does not need palliative medical care" seems largely refuted (Husebo-Sandgathe and Husebo 2001).

"Why did father (and mother) have to suffer unnecessarily and infinitely?" Do we believe that patients with dementia have no pain because they cannot describe pain, a seasoned British doctor described (Ascolon 1998).

The following criteria for pain and discomfort should be observed in dying persons with dementia (Husebo-Sandgathe and Husebo 2017):

- Rapid shallow breathing and rapid pulse
- Tense expression on the face
- Uncontrolled moaning and calling
- Restlessness in certain positions
- Defensive reactions
- Intensification of these reactions during care or under movements

The first palliative care units were primarily set up for patients with advanced cancer. Many cancers are now curable or at least more manageable. In the routine treatment of elderly oncological patients, it is occasionally forgotten that palliative therapies have always been carried out in the field of oncology!

> ▶ The non-word "therapeutically exhausted" has "served its time!"

Decades ago, Supportive Care was introduced almost simultaneously with the first successful chemotherapies. Good supportive care is considered a prerequisite for good studies, with its goals being (Mathis 2017):

- Improvement of the prerequisites for the feasibility of oncological therapies
- Reduction of the occurrence of unwanted side effects from potentially toxic therapies
- Maintenance or enhancement of the patients' quality of life
- Relief of disease-related symptoms
- Prognostic improvement of treatment outcomes

While in some European countries half of the population dies in nursing homes, this is the exception in African countries, especially since there are only a few nursing homes there. This is not only due to the significantly lower proportion of people over 65 years of age, but above all to the willingness of the African extended family to care for the mother and father at home, even outdoors "in the sacred palm grove" of the village. There are no studies available to us yet about the real life reality of the elderly in Africa, but the admittedly subjective impression of a former development aid worker recalls old, contented women and men who—sitting in front of the hut under palm trees or under the baobab—have a chat. The elderly patients whom we could no longer help at CHR Dori usually sensed their impending death and called their relatives to them. Our primitive palliative care station consisted of a larger room where the family could say goodbye to their elderly parents and grandparents. Due to the remoteness and the resulting long distances to the individual villages in the Seno province, transport for the seriously ill patients was impossible. The relatives of the patients knew this and did not leave the deathbed of their mothers and fathers in this situation. In the almost always prevailing great heat, they fanned cooling air to the dying and touched their arms and legs. We did not need air conditioning or physiotherapists on our primitive palliative care station! The care and treatment of our "palliative patients" was in the hands of the family, and their practiced love for the dying family member was the only therapy possible for us, our form of "Primitive Palliative Care"!

Can we learn humility, harmony with nature, and resignation to the fate of aging from these wise women and men in the African villages?

As shown in Chap. 15 (Effects of modern obstetrics on human development using the example of premature termination of pregnancy), we as obstetricians have learned a lot and scientifically investigated during our work in Africa as a Tropical Doctor. I am convinced that we can still learn a lot in the field of palliative medicine and apply it to us!

On one of our forays, between 1986 and 1988, through the Sahel, between Markoye and Tin-a-Koff, on the banks of the Beli, a tributary of the Niger, in the north of Burkina Faso, we met Abou, the Tuareg, who invited us to a tea ceremony in front of his tent. He boiled the ornate tin teapot three times with the charcoal stove, then poured the hot tea from a great height into the ready tea glasses. He explained to us what each tea infusion stands for:

> The first glass is bitter like life,
> the second sweet like love

and the third gentle like death.
Tuareg—Tea Wisdom from Africa

Attempt to answer the five initial questions

1. We know that for a healthy pregnancy and a healthy child, the health of the parents at the time of conception and, of course, throughout the entire pregnancy, a healthy lifestyle are important prerequisites for a good and healthy development of the child.
2. **"Therapy has served its purpose"**! We must never disappoint hopes, but on the other hand, we must not raise false hopes! The most important principle in any form of treatment is to gain and maintain the trust of the patients!
3. Cicely Saunders and Albert Schweitzer oppose any form of euthanasia out of reverence for life. I can only share their attitude, knowing that modern palliative medicine can help patients alleviate severe symptoms of their respective serious illness, with few exceptions, and usually also control them.
4. When a doctor is called to a life-threatening emergency of a patient unknown to him, he must act and resuscitate the patient if necessary! This does not apply if the patient has expressly, in writing or credibly informed the treating doctor that he does not wish any intensive medical, potentially life-saving measures, even in an emergency!
5. What does the ethical principle of Albert Schweitzer mean for modern, global medicine: "**I am life that wants to live, in the midst of life that wants to live!**" This quote from Albert Schweitzer continues to apply unchanged and is for me the modern addition to the old Hippocratic Oath! In the meantime, it stands for all of humanity on our earth. Global gender-equitable health is based on the fact that the individual person, the individual nation and the individual continent understand that we ourselves cannot be well if the neighbor is sick, the other nation of Ukraine is invaded by a war of aggression, and the neighboring continent Africa continues to live in poverty and economic dependence!

References

Ascolon CM (1998) Why? Pall Med 12:195–196

Husebo S, Mathis G (2017) Palliativmedizin, 6. ed. Springer, Heidelberg

Husebo-Sandgathe B, Husebo S (2001) Palliativmedizin – auch im hohen Alter? Der Schmerz 5:350–357

Husebo-Sandgathe B, Husebo S (2017) Palliativmedizin im Pflegeheim – wie alte, schwer kranke Menschen leben und sterben. In: Husebo S, Mathis G (Eds) Palliativmedizin, 6. ed. Springer, Heidelberg

Klingholz R (2019) Alternde Gesellschaften. In: Mahlke S (Hrsg) Atlas der Globalisierung. Welt in Bewegung Le Monde diplomatique, Paris p 52
Mathis G (2017) Palliative Onkologie – Möglichkeiten und Herausforderungen. In: Husebo S, Mathis G (Eds) Palliativmedizin, 6. ed. Springer, Heidelberg
Saunders C (1996) A personal therapeutic journey. BMJ 313:1599–1601
Smeding R Aulberg E (2012) Trauer in der Palliativmedizin. In Aulbert, Nauck und Radbruch: Lehrbuch der Palliativmedizin pp 1173–1188. Schattauer, Stuttgart
Wacker J (2011) Isaaks Schwestern. Westkreuz, Berlin/Bonn, pp 161 ff
Watzke H (2017) Symptomkontrolle. In: Husebo S, Mathis G (Eds) Palliativmedizin, 6. ed. Springer, Heidelberg
World Health Organization (1996) Cancer pain relief: with a guide to opioid availability, 2. ed. World Health Organization, Genf
Zebraski SE, Kochenash SM, Raffa RB (2000) Lung opioid receptors pharmacology and possible target for nebulized morphine in dyspnoe. Lif Sci 66:2221–2231

Further Reading

Arzneimittelkommission der Deutschen Ärzteschaft (2007) Empfehlungen zur Therapie von Tumorschmerzen. Arzneiverordnung in der Praxis. 3. ed. Berlin, Deutscher Ärzte Verlag
Aulbert E, Nauck F, Radbruch L (2012) Lehrbuch der Palliativmedizin, 3., Akt. ed. Schattauer, Stuttgart
Bugen LA (1977) Human grief: a model for prediction and intervention. Am J Orthopsychiatry 2:196–206
Clemens KE, Klaschik E (2012) Respiratorische Symptome pp 366–383. In Aulbert, Nauck und Radbruch: Lehrbuch der Palliativmedizin, Schattauer, Stuttgart, pp 1173–1188
Jonen-Thielemann I (2012) Sterbephase in der Palliativmedizin, pp 989–997. In Aulbert, Nauck und Radbruch: Lehrbuch der Palliativmedizin, Schattauer, Stuttgart, pp 1173–1188
Klaschik E (2003) Schmerztherapie und Symptomkontrolle in der Palliativmedizin. In: Husebo S, Klaschik E (Eds) Palliativmedizin, 3. ed. Springer, Heidelberg, pp 256–259
Kübler-Ross E (1969a) The dying patient as teacher. Chikago Theol Register 3:1–14
Kübler-Ross E (1969b) Interviews mit Sterbenden. Kreuz, Stuttgart
Lunzen J, Albrecht H (2012) Erworbene Immunschwäche (AIDS): Therapie opportunistischer Erkrankungen in Aulbert, Nauck und Radbruch: Lehrbuch der Palliativmedizin, Schattauer Verlag Stuttgart, pp 710–737
Mahlke S (2019) Atlas der Globalisierung; Welt in Bewegung. Le Monde diplomatique
Morita T, Tsunoda J, Inoue S, Chihara S (1999) Contributing factors to physical symptoms in terminally ill cancer patients. J Pain Symptom Manage 18:338–346
Nauck F Radbruch L (2012) Systemische medikamentöse Schmerztherapie, pp 175–207. In Aulbert, Nauck und Radbruch: Lehrbuch der Palliativmedizin, Schattauer, Stuttgart, pp 1173–1188
Peters U, Maschmeyer G (2012) Fieber und Infektionen. pp 410–418. In Aulbert, Nauck und Radbruch: Lehrbuch der Palliativmedizin, Schattauer, Stuttgart, pp 1173–1188
Saunders C (2009) Sterben und Leben; Spititualität in der Palliative Care; Theologischer, Zürich; Übersetzung der englischen Originalausgabe von 2003: „Watch with me – inspiration for a life in hospice care" Mortal press
White PH, Kuhlenschmidt HL, Vancura BG, Navarin RM (2003) Antimicrobial use in patients with advanced cancer receiving hospice care. J Pain Symptome Manage 25:438–443
Worden JW (2009) Grief counseling and grief therapy, 4. ed. Routledge, London

Creating Guidelines for Poor and Rich Countries—What is Indispensable?

19

Rosemarie Burian, Eva J. Kantelhardt and Jürgen Wacker

Contents

R. Burian (✉)
Basel, Switzerland

E. J. Kantelhardt
Global & Planetary Health AG; Klinik und Poliklinik für Gynäkologie, Medizinische Fakultät der Martin-Luther-Universität Halle-Wittenberg, Universitätsklinikum Halle (Saale), Halle (Saale), Germany
e-mail: eva.kantelhardt@medizin.uni-halle.de

J. Wacker
ehemaliger Chefarzt der Frauenklinik Bruchsal, Bruchsal, Germany
e-mail: wacker@menschenfuerfrauen.de

J. Wacker et al. (eds.), *Global Women's Health*,
https://doi.org/10.1007/978-3-662-69700-9_19

Introductory Questions

1. What distinguishes **guidelines from directives**?
   A. There is no difference, both terms mean the same thing and can be used interchangeably.
   B. Directives are a guideline that one can follow; guidelines guide a process and must be followed.
   C. Guidelines are medical decision aids that can be deviated from, directives are legally binding.
2. For which **target groups** are guidelines written?
   A. For private individuals
   B. For non-governmental organizations
   C. For medical professionals and political decision-makers in healthcare
3. What is **indispensable in the creation** of guidelines?
   A. From the beginning, consider the target group and their needs and integrate them into the decision-making process
   B. Eminence is rated higher than evidence
   C. In addition to transparent and systematic creation, implementation and continuous evaluation are also part of the guideline creation process

Guidelines have continuously increased in importance and number worldwide over the last three decades. Developed for mostly medical decision-making in specific clinical situations, they have now gained both clinical and health policy significance. In German-speaking countries, these are the basis for disease management programs, e.g., for breast cancer patients, as well as the nationwide certification process for breast centers of the German Cancer Society (Nothacker et al. 2014). In a global setting, the guidelines provide a basis for economically realistic and sustainable planning for the infrastructures, medications, consumables, and personnel required for the respective disease spectrum.

Well and systematically developed guidelines contain information and decision aids, offer valuable communication aids in dialogue with patients, and increase decision transparency. For the high-quality, generally accepted, and easily accessible guidelines required for this, development always includes a plan for their implementation and ongoing evaluation. Therefore, in addition to rigorous methodology, early involvement of the target groups is indispensable: for national guidelines, the involvement of various professional groups and patient representatives, for international guidelines, the involvement of representatives of various countries and regions and the relevant non-governmental organizations for implementation.

In Germany, the Association of Scientific Medical Societies (AWMF), currently with over 179 different medical societies, has established itself as a forum for guidelines (MacDonald et al. 1985). Since 1992, it has been active in guideline work with the aim of improving the quality of clinical practice and research. Currently, over 805 guidelines from various professional societies are published on its website. The German Society for Gynecology and Obstetrics, the DGGG, has been represented here since 1998 with its own guideline commission, which is supposed to advance the quality of guideline development and ensure coordination with the recommendations of the AWMF. Since 2015, this has been a cross-border guideline commission with representatives of the Austrian Society for Gynecology and Obstetrics, the OEGGG, and the Swiss Society for Gynecology and Obstetrics, the SGGG.

The Institute of Medicine (IOM), since 2015 National Academy of Medicine, a US institution, published its clinical practice guidelines in the same year that the AWMF began its guideline work (Field and Lohr 1992). At that time, the IOM already recommended indicating the cost relevance of the clinical recommendations. This recommendation takes on special relevance in a global context when, in addition to what is clinically possible, it is also about what is financially feasible and sensible in the respective country context and the guidelines serve the Ministries of Health and Finance as a decision-making tool.

In 2016, "The African Cancer Coalition (ACC)" was founded to serve as a regional cooperation of 12 African countries to draft oncological guidelines for the African countries south of the Sahara (Mutebi et al. 2020). The guidelines were developed in collaboration with the American National Comprehensive Cancer Network (NCCN), taking into account local needs and the typical pre-existing conditions of the regions (Anderson 2020). In August 2020, 46 NCNN Harmonized Guidelines for Sub-Saharan Africa (SSA) were published on the NCCN website, all of which have since been updated without exception. In addition to this project, seven oncological NCCN Harmonized Guidelines for the Caribbean were also published in 2018, taking into account the needs and resources of this region.

The World Health Organization (WHO) has been drafting and publishing guidelines on medically relevant topics worldwide for decades. Some guidelines are drafted by the WHO regional offices for the respective region, e.g. the two EMRO (Regional Office for the Eastern Mediterranean) guidelines on the subject of breast cancer (WHO EMRO 2006); others, like the guideline from 2018 on "Care during normal childbirth for a positive birth experience", are explicitly not written for specific countries or regions, but are designed for worldwide application (WHO 2018a, b).

This chapter first explains the concept of a guideline and the process of guideline development using the tools used by the German AWMF, the American NCCN, and the WHO, thus providing an insight into the methodology of guideline development and evaluation.

The global aspect is illustrated by a synopsis of three guidelines on the topic of "Hypertensive disorders in pregnancy": the joint one of the German-speaking area, the DGGG, OEGGG and the SGGG, the country-specific guideline from Cameroon and the three guidelines on this topic written by the WHO for worldwide use: Prevention and treatment of preeclampsia and eclampsia; drug therapy for severe hypertension in pregnancy and drug therapy for non-severe hypertension in pregnancy.

19.1 Definition and Delimitation

Guideline Guidelines ("guidelines") are developed systematically and support the decision-making of doctors and patients regarding the appropriate course of action for specific health problems and decision-makers in the health and finance sector in providing and financing the necessary infrastructure.

Guidelines support all professional groups involved in medical treatment and patients in making decisions in specific situations of prevention, diagnosis, therapy, and aftercare. They thus accelerate, among other things, the transfer of the best available evidence into everyday care and promote the transparency of medical decisions. They are developed by gathering knowledge from different sources on specific questions and evaluating it in consideration of existing resources. The identification of conflicts of interest, the discussion of opposing viewpoints, and special situational requirements are important components of this process.

AWMF guidelines are divided into three development stages (Table 19.1). Only stage 3 guidelines are considered evidence-based. The following Table 19.1 shows the development stages of guidelines.

> **Important** **Guidelines** are created and published by medical professional societies and not by the legislator. They do not exempt from the verification of individual applicability in the specific case. They are not legally binding, but serve as decision aids, from which deviations can and even must be made in justified cases.

This distinguishes them from **directives**, which are issued by the legislator or sub-legislative standard setters such as the Joint Federal Committee (G-BA) or the German Medical Association (Muche-Borowski and Kopp 2015). The G-BA has issued the Maternity and Cancer Early Detection Directive; the German Medical Association has published directives on assisted reproduction and transfusion and transplantation medicine. The American usage of language promotes the confusion

Table 19.1 Development stages of guidelines. (Stage scheme according to AWMF rules)

Stage	Characteristics
Stage 3	**Evidence- and consensus-based** guideline with all elements of systematic development (logic/clinical algorithms, representative body, systematic research, selection and evaluation of literature, structured consensus finding)
Stage 2 S2e S2k	Constructs of systematic consensus processes **Evidence-based** guideline through systematic research, selection, and evaluation of literature **Consensus-based** guideline through a representative body, structured consensus finding
Stage 1	Recommendations for action by expert groups

of the two terms: Here, the term "guideline" is used for both guidelines and directives. In the official language of the EU, however, a distinction is made according to bindingness:

- "guideline" = "guideline"
- "directive" = "directive"

▶ **Directive** Directives ("directives") are regulations of action or omission, which have been consented, written down and published by a legally legitimized institution. They are binding for the legal area of this institution. Non-compliance results in defined sanctions [Medical Center for Quality in Medicine (ÄZQ), 1997].

To what extent principles of guideline development can be applied to the formulation of directives is questionable.

How different the respective specifications can be was shown until 2012 by the example of hyperglycemia screening in pregnancy. While the German Maternity Directive prescribed the urine test for screening for gestational diabetes, this was no longer recommended in any current guideline. In March 2012, the guideline-compliant blood glucose test for screening for gestational diabetes was included in the German Maternity Directive.

19.2 Guideline Development

The supreme commandments of evidence-based guideline development are systematic and transparency. In the national and international context, in addition to methodological transparency, the disclosure of personal conflicts of interest of those involved in guideline development also plays an important role. With regard to transparency, for example, the NCCN requires a six-monthly update of conflicts of interest, which are published together with the guidelines, and prohibits further participation in the development of the respective guideline in the case of conflicts of interest. The AWMF guidelines also contain a published overview of possible conflicts of interest of the guideline authors in the methodology section.

All steps of development, from the composition of the panels, identification and evaluation of the evidence, consensus finding and formulation to implementation (overview "Summary of the flowchart of guideline development"), are based on systematic and pre-defined methodology. An important characteristic of evidence-based guidelines is their limited validity and their regular revision. There is a certain range here: The validity of the AWMF guidelines is limited to five years. The guideline commission of the DGGG, SGGG and OEGGG has developed a flowchart for updating, which groups the update according to low urgency and high urgency and provides and enables a timely update before the actual 5-year period expires. The NCCN standardly provides for an annual review of the evidence of its oncological guidelines, with a necessary update if required. The WHO does not specify a specific validity period, but reviews the evidence annually and recommends an update as soon as relevant new findings are identified.

Summary of the flowchart of guideline development using the example of the WHO Handbook for Guideline Development

1. Identification of relevant questions and outcomes
2. Search for evidence
3. Assessment and synthesis of evidence
4. Formulation of recommendations
5. Planning of dissemination, implementation, evaluation and updating

19.2.1 Initiative and Preparation

19.2.1.1 Identifying and Prioritizing Questions

Classical evidence-based medicine deals with a specific clinical question of an individual patient. In contrast, guidelines provide decision aids for a multitude of related clinical questions and patient groups. The topics to be addressed are determined by the professional societies or guideline publishers.

Under the keyword "logic", the AWMF recommends the use of clinical algorithms for formulating the initial questions: Clinical questions should be broken down into "finite steps using if-then conditions" and should consider both typical and special patient groups.

19.2.1.2 Composition of Guideline Groups

For AWMF S3-, NCCN- and WHO-guidelines, an interdisciplinary composition of the guideline group is made with representatives of all professional societies relevant to the clinical problem, possibly also from different geographical regions. The participation of research specialists, epidemiologists and possibly also social psychologists is planned. In addition, with a view to implementation, patient representatives, representatives of other professional and interest groups, and in the global context also non-governmental organizations are involved. Beyond the professional enrichment, this is expected to improve the general acceptance of the guidelines.

In the current WHO guideline on "Care for a normal birth for a positive birth experience", which was designed for worldwide use, there were four groups involved in the development and a fifth with observer status. The backbone was the WHO steering committee with representatives from the three WHO departments for reproductive health and research (RHR), for maternal, newborn, child and adolescent health (MCA) and family, women's and children's health (FWC).

This steering committee appointed 18 experts from the six WHO regions to the second group, the "Guideline Development Group". For the later peer review, six experts were appointed to a third, the external review group, who were balanced in terms of geographical origin and gender and had no relevant conflicts of interest. The fourth, the technical working group (Technical working group) consisted of two teams, one from the northern hemisphere (England) and one from the southern hemisphere (Argentina). The last and fifth group, which only had observer status, consisted of international partners relevant for publication and implementation: representatives of the International Federation of Gynecology and Obstetrics (FIGO), the International Confederation of Midwives (IMC); the Royal College of Obstetricians and Gynaecology (RCOG) as well as the United Nations Population Fund (UNFPA) and the US Agency for International Development (USAID).

Concrete action recommendations are the goal of developing a guideline. For this, different viewpoints, discrepancies in the data situation and divergent positions in the weighting must be led to a consensus. For consensus finding, various scientifically based forms are available from social psychology (overview "Methods of consensus finding"). The type of decision-making must be determined before the start of group work and described in the guideline to ensure the traceability of the decisions (Koop 2010). In the S3 guideline on breast cancer, which in its current form covers both early detection and diagnosis, therapy and aftercare of breast cancer, a nominal group process was chosen under the direction of independent moderators, and for the S2k guideline on hypertensive pregnancy diseases: diagnosis and therapy, the method of consensus conference was chosen.

Methods of Consensus Finding

- **Nominal Group Process**
  - Group decision-making process in which written answers to predefined problems are first composed by all participants
  - Subsequent publication of individual opinions as an anonymous list, statements of all participants one after the other in a discussion round
  - Possibly repeated repetition of these steps
- **Delphi Method**
  - Interactive survey method with controlled feedback and questioning of anonymized experts
  - Typically, there are several rounds of questioning with interim systematic summarization, modification and criticism of individual opinions
- **Consensus Conference**
  - Open discussion, e.g. in working groups, after extensive preparation
  - Attempt at consensus finding, followed by official announcement, also in the form of a publication in peer reviewed journals

19.2.2 Review and Assessment of Evidence

19.2.2.1 Literature Search

Comparable to the Literature search for systematic reviews, the evidence review for guidelines also requires a comprehensive search for studies on all essential questions that are formulated in the clinical algorithms to ensure an unbiased view. In contrast to the classic guideline round, where the protagonists can contribute study material of their own choice, S3 guidelines require disclosure of the sources including an electronic search strategy. It is recommended to involve search experts for this purpose.

19.2.2.2 Evidence Evaluation and Classification of Evidence Quality

The hierarchy of Evidence is one of the central characteristics of an evidence-based guideline. There has been significant development over the years. Several classification systems now exist side by side. A typical example of a "1st generation" evidence classification can be found in Table 19.2 (McCormick and Fleming 1992). The following Table 19.2 shows an example of an evidence classification.

This classification refers to the basic suitability of a study design to achieve valid results by avoiding systematic errors (bias). For questions of therapy or prevention, the randomized clinical study is theoretically the optimal design. Other criteria apply to other questions. Therefore, the shown scheme is not directly transferable to problems of diagnosis, prognosis or adverse effects. It also remains unclear how to classify evidence when studies have significant methodological weaknesses or multiple studies on the same question show inconsistent results (heterogeneity).

While the first version of the breast cancer early detection guideline used a similar classification, the updated version of the breast cancer guideline uses the much more differentiated recommendations of the Oxford Centre for Evidence-based Medicine (CEBM). These take into account the requirements of different questions, allow deductions for methodological weaknesses or heterogeneity of study results, and distinguish ten levels of evidence in their current version from 2009. The detailed scheme can be found on www.cebm.net.

Table 19.2 Example of an evidence classification

Level	Type of Evidence
Ia	At least one systematic review based on methodologically high-quality randomized, controlled studies (RCT)
Ib	At least one sufficiently large, methodologically high-quality RCT
IIa	At least one high-quality study without randomization
IIb	At least one high-quality study of another type of quasi-experimental studies
III	More than one methodologically high-quality non-experimental study
IV	Opinions and beliefs of respected authorities (from clinical experience); expert committees; descriptive studies

19.2.2.3 Strength of Recommendations

Classifications of evidence quality refer to the methodological quality of the existing evidence. However, the strength of a recommendation also depends on other factors. For this reason, many guideline developers make an additional classification of recommendation strength. The classification in Table 19.3 is often used in combination with the simple classification in Table 19.2. The following Table 19.3 shows the classification of the American Society of Clinical Oncology.

Still not taken into account are the strength of the effect, the relevance of the endpoint examined, and the weighing of efficacy and possible side effects. In addition, available resources, ethical considerations, and the practicability and applicability in the specific environment are conceivable as possible influencing factors (value level).

19.2.3 Decision Making and Formulation of Guidelines

19.2.3.1 Integration of the Value Level

The SIGN Group (Scottish Intercollegiate Guidelines Network) summarizes the aspects that must be considered in the formulation of guidelines as follows (overview): In 2013, SIGN decided to use the GRADE system (Sect. 19.2.3.2) in the development of guidelines, instead of the ABCD classification used until then (Table 19.3). This system is also used in the development of WHO guidelines.

Relevant Aspects of Guideline Development (according to SIGN)

- Scope, quality, and consistency of the evidence
- Generalizability of the study results
- Direct relevance to the target group of the guideline
- Clinical impact—extent of the effect and resources needed in the target group
- Feasibility—how practical is the implementation of the guideline in the context of the respective health system?

Table 19.3 Classification of the American Society of Clinical Oncology (ASCO). (After Desch et al. 1999)

Grade	Grade of recommendation
A	Evidence of quality class I or consistent results from many studies of class II, III or IV
B	Evidence of quality class II, III or IV with largely consistent results
C	Evidence of quality class II, III or IV with inconsistent results
D	Little or no systematic empirical evidence

19.2.3.2 GRADE System

To meet the complexity of integrating methodological quality, effect size, and value level, a standardized approach is needed that takes into account the different aspects. Since the year 2000, the international GRADE working group (**G**rading of **R**ecommendations **A**ssessment, **D**evelopment and **E**valuation) has set itself the task of organizing the previously existing classifications and considering other important aspects such as relevance and feasibility (Atkins et al. 2005; Guyatt et al. 2008, 2011).

Since then, the GRADE working group has developed three important tools:

1. The GRADE system, which is now used by over 100 organizations worldwide, including the WHO, the Cochrane Collaboration, and the English National Institute for Health and Care Excellence (NICE), allows the quality of evidence to be adjusted to the quality and overall study situation, taking into account the value level in relation to quantitative evidence. Here too, the quality of evidence for a problem is initially classified as high if RCTs are available. The evidence from observational studies is classified as low, other sources of evidence are classified as very low. Adjustments are also planned depending on the quality of the study, the strength of the effect, and the extent of the data situation. Deductions are made for errors in study design and execution, for uncertainties in implementation and transferability of results, and for inconsistent results of the studies considered. Conversely, pronounced effects (very strong: RR >5.0 or <0.2, strong: RR >2.0 or <0.5) or the demonstration of a dose-effect relationship each lead to a corresponding upgrade of the evidence class. After integrating classifications of clinical relevance, economic circumstances, and practicability, concrete weighted recommendations result.
2. In the WHO guideline for "Care for normal birth for a positive birth experience", in addition to GRADE for the assessment of quantitative studies, the GRADE-CERQual tool (Confidence in the Evidence from Reviews of Qualitative research) is used for the assessment of qualitative reviews, with a comparable approach to GRADE (Lewin et al. 2015).
3. In 2016, the GRADE working group, supported by the European Union, also developed the GRADE-based tool "Evidence to decision" framework, which is intended to help clinicians, guideline developers, and policy makers use the best available evidence for their decisions. This is used, for example, in the WHO guideline "Drug therapy for severe hypertension in pregnancy" (Alonso-Coello et al. 2016)

19.3 Dissemination and Implementation of Guidelines

It is essential to promote the attractiveness and widespread implementation of guidelines. Therefore, the guidelines are adapted to the needs of different users and published in user-specific versions.

The AWMF guideline on hypertensive pregnancy disorders: Diagnosis and therapy is available as a long version and a short version and slide version are planned. The AWMF guideline on gestational diabetes is available as a long version, patient guideline, and as a slide version. In addition, a guideline report, an evidence report, a practice aid, and insert sheets for the maternity record as well as BMI percentiles have been made available. Other guidelines are also available as a pocket version and from the German Society for Internal Medicine (DGIM) also as an app.

On the WHO website "iris—Institutional Repository for Information Sharing", all WHO publications including the guidelines are stored; depending on the target group, there are versions in different languages.

The WHO guideline "Care of normal childbirth for a positive birth experience" was distributed to the WHO regional and country offices, health ministries, WHO cooperation centers, non-governmental organizations, and professional societies in addition to the online version. Furthermore, there were two separate compilations of scientific evidence, which also presents the main recommendations and their possible implementations: one for policy makers and a second for medical professionals. A short version including an overview of the recommendations was translated into the six official UN languages.

To support wide implementation and application, the WHO works with the GREAT Network (Guideline-driven, Research priorities, Evidence synthesis, Application of evidence, and Transfer of Knowledge). This facilitates the adaptation and implementation of the guidelines to various local needs.

On the NCCN website, the original oncological NCCN guidelines can be found, as well as pure translations of these existing NCCN guidelines and versions of these guidelines adapted for specific countries. In addition, there are the "Harmonized Guidelines" developed in collaboration with the target regions for Sub-Saharan Africa and the Caribbean (Carlson et al. 2016).

The current guidelines of the DGGG are published on the AWMF page. There, the guidelines are deleted one year after the expiration of their validity. To ensure long-term access to the guidelines, the DGGG archives all guidelines and statements and allows public access via its website. In the first years, short versions of the guidelines were published in the journal *Der Frauenarzt*, in 2014 the switch to the peer-review journal *Geburtshilfe und Frauenheilkunde (GebFra)* was decided. Since then, published guidelines are now also listed internationally in MEDLINE in English and can be cited.

The publication of a guideline is the first step. The subsequent continuous evaluation is indispensable. Together with a WHO guideline, an evaluation module based on the AGREE concept (Appraisal of Guidelines for Research and Evaluation) is also published. This evaluation tool, initially developed in 2003 by international researchers and guideline developers, was last updated in 2013 under the leadership of Canadian scientists and translated into German. Since 2009 it is called AGREE II and provides a framework for the quality assessment of guidelines, the methodologically sound development of guidelines, and the selection and presentation of information in guidelines.

In June 2005, the **G**erman **G**uideline **A**ppraisal **I**nstrument (DELBI) was published. It was developed on the basis of the initial AGREE in collaboration with the Association of the Scientific Medical Societies (AWMF) and the Medical Center for Quality in Medicine (ÄZQ) and replaced the checklist "Methodological Quality of Guidelines" published in the *Deutsches Ärzteblatt* in 2000. In 2008, the initial seven DELBI domains were expanded by domain 8 "Methodological accuracy of guideline development when using existing guidelines". The long version can be viewed at www.guidelines.de/guidelines-basics/guidelines-evaluation/delbi.

Criteria of guideline quality according to AGREE II (Update: September 2013)

1. Scope and Purpose
2. Involvement of interest groups
3. Accuracy of guideline development
4. Clarity of presentation
5. Applicability
6. Editorial independence
7. Overall assessment

19.4 Synopsis of Guidelines on Hypertensive Diseases in Pregnancy in the German-Speaking Area, the Central African Country of Cameroon, and the WHO

The German-language guideline on hypertensive pregnancy diseases: Diagnosis and therapy was completely revised in 2019 as part of the guideline collaboration of the DGGG, OEGGG and SGGG, which has existed since 2015, and published as a 2Sk guideline by the AWMF. This guideline covers all topics in this area that are dealt with by the WHO in three different guidelines: drug therapy for non-severe hypertension in pregnancy (WHO 2020), drug therapy for severe hypertension in pregnancy (WHO 2018a, b) and prevention and treatment of preeclampsia and eclampsia (WHO 2011). The guideline of the Central African French-speaking country Cameroon, like the AWMF, summarizes the three areas in one guideline under the title Preeclampsia and Eclampsia.

All three guidelines share the detailed presentation of the various hypertensive disease patterns and the precise definition of the respective diagnoses.

The WHO guideline Prevention and Treatment of Preeclampsia and Eclampsia includes a tabular overview of its 23 recommendations. In this table, each of these recommendations receives a classification of the quality of the evidence on which it is based, into the four categories: very low, low, moderate, and high, as well as an assessment according to GRADE into weak and strong recommendation.

The two WHO guidelines on the subject of drug therapy for non-severe and severe hypertension in pregnancy summarize their respective two recommendations also in tabular form and provide them with a strength of recommendation and assessment of the safety of the evidence supplemented by a detailed justification of the classification. Both recommendations for drug therapy of non-severe hypertension in pregnancy receive the recommendation to assess the implementation of a possible oral antihypertensive therapy only in the country context. The two recommendations for drug therapy of severe pregnancy-related hypertension are both based on very low evidence. The recommendation to treat severe hypertension is strong, the recommendation on the method, whether oral or i.v., should be decided country-specifically depending on available resources.

In the diagnostic and therapeutic recommendations, the guidelines largely agree on diagnostics, assessment of the anamnestic and clinical risk factors for preeclampsia and the indicated antihypertensive and anticonvulsive therapy. The AWMF guideline also includes a recommendation on the sFlt-1/PIGF ratio: While it advises against its use in general screening, the determination of angiogenic factors can be used to secure and exclude the diagnosis of preeclampsia. The overview from Cameroon also includes the note that the recommendation for hospital admission is observed depending on the patient's financial capabilities. The following Fig. 19.1 shows the standard for diagnosis and therapy of preeclampsia in Cameroon.

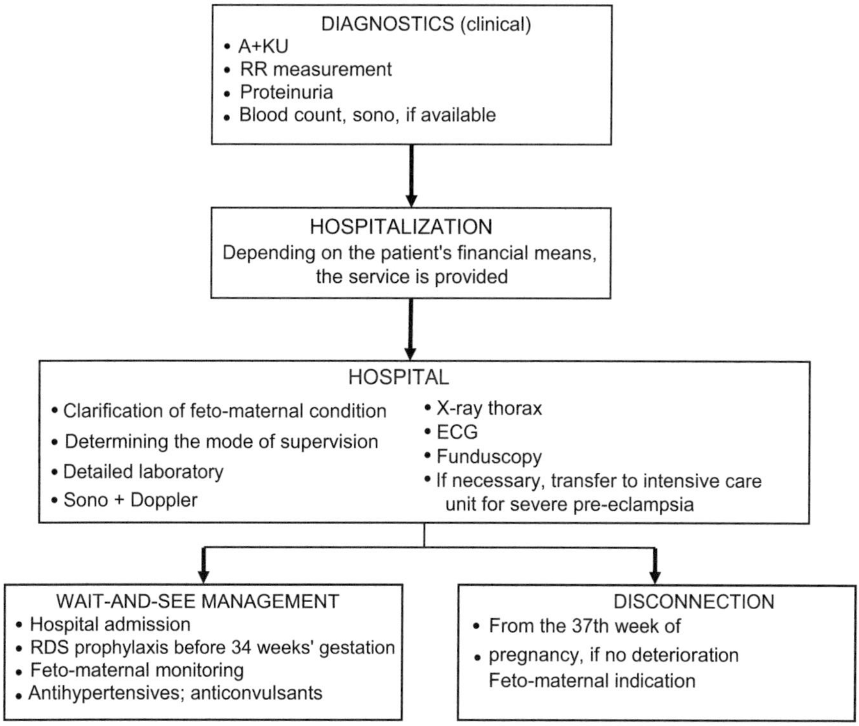

Fig. 19.1 Standard for diagnosis and therapy of preeclampsia in Cameroon

19.5 Summary

Essential for the creation of guidelines for poor and rich countries is to develop them systematically and transparently and to include the respective target groups of the guideline, whether they are patients, clinicians, non-governmental organizations and all groups relevant for implementation, from the outset.

Once the guideline has been developed taking into account the respective target group—worldwide, regionally or country-specific—quality assurance includes accompanying the distribution and implementation with continuous evaluation and reviewing the current evidence at previously defined intervals and updating the guideline.

19.6 Resources—Useful Web Links

The following Table 19.4 lists useful web links.

Table 19.4 Useful Web Links

Association of the Scientific Medical Societies (AWMF)	www.awmf.org/leitlinien
German Society for Gynecology and Obstetrics (DGGG)	www.dggg.de
Swiss Society for Gynecology and Obstetrics (SGGG)	www.sggg.ch
Scottish Intercollegiate Guidelines Network (SIGN)	https://www.sign.ac.uk
Grading of Recommendations Assessment, Development and Evaluation (GRADE)	https://www.gradeworkinggroup.org
Confidence in the Evidence from Reviews of Qualitative research (CERQual)	www.cerqual.org
Appraisal of Guidelines for Research and Evaluation in Europe (AGREE II)	www.agreetrust.org
German Guideline Evaluation Instrument (DELBI)	www.leitlinien.de/leitlinien-grundlagen/leitlinienbewertung/delbi
Guidelines International Network	https://g-i-n.net
WHO handbook for guideline development	https://www.who.int/publications/i/item/9789241548960
Institutional Repository for Information Sharing (WHO) (iris)	https://apps.who.int/iris
National Comprehensive Cancer Network (NCCN)	https://www.nccn.org/guidelines/guidelines-process/development-and-update-of-guidelines
Guideline-driven, Research priorities, Evidence synthesis, Application of evidence, and Transfer of Knowledge (GREAT network)	https://greatnetworkglobal.org

Answers to the Initial Questions

1. C is correct
2. A, B and C are correct
3. A and C are correct

References

Alonso-Coello P, Schünemann HJ, Moberg J, Brignardello-Petersen R, Akl EA, Davoli M et al (2016) GRADE Evidence to Decision (EtD) frameworks: a systematic and transparent approach to making well informed healthcare choices. 1: Introduction. BMJ 353:i2016

Anderson BO (2020) NCCN harmonized guidelines for sub-saharan Africa: a collaborative methodology for translating resource-adapted guidelines into actionable in-country cancer control plans. JCO Glob Oncol 6(2020):1419–1421

Atkins D, Briss PA, Eccles M et al (2005) Systems for grading the quality of evidence and the strength of recommendations II: pilot study of a new system. BMC Health Serv Res 5(1):25

Carlson RW, Scavone JL, Koh WJ et al (2016) NCCN framework for resource stratification: a framework for providing and improving global quality oncology care. J Natl Compr Canc Netw 14:961–969

Desch CE, Benson AB III, Smith TJ et al (1999) Recommended colorectal cancer surveillance guidelines by the American Society of Clinical Oncology. J Clin Oncol 17(4):1312

Field M, Lohr K (1992) Clinical practice guidelines: directions for a new program; Committee to Advise the Public Health Service on Clinical Practice Guidelines, Institute of Medicine. National Academies Press (US), Washington, DC. ISBN: 0-309-56001-2

Guyatt G, Oxman A, Akl E, Kunz R, Vist G, Brozek J, Norris S, Falck-Ytter Y, Glasziou P, deBeer H, Jaeschke R, Rind D, Meerpohl J, Dahm P, Schünemann H (2011) GRADE guidelines: 1. Introduction – GRADE evidence profiles and summary of findings tables. J Clin Epidemiol 64(4):383–394

Guyatt GH, Oxman AD, Vist GE et al (2008) GRADE: an emerging consensus on rating quality of evidence and strength of recommendations. BMJ 336(7650):924–926

Hypertensive Pregnancy Disorders: Diagnosis and Therapy. Guideline of the German Society of Gynecology and Obstetrics (S2k-Level, AWMF-Registry No. 015/018, March 2019). http://www.awmf.org/leitlinien/detail/II/015-018.html

Koop I (2010) Konsensusfindung in evidenzbasierten Leitlinien – vom Mythos zur rationalen Strategie. Z Ärztl Fortbild Qual Gesundheitswesen (ZaeFQ) 101(2007):89–95

Lewin S, Glenton C, Munthe-Kaas H et al (2015) Using qualitative evidence in decision making for health and social interventions: an approach to assess confidence in findings from qualitative evidence syntheses (GRADE-CERQual). PLoS Med 12(10):e1001895

MacDonald D, Grant A, Sheridan-Pereira M, Boylan P, Chalmers I (1985) The Dublin randomized controlled trial of intrapartum fetal heart rate monitoring. Am J Obstet Gynecol 152(5):524–539

McCormick KA, Fleming B (1992) Clinical practice guidelines. The Agency for Health Care Policy and Research fosters the development of evidence-based guidelines. Health Prog 73(10):30–34

Muche-Borowski C, Kopp I (2015) Medizinische und rechtliche Verbindlichkeit von Leitlinien. Z Herz- Thorax- Gefäßchirurgie 29:116–120

Mutebi M, Koh WJ, Carlson R (2020) Toward optimization of cancer care in sub-Saharan Africa: Development of National Comprehensive Cancer Network harmonized guidelines for sub-Saharan Africa. JCO Glob Oncol 6(2020):1412–1418

National Comprehensive Cancer Network (NCCN): NCCN Harmonized Guidelines for Sub-Saharan Africa. https://www.nccn.org/harmonized/default.aspx

National Comprehensive Cancer Network (NCCN): NCCN Framework for Resource Stratification of NCCN Guidelines. https://www.nccn.org/framework/default.aspx. Zugegriffen: 18. Mai 2022

Nothacker M, Muche-Borowski C, Kopp I (2014) 20 Jahre ärztliche Leitlinien in Deutschland – was haben sie bewirkt? Z Evid Fortbild Qual Gesundh wesen (ZEFQ) 108:550–559

World Health Organization (2011) WHO recommendations for prevention and treatment of pre-eclampsia and eclampsia. World Health Organization. https://apps.who.int/iris/handle/10665/44703

World Health Organization (2018a) WHO recommendations: intrapartum care for a positive childbirth experience. World Health Organization. https://apps.who.int/iris/handle/10665/260178. License: CC BY-NC-SA 3.0 IGO

World Health Organization (2018b) WHO recommendations: drug treatment for severe hypertension in pregnancy. World Health Organization. https://apps.who.int/iris/handle/10665/277234. License: CC BY-NC-SA 3.0 IGO

World Health Organization (2020) WHO recommendations on drug treatment for non-severe hypertension in pregnancy. World Health Organization. https://apps.who.int/iris/handle/10665/333816. License: CC BY-NC-SA 3.0 IGO

World Health Organization. Regional Office for the Eastern Mediterranean (2006) Guidelines for management of breast cancer. https://apps.who.int/iris/handle/10665/119806

Quality Improvement and Patient Safety: Systemic Approaches and Processes

20

Michael Marx

Contents

20.1 Problem Quality

The healthcare in the 21st century is characterized by increasing complexity and specialization. The following quote expresses this development in a pointed form:

> "Medicine used to be simple, ineffective, and relatively safe—today it has become complex, effective, and dangerous" (Chantler 1999). In 2018, the Lancet Global Health Commission, a coalition of WHO, OSCE and WB, as well as the US National Academies of Sciences, Engineering and Medicine, urgently appealed in three groundbreaking reports

M. Marx (✉)
Heidelberger Institut für Global Health, Universitätsklinikum Heidelberg, Heidelberg, Germany
e-mail: michael.marx@uni-heidelberg.de

J. Wacker et al. (eds.), *Global Women's Health*,
https://doi.org/10.1007/978-3-662-69700-9_20

> to improve the **quality** of care in health systems of poor and rich countries, to avoid adverse events and harm to patients, and to ensure universal **healthcare** in all countries, especially in low and middle-income countries (Braithwaite et al. 2020).

Despite various approaches and models for quality improvement, mortality and morbidity rates have not decreased accordingly (Das 2011), even though the use of healthcare in some low and middle-income countries (LMIC) has increased (Makinen et al. 2000; Banerjee et al. 2004). This discrepancy could be due to the low quality of care in both the public and private sectors (Berendes et al. 2011). Globally, there are large and often unexplained differences in quality assessment between hospitals, facilities, and providers (Marx et al. 2018).

The Lancet Global Health Commission defines the various determinants of good quality care as follows: … "*the foundations of high-quality health systems include the population and their health needs and expectations, governance of the health sector and partnerships across sectors, platforms for care delivery, workforce numbers and skills, tools and resources, from medicines to data. In addition to strong foundations, health systems need to develop the capacity to measure and use data to learn*" (Kruk et al. 2018).

In this statement, we also see fundamental elements and characteristics of a health system, the so-called *building blocs* of the WHO, represented: human resources, patients with their needs and expectations, leadership (*governance*), infrastructure and tools, resources such as medicines, but also processes, information, and data.

Quality in medical care is therefore a cross-cutting concept that transcends sectors and the classic silo thinking, but also professional boundaries.

Today, we also speak—in analogy to the model of Donabedian[1]—of structure, process, and outcome quality as frequently used categories or dimensions of quality. In addition to structural quality in the area of basic technical equipment and maintenance, standards, such as guidelines, and processes play a paramount role for the quality of care, both in **LMIC** and in high-income countries (HIC). We also speak here of process quality of clinical work. Outcome quality is reflected in corresponding outcome and impact indicators, such as facility-related treatment data, morbidity, and mortality data.

When looking at the situation worldwide, alarming numbers are still being reported from hospitals, not only in LMICs, but also in HICs:

- Of 421 million annual hospital stays worldwide, approximately 42.7 million lead to undesirable outcomes, resulting in a loss of 23 million "disability

[1] "The quality development in healthcare is closely associated with the name Avedis Donabedian (* 1919; † 2000). In 1966, he introduced the concept of quality into the fields of medicine and nursing for the first time with a publication on the quality assessment of medical performance. He presents the necessary distinction between structure, process, and outcome quality as central dimensions of quality in healthcare." (Wikipedia, 25.03.2022).

adjusted-life years" (DALYs). 2/3 of these are attributable to low- and middle-income countries (Jha et al. 2013).
- The results of a WHO "systematic review" of 900 studies between 1990–2009 show that only 40% of patients in public health facilities and only 6–19% of patients in private facilities were treated according to standard guidelines (Holloway et al. 2013).
- In Germany, 5–10% of all hospital patients experience an undesirable event; half of these events could have been avoided.
- 0.1% of all hospital patients die as a result of a preventable undesirable event = 17,000–18,000 people/year (with 17–18 million hospital treatments per year) (APS (Action Alliance for Patient Safety) 2016).
- In a survey of the population, however, the risk is perceived as much higher (up to 30%) of being harmed during hospital treatment (Europe-wide 2009).

The main causes of these undesirable events are medication errors, nosocomial infections, diagnostic errors, and patient accidents (e.g., falls) (APS (Action Alliance for Patient Safety) 2016).

The most tangible way to derive current requirements for **quality of care** is from problems that are almost ubiquitously observed and not limited to resource-poor health systems:

- Not all patients receive the recommended (evidence-based) care.
- Not all patients have access to adequate medical care.
- The implementation of evidence-based guidelines is slow.
- A number of diagnostic tests or prescribed medications are not evidence-based, unnecessary, or potentially harmful.
- Patients can be harmed by undesirable events (medication errors, complications, infections, etc.).
- There are large, sometimes unexplained differences in quality and safety between hospitals, facilities, and providers of health services.
- We are experiencing a global demographic change with a significant increase in chronic diseases and multimorbidity. This will place enormous demands on medical care in the future.
- To meet the personnel needs for this, 40–50 million new health professionals will need to be trained and deployed over the next twenty years.

20.2 Dimensions of Quality in Care

Due to its complexity, improving the quality of care requires system-wide measures. But where is the evidence that our approaches and methods work, are effective and efficient? For this, scientifically based, e.g., indicator-based measurement models are needed, not only to ensure quality standards, but also to make them comparable. This is demanded for all **dimensions of quality**, i.e., for structure, process, and outcome quality.

In the past, quality in the German health system was often seen as a bothersome exercise under the term quality management (QM), almost synonymous with bloated bureaucracy in clinical everyday life without any real effect on the quality of care. Quality improvement in medical care is now widely recognized as a concept, even by the most skeptical and hesitant physicians. Methods and tools for quality improvement or procedures to objectively measure them are legally anchored in Germany. Guidelines for both outpatient and inpatient care have been issued by the legislator.

A number of accredited procedures are approved. Examples include: for the inpatient sector: KTQ (Cooperation for Transparency and Quality in Healthcare); DIN ISO 9001:2015 incl. derivatives; in the outpatient sector: EPA (European Practice Assessment); QEP (Quality and Development in Practices); EFQM (European Foundation for Quality Management).

In LMICs, different models and procedures are now also being used, partly introduced and propagated by development cooperation organizations. Due to the sometimes confusing multitude of different instruments and measurement methods, the objectification and comparability of the data is often not possible. Overall, there is a lack of scientific evidence in the measurement of quality, with a few exceptions.

The problems listed above, as far as they concern the political level, may still be too abstract, not really connected with the daily reality of patients and healthcare staff. At the heart of quality assurance is the well-being of patients. Here, the principle of avoiding risks and not causing harm to patients is paramount. Under the term **patient safety**, a multitude of quality standards are summarized, which should have the highest priority for a **patient-centered care** in all countries.

Two case studies, one from the German health system and one from a hospital in Tanzania, are intended to illustrate the relationship between quality of care and patient safety and the complexity of quality improvement.

Case Study 1 (Germany)

In 2013, the following case was heard before a German regional court: A medical student, who was doing his practical year in a public hospital, injected an infant with an antibiotic for oral administration; the child suffered an anaphylactic shock and died a few hours later. The focus of media coverage was the young man's mistakes and the question of how this could have happened. The student was alone in the room with the baby's mother and was supposed to draw blood from the child. He thought he should administer the medication, even though he should not have done this alone. This was the basis for the penalty assessment.

Case Analysis: The error was facilitated by factors at various levels of the hospital: Apparently, there was no **written training manual** for medical students in their practical year regarding the activities they were allowed to perform. A nurse had filled a syringe with the **orally administered** medication, but had **not labeled** it, and placed it on the child's bed. The **equipment** also contributed to this **fatal medication error**: The **syringe**, which was supposed to be used to drip the antibiotic into the child's mouth, **fit into the perfusor**. Cases of such confusion have been known for several years from studies, especially in the USA (The Joint Commission 2006). According to media reports, the hospital introduced unmistakable syringes in the relevant department only the day after the accident. In addition, there is the position of the students: In many hospitals, they are used as health assistants, without being accompanied by a supervisor. It is **silently assumed** that they will take over activities such as taking blood samples or administering medication. The students are often **uncertain** about **what they are allowed to do independently and what they are not**.

Conclusion: Asking questions or refusing activities is often difficult for students. Singh et al. (2007) showed in data from insurers from 2007 that in almost three quarters of the cases where treatment errors were made by medical interns and trainees, errors in the assessment of the situation and lack of supervision contributed to the treatment error. The sad example shows how patient safety is endangered by the **behavior of several people**, the **organization of workflows and the design of work tools** (Gesine Hofinger 2015). ◄

The factors listed above are neither unique nor limited to this one case or one hospital. The mentioned factors—suitable connections, unlabeled syringes, no questioning of unclear orders, lack of supervision—belong to the human factors. We see that it is not just about technical solutions, but also about a cultural change.

Case Study 2 (Tanzania)

Mrs. Y., a primigravida, 28 years old, in the 37th week of pregnancy (SS), was admitted to the regional hospital at 8 pm. The vital parameters at admission were: BP 110/70 mmHg, pulse 110 per minute, respiratory rate 22 breaths per minute, fully conscious and well oriented.

The woman had been complaining of breathing difficulties for a month and chest pain for a week. Further history revealed that the woman had started antenatal care in a neighboring health center in the 18th week of pregnancy and had so far made three visits.

During the visits, it was not possible to administer iron sulfate due to clinically manifest anemia, as it had been sold out for weeks. The only hemoglobin test was performed two weeks earlier, when she was told that she was severely anemic, and she was referred to the district hospital for appropriate treatment. After consulting with the family, money was collected to enable her hospital treatment. Further examination revealed that the woman was in labor with at least two contractions every 10 minutes, which were classified as moderate, the cervix dilated 5 cm. The Hb control on the delivery ward showed a threatening anemia with an HB value of 6 g/dl; blood was taken for blood group determination and two units of whole blood were requested for transfusion, as the hospital did not have erythrocyte concentrates. The laboratory report indicated that no standby blood was available, as the refrigerator for blood storage had been out of operation for the last 3 months and no blood had been available for 3 months. The delivery ward team was instructed to wait until the next morning until the blood would be picked up from the blood donation center of the reference hospital. Labor progressed, the patient's condition continued to deteriorate. At midnight, the patient's pulse rate was 120/min, blood pressure 100/60, 28 breaths per minute, the breathing sounds described as crepitant. Lasix 40 mg i.v. was administered. The contractions were classified as strong, the cervix dilated 8 cm. An hour later, the mother gave birth to a normal vital girl weighing 2.5 kg.

Shortly after delivery, however, the woman began to bleed heavily; within half an hour, she reportedly lost almost 600 ml of blood. Oxytocin drops were administered. However, her vital signs deteriorated rapidly with pulse 140/min, BP 80/30 and 34 breaths per minute. Despite life-sustaining measures including oxygen administration, the woman died at 4 am (Irmgard Marx 2013). ◄

20.3 Error Analysis, Factors and Causal Chains

An **error analysis** of Case Study 2 revealed a **causal chain** with various **system factors** that ultimately led to this avoidable disaster: late start of SS care; no treatment of clinically manifest anemia; no iron substitution possible; delayed referral to the hospital; no functioning transfusion system there; no emergency plans available, no SOPs (Standard Operating Procedures), e.g. quick procurement of fresh blood, pool of blood donors for acute transfusion, inadequate maintenance (refrigerator not functional).

Such catastrophic events are unfortunately not uncommon in many resource-poor health systems and contribute significantly to the high maternal mortality worldwide. To break this fatal chain of errors and avoid such severe treatment consequences, corrective measures must be taken at various levels of the health system. Above all, structures and processes must be improved to achieve good and acceptable quality of results for all involved.

Errors can occur at any point in the system. Hospitals are high-risk organizations, so they should be sensitized to errors in order to establish effective corrective and preventive measures. As the case studies show, errors usually have not just one cause, but are caused by a chain of causes.

The "**Human Factor**" plays a central role here, the human factor. People have different abilities, physical characteristics and other features and limitations, which leads to differences in behavior and understanding of systems, processes and tasks. A challenge is to design tools and machines, systems, environments, processes and workplaces in such a way that people can achieve productive, safe, comfortable and effective results. As Sarah H Parker says: "We don't redesign people, but the system in which people work" (Henrickson Parker et al. 2014).

We talk about human factors involving engineering, ergonomics and psychology. All these sciences deal with the relationship between human, technical and organizational factors and aim to ensure the efficiency and safety of work systems as well as the health and well-being of the people involved. The discipline deals with uncovering and eliminating mismatches between people, the tools available to them and the systems in which they work. By eliminating these discrepancies, patient safety, efficiency, staff and patient satisfaction and technology acceptance can be improved and the need for user training can be reduced.

The human-factor approach leads to a multitude of consequences for clinical care.

However, it often remains unclear what exactly is meant by human factors. Sometimes the term is used to describe the systemic causation of errors, sometimes as a synonym for errors, sometimes as a generic term for psychological measures. Human factor experts are very pleased that since the turn of the millennium, the concepts of their sciences have increasingly influenced efforts to improve patient safety. There is even talk of a "broad recognition of the value of a human-centered system thinking in healthcare". Thus, in many case studies, human factors are cited as the cause in about 80% of **avoidable adverse events** and patient accidents.

In medicine, there seems to be a one-sided emphasis on errors and the behavior of individuals so far. Thus, human factors are often used as a substitute for the word "error". This reduces the importance of "human factors" to wrong behavior and its avoidance—a view that is perhaps typical for doctors with their focus on personal responsibility. However, reducing the "**Human Factors**" to behavioral aspects prevents the potential for system changes for more patient safety from being fully exploited (APS (Action Alliance for Patient Safety) 2016). Thus, the often lamented "name-blame-shame" culture is only superficially changed. Quote Catchpole: "*When individual people make mistakes, they should no longer be pilloried, but if the response to mistakes is more training, more education and 'more effort', then the mechanisms underlying the mistakes are hidden. If human factors are equated with errors, then the term is just a semantic substitute for 'guilt'*" (Catchpole 2013).

Patient safety is one of the central tasks for which the management of non-medical areas such as purchasing or personnel administration is also responsible. Areas of system design that include human-factor aspects are, for example, the design of devices, the design of the workplace, the design of processes, continuous professional development and, if necessary, targeted training.

20.4 What Does Patient Safety Mean in Clinical Care?

20.4.1 Definition

The essence of patient safety is to "do no harm to patients", according to the postulate of the Hippocratic Oath: "*primum non nocere.*"

However, this assumption is not supported by statistics. Due to the difficulties in measuring medical errors, the numbers, both in HIC and LMIC, only show the tip of the iceberg. Hospitals and clinics where many errors, near misses, and adverse events occur must introduce procedures, mechanisms, and regulations to ensure that patient safety standards are met.

In clinical care, the complex design of services and the increasing number of comorbidities in people with chronic diseases require **cross-team work.** Healthcare is provided in many different scenarios, from community and primary care to secondary or tertiary care. Many actors from different layers of the treatment pyramid are involved. Within a hospital, clinical teams often work in isolation, almost in silos, and the patient is seen more as a disease unit than as a person with multiple problems requiring integration. The lack of integrated care can lead to safety and quality issues.

20.4.2 Patient-Centered Care (Patient Centred Care)

An important element of patient safety is **patient-centered care**. Patient-centered care means putting the patient and their medical needs at the center and making them a partner in decision-making in all aspects of the treatment process.

Illness and hospitalization can cause anxiety in patients and their families. Therefore, there should be open communication between the patient and the treatment team about what treatment is being carried out, what consequences it will have, what medications need to be taken, etc. Only when patients receive this important information can they participate in their own care and pay attention to it, thus contributing to error prevention.

Main Issues

From the patient's perspective, the following main issues are at the forefront:

- the lack of coordinated care;
- exclusion in decision-making;
- communication problems;
- lack of medication coordination;
- delays in treatment;
- confusing and contradictory messages.

From a safety perspective, given the increasingly complex chronic diseases, the traditional way of care by a single doctor can pose a safety problem. **Multidisciplinary teams** (MDT) aim to integrate care and put the patient and their family at the center of all decisions. Core MDTs usually consist of team leaders and members who provide direct care services, e.g., nurses, dentists, pharmacists, doctors, other professionals, and case managers. The MDT aims to develop a common understanding to achieve the desired outcomes. Despite the widespread recognition of the value of person-centered thinking in healthcare, there is still a pronounced hierarchy in this area with doctors at the top of the pyramid. This can prevent staff collaboration both within a team and across teams and promotes silo thinking, which negatively affects healthcare. Often the focus still seems to be on individual behavior, as clinicians and team members act as individuals and not as integrated members of a team with a **common understanding of the treatment process.**

A good example is the care of a cancer patient, which involves numerous specialties, from the primary care team to the internist and surgeon to the radiation therapist and oncologists. They can work in different departments and hospitals. Once they are involved in the patient's care, they form the core team. However, without a formal MDT process, there is a risk of falling back into old patterns characterized by silo thinking.

Team members with very different training, experiences, backgrounds (both personal and professional), and skills can complement each other well. But regardless of whether they provide care for chronic diseases in the community or manage a cardiac arrest in the intensive care unit, it is crucial that healthcare providers work together, function as an effective MDT, and avoid harmful behaviors like the silo or halo effect[2] , where individuals can be held responsible for the team's failure.

20.4.3 Case and Error Analysis

A number of tools are available for case or **error analysis**, with the aim of capturing a common understanding in the MDT of the complexity of causal chains, in addition to error detection, and initiating corresponding corrective and preventive measures. Structured quality circles, supervision, and error reporting systems are to be mentioned here as exemplary procedures. Undesired events can be systematically recorded and evaluated using "**Critical Incident Reporting Systems**" (CIRS). This can prevent errors and their repetition and objectify quality problems.

In addition to the Ishikawa or Fishbone diagram, the ***5-Why analysis*** has proven to be a simple method. Ask your team why the problem occurs or has occurred. The question "why?" the problem occurs or has occurred sounds simple, but answering it requires thought and intelligent application. Answers should be sought that are based on facts: they must be reports about things that have actually happened—not assumptions about what might have happened. This prevents

---

[2] The halo effect is understood as the tendency to perceive factually independent or only moderately correlating properties of people or things as interconnected (Manfred Schmitt, Beauty and Talent: Studies on the Disappearance of the Halo Effect, Journal of Experimental and Applied Psychology 1992, 475–492, 493).

the "5-Whys" from becoming a purely deductive thought process that produces a large number of possible causes and sometimes creates even more confusion when pursuing hypothetical problems. Figure 20.1 illustrates the step-by-step approach.

20.4.4 Risk Assessment

For acute **risk assessment**, algorithms and so-called *"Red-Flags-Matrices"* are increasingly being used. "Numerous symptoms in emergency medicine are referred to as ***"Red Flags"***. *"Red Flags"* are understood to be warning or alarm signs and symptoms that indicate an underlying treatable acute disease before it is fully developed. Therefore, recognizing the "Red Flags" is of great importance in the field of emergency medicine, as a timely correct interpretation and initiation of therapy can positively influence the course of the disease" (Koppenberg et al. 2019).

The transfer of risks into a *Red-Flag-Matrix* is intended to visualize the urgency of the need for action through the four defined color areas red—orange—yellow—green.

The numbers in the individual risk fields result from the multiplication of the coordinates of the estimated probability of occurrence and the assumed impact (Patient Safety in Resource Poor Settings n.d.).

20.4.5 "Hotspots" in the Hospital

There are typical **critical points, so-called "hotspots,"** for patient safety in the hospital.

These can be assumed to be universally relevant for all hospitals worldwide (Table 20.1).

20.4.6 Correction and Prevention Measures

Measures should be selected, implemented, and evaluated based on a recognizable cause-effect relationship. In the safety research of work and organizational psychology and ***Human Engineering***, it has been found that there is a certain hierarchy in the **effectiveness of measures** that are implemented to make processes safer. Some measures have a stronger influence on patient safety than others. The stronger the effect of a measure, the less it depends on the individual person carrying out the process. It is also important that the activity or process can only be carried out in a certain way, e.g., with device connections: If there is only one suitable connection for a specific device, an incompatible connection to another device cannot be established, which limits the possibility of human error (National Patient Safety Foundation 2016).

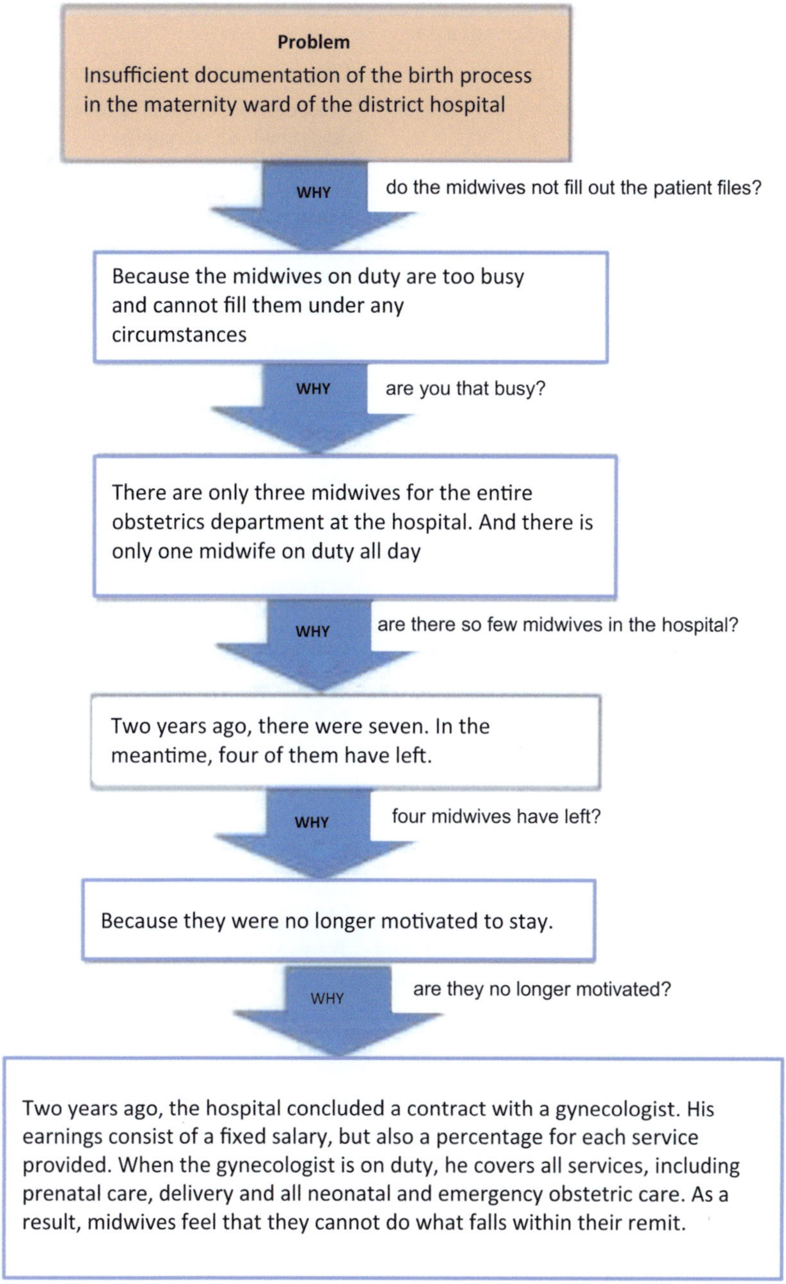

Fig. 20.1 Why-analysis. (Patient Safety in Resource Poor Settings n.d.)

Table 20.1 Exemplary central areas of patient safety in the hospital (so-called "*hotspots*"). (Patient Safety in Resource Poor Settings n.d.)

Central Patient Reception Area	**Pharmacy and Supply Warehouse**
• Patient orientation • Reception area • Triage of patients • Infection screening • Emergency management • Discharge of the patient and further care	• Processes for controlling the delivery of drugs and medical supplies • Ordering, storage, arrangement, and labeling of drugs and medical supplies • Dispensing of drugs and medical supplies
Intensive Care Unit	**Infection Prevention and Hospital Hygiene Management**
• Intravenous devices • Interdisciplinary care • Monitoring and care of multimorbid patients • Infection prevention	• Overall concept for infection prevention in the hospital, hygiene plan, and disinfection plans • General hygiene measures including hand hygiene and protective equipment • Ward-related sterilization procedures • Leadership and staff competencies • Management of statistics on nosocomial infections and antibiotic therapy • Prevention and management of epidemics (Norovirus, Ebola, Covid 19)
Operating Room	**Gynecological and Obstetric Care**
• Patient handover in the OR • Standard processes, according to OR • Hygiene management in the OR	• Emergency cesarean section • Emergency care of newborns • Diagnosis and management of high-risk pregnancies • Diagnosis and management of obstetric emergencies • Management of delivery • Breastfeeding management
Ward Management	**Central Sterilization**
• Admission process or referral from another ward (e.g., intensive care unit) or central emergency room or another hospital • Documentation in the patient file • Implementation of standards in care including risk assessment and prevention • Application of SOPs • Medication management including pain management • Patient information and confidentiality • General aspects of ward management and conducting ward rounds • Communication on the ward • Continuous medical education (CME) and on-job trainings • Discharge planning (transfer to another ward, referral to another facility or discharge to home) • Transfusion management	**Waste Management**

Effectiveness of Measures (National Patient Safety Foundation 2016)

Examples of strong measures

- Technical obstacles of technical solutions (buildings, equipment, design), e.g., designing the premises for central sterilization in such a way that dirty instruments can never enter the clean zone
- Standardization of processes or equipment (as uniform design and construction of important devices and equipment as possible, e.g., perfusors, ventilators, infusion sets, blood pressure monitors, offer in the central admission area (e.g., streptococcal rapid tests) of the hospital, instead of sending the patient through the hospital to the central laboratory).
- Tangible support from the management level in establishing a safety culture

Examples of measures of medium effectiveness:

- Redundancy (independent double check, i.e., information from different sources is independently checked, e.g., by two different people, and the results are compared with each other)
- Improvement of staffing, reduction of workload, software support (warning notices)
- Reduction of distraction (reducing a distracting environment for work steps that require high concentration)
- Simulation-based training with debriefing and refreshment
- Checklists, cognitive aids that, for example, prevent important process steps from being forgotten
- Elimination of noise, look-alikes
- Reduce handovers, transmissions
- Simplified reduced handovers, e.g., written transfer from one document to the patient file
- Standardized communication tools

Examples of weaker measures:

- Dependent double check
- Audible, visible warnings
- Reminding of the application of standards and protocols
- Increased use of feedback
- Train employees (impart knowledge, improve access to information)

20.5 Conclusive Conclusions

The mentioned measures for quality improvement and patient safety can be applied in all medical care systems. A change plan adapted to the conditions of the respective country should be developed, standards defined, and concrete steps to reduce inequalities within a health system, including the redistribution of resources to areas with the greatest need, should be initiated (Braithwaite et al. 2020).

The following measures contribute to improving the quality of care and to **minimizing risks and harm** to patients:

- Introduction of a data- and indicator-supported procedure for quality improvement
- Introduce binding guidelines (SOPs)
- Establish structured quality circles taking into account MDT
- Recognize what can go wrong in care and what cannot. Develop an understanding of influencing factors.
- Set up systems for risk reduction, e.g. error reporting systems (CIRS)
- Ensure that measures are taken to prevent a recurrence
- Tangible support from the management level in establishing quality assurance and a safety culture

In the 21st century, medicine has advanced IT systems and telecommunication technologies, genetic technology, high-resolution imaging procedures, artificial intelligence, new vaccines and pharmaceuticals. This toolkit greatly expands both diagnostics and therapy options, but due to high costs, it is only available to a limited extent in LMIC. Therefore, only limited resources are available for so-called high-tech medicine in poorer countries. To work more cost-effectively and still have access to "*state-of-the-art medicine*", IT tools and telecommunication technologies, micro networks instead of large computer systems can be used as bridge technology.

In HIC, research is increasingly being conducted on care quality and patient safety. However, for the transition from poor quality to high quality health systems, reliable data and a corresponding focus of implementation research are urgently needed.

References

APS (Aktionsbündnis Patientensicherheit) (2016). https://www.aps-ev.de/wp-content/uploads/2016/10/Agenda_2008. 15.06.2019

Banerjee A, Deaton A, Duflo E (2004) Health care delivery in rural Rajasthan. Econ Polit Weekly 944–949. February 28, 2004

Berendes S, Heywood P, Oliver S, Garner P (2011) Quality of private and public ambulatory health care in low and middle income countries: systematic review of comparative studies. PLoS Med. https://doi.org/10.1371/journal.pmed.1000433

Braithwaite J et al (2020) Transformational improvement in quality care and health systems: the next decade. BMC Med 18:340. https://doi.org/10.1186/s12916-020-01739-y

Catchpole K (2013) Spreading human factors expertise in healthcare: Untangling the knots in people and systems. BMJ Qual Saf 22(10):793–797. PubMed-ID: 23592761

Chantler C (1999) The role and education of doctors in the delivery of health care. Lancet 353(9159):1178–1181

Das J (2011) The quality of medical care in low-income countries: from providers to markets. PLoS Med. https://doi.org/10.1371/journal.pmed.1000432

Europaweite (2009) Befragung zu Patientensicherheit und Qualität der Versorgung in 2009. http://ec.europa.eu/public_opinion/archives/ebs/ebs_327_en.pdf

Gesine Hofinger (2015) Human Factors im Krankenhaus- Konzepte und Konsequenzen. 2015. CLINOTEL-Journal – Interdisziplinäre Beiträge zum Krankenhaus-Management I Artikel-ID 016 I 25.11.2013

Henrickson Parker S, Flin R, McKinley A, Yule S (2014) Factors influencing surgeons' intraoperative leadership: video analysis of unanticipated events in the operating room. World J Surg 38(1):4–10

Holloway KA, Ivanovska V, Wagner AK, Vialle-Valentin C, Ross-Degnan D (2013) Have we improved use of medicines in developing and transitional countries and do we know how to? Two decades of evidence. Trop Med Int Health 18(6):656–664

Irmgard Marx (2013) Klinische Fallanalysen 3; 2013. Curtesy

Jha AK, Larizgoitia I, Audera-Lopez C, Prasopa-Plaizier N, Waters H, Bates DW (2013) The global burden of unsafe medical care: analytic modelling of observational studies. BMJ Qual Saf 22(10):809–815

Koppenberg J et al. Red Flags und Schocksymptome. Published Online: 1 Oct 2019. https://doi.org/10.1024/1661-8157/a003313

Kruk ME, Gage AD, Arsenault C, Jordan K, Leslie HH, Roder-DeWan S et al (2018) High-quality health systems in the sustainable development goals era: time for revolution. Lancet Glob Health 6:E1196–E1252

Makinen M, Waters H, Rauch M, Almagambetova N, Bitrán R, Gilson L, McIntyre D, Pannarunothai S, Prieto AL, Ubilla G (2000) Inequalities in health care use and expenditures: empirical data from eight developing countries and countries in transition. Bull World Health Organ 78(1):55–65

Marx M et al (2018) If you can't measure it- you can't change it – a longitudinal study on improving quality of care in hospitals and health centers in rural Kenya. BMC Health Serv Res 18:246. https://doi.org/10.1186/s12913-018-3052-7

National Patient Safety Foundation (2016) RCA2 – improving root cause analyses and actions to prevent harm. Version 2 http://c.ymcdn.com/sites/www.npsf.org/resource/resmgr/PDF/RCA2_v2-online-pub_010816.pdf

Patient Safety in Resource Poor Settings. Online-Trainingskurs. Heidelberg Institut für Global Health & evaplan am Universitätsklinikum Heidelberg. https://evaplan-training.org

Singh H, Thomas EJ, Petersen LA, Studdert DM (2007) Medical errors involving trainees: a study of closed mal-practice claims from 5 insurers. Arch Intern Med 167(19):2030–2036. PubMed-ID: 17954795

The Joint Commission (2006) Sentinel event alert: tubing misconnections – a persistent and potentially deadly occurrence. Quelle: http://www.jointcommission.org/assets/1/18/SEA_36.PDF. Zugegriffen am 12.09.2013

Female Genital Mutilation

21

Maryam En-Nosse and Jürgen Wacker

Contents

Introductory Questions

1. Where does FGM occur?
   A. Only in Africa
   B. Only in Asia
   C. FGM does not occur in Europe
   D. Worldwide

M. En-Nosse (✉)
Oberärztin Klinik für Gynäkologie und Geburtshilfe, Universitätsklinikum Gießen und Marburg, Gießen, Germany
e-mail: maryam.en-nosse@uk-gm.de

J. Wacker
ehemaliger Chefarzt der Frauenklinik Bruchsal, Bruchsal, Germany
e-mail: wacker@menschenfuerfrauen.de

J. Wacker et al. (eds.), *Global Women's Health*,
https://doi.org/10.1007/978-3-662-69700-9_21

2. What is not a health consequence of FGM?
   A. Menstrual disorders
   B. Complications during childbirth
   C. Schizophrenia
   D. Death from bleeding out
3. How many forms of FGM are there according to the WHO classification?
   A. 1
   B. 2
   C. 3
   D. 4

21.1 Definition and Use of Terms

The WHO defines Female Genital Mutilation as a partial or complete removal of the external female genitalia without any medical background (WHO 2018). In this chapter, we use the term Female Genital Mutilation (FGM) as is common in the scientific context. Context-dependent use of terms is particularly important when dealing with affected individuals to avoid stigmatization and to approach the affected individuals respectfully. The term "mutilation" should be avoided in conversation with affected women and girls, instead, the often self-used terms "Cutting" or "Excision" should be used (Plan international 2018).

21.2 Global Occurrence

FGM is a global problem. The UN and WHO cite current figures of at least 230 million affected girls and women in 32 countries worldwide. The figures are based on large-scale representative surveys. However, it is assumed that the actual number of those affected is much higher. Other sources suggest that FGM is practiced in at least 60 other countries on all continents (End FGM European Network 2020). The countries with the highest prevalence rates are in Africa and Asia: e.g., Somalia (approx. 97–99%), Gambia (approx. 75%), Indonesia (approx. 50% of those under 12) (Terre des Femmes 2021; UNICEF 2021). In Europe and countries of the global North, more and more girls and women affected by FGM are living due to global migration movements (Momoh et al. 2001; Wacker and Zerm 2020). In Germany, according to current estimates, about 80,000 affected individuals live (Terre des Femmes 2022).

It is important to note that FGM is not just an African problem. FGM is also practiced in countries not primarily associated with FGM, such as Colombia, Sri Lanka, Dagestan, and the Maldives (Plan International 2018; End FGM European Network 2020). Likewise, the respective region or ethnic affiliation in the respective country should always be considered: In Northern Iraq and Kurdistan, FGM is relatively common at 38%, but almost non-existent in the rest of the country at 1% (Fig. 21.1).

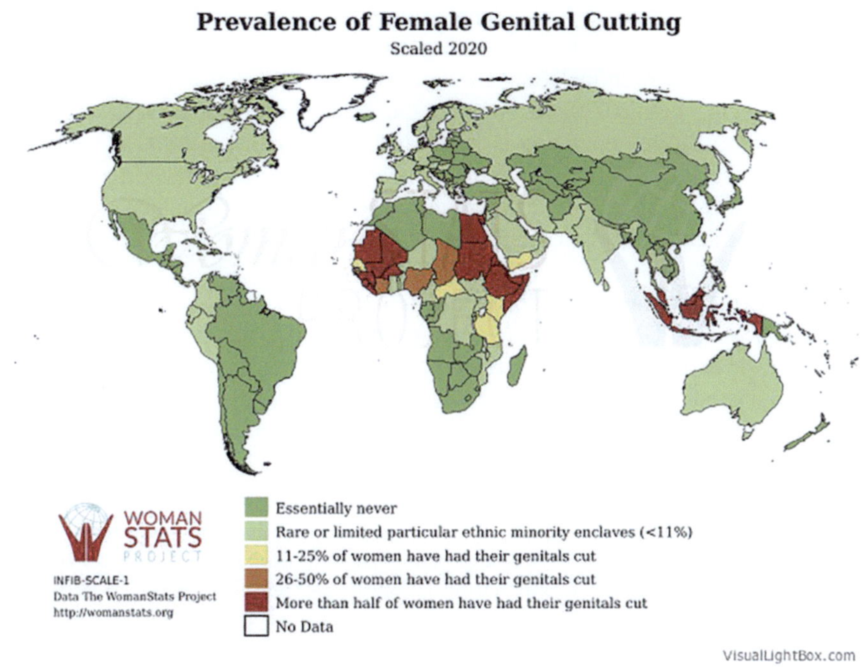

Fig. 21.1 Global distribution of FGM. *Source* The WomanStats Project 2020

21.3 Sociocultural Backgrounds

To understand the backgrounds and causes of FGM, the topic should be considered in the context of family, society, culture, and history.

There exist various explanatory patterns, and it must be emphasized that FGM is often justified by religious motives, but actually has no religious origin.

In practicing communities, FGM is a deeply rooted tradition that is embedded in a culturally shaped understanding of women, sexuality, family, and marriage (Plan International 2018).

Common myths are based on a harmful or masculinizing understanding of the clitoris. It often involves preserving the virginity before marriage and maintaining the fidelity of a married woman, as well as control through seemingly reduced sexual desire. FGM is also performed as an initiation rite and stands for purity, cleanliness, and appropriate social status in society (Plan International 2018).

FGM is performed depending on the country and region in infancy and early childhood, often also at the age of 6–8 years, but also in adolescents and adults, e.g., before marriage.

Second circumcisions also occur if the first circumcision was not "sufficient" according to cultural norms. As a rule, circumcisers have high social status.

Families are often under high social pressure to have their daughters circumcised. Depending on the culture, after an opening of the scars during childbirth (defibulation), the so-called re-infibulation, the re-closure of the vaginal opening, occurs (Von Fritschen et al. 2020). In Nigeria, the "Gishiri cut" often follows FGM during childbirth. This operation is performed by a traditional birth attendant in women with prolonged labor. The birth attendant uses a knife to make a soft tissue cut with the aim of enlarging the birth canal. The Gishiri cut is a major risk for the occurrence of genital fistulas (Ampofo et al. 1990).

Historical and geographical backgrounds

The origins of the FGM practice are unknown and little researched (Abdallah et al. 1996). However, it is assumed based on the Greek historians Herodotus and Strabo that it originated in ancient Egypt and spread from there, due to the migration of the Fulani ethnic group, to West Africa and the Arabian Peninsula (Assad 1980).

In a survey of village midwives in northern Burkina Faso, the following explanations for the performance of FGM were named: tradition, religion, facilitation of childbirth, cleanliness of the female genitalia, "rite de passage" (initiation rite) (Dehne et al. 1997). Another explanation is mentioned with remarkable agreement by women from different regions and ethnicities: Fulani, Gourmantsche, Rimaibe, Mossi. The circumcision is supposed to prevent a worm disease, which is referred to as "Bourouwel" (Dehne et al. 1997).

Much suggests a common origin of these traditional justifications. There were and are strong connections between the Fulani in Burkina Faso and Sudan and Egypt.

Various indications suggest that due to the characteristic lesions on the external female genitalia, schistosomiasis (Female Genital Schistosomiasis, FGS) must be considered as the cause of "Bourouwel" (Wacker et al. 2013). In addition to the clinical presentation, the geographical distribution of FGM and the pathogen Schistosoma haematobium and the sources on the origin of FGM also suggest this. The geographical spread of FGM and the pathogen Schistosoma haematobium, which primarily causes urogenital infections, is strikingly similar. The two small differences in the distribution of FGM and FGS can be explained by migration movements. The Bantus settled in eastern South Africa originally come from the Kalahari Desert, where neither FGS exists nor FGM is practiced. The inhabitants of Madagascar, where FGS is widespread but FGM is not practiced, have migrated from Asia (Wacker et al. 2013).

In Egypt, a high prevalence of Schistosoma-haematobium infections is already documented for antiquity. Eggs of schistosomes were found in mummies from the 20th Dynasty (1250–1000 BC). The prevalence likely increased even further when the irrigation culture along the Nile was expanded.

The connection between FGS and FGM presented here may possibly contribute to a better understanding of the origins of the practice of FGM. (Wacker et al. 2013). However, there is no clear evidence for this, and it must still be assumed that this practice has multifactorial origins.

21.4 FGM Forms: The WHO Classification

The WHO defines four different FGM types, each with subforms (Table 21.1).

WHO Type I (removal of the clitoral tip with or without prepuce) and Type II (removal of the labia with or without removal of clitoral tip/prepuce) are the most common worldwide. Type I and also Type II can sometimes be extremely difficult to recognize and are quickly overlooked if FGM is not explicitly considered (En-Nosse et al. 2022). Type III (infibulation, removal of the labia with or without removal of the clitoral tip/prepuce and almost complete closure of the genitals) occurs less frequently, at about 30% (WHO 2018). In Somalia, for example, Type III is almost exclusively practiced (Terre de Femmes 2021).

A finding cannot always be assigned to a single type. There can also be fluid transitions and mixed forms.

Figures 21.2, 21.3, 21.4 and 21.5 show examples of the respective FGM types. The photos were taken with the consent of the patients during the FGM consultation at the University Hospital Freiburg, Clinic for Gynecology and Obstetrics.

Table 21.1 WHO classification of FGM types. (En-Nosse et al. 2022)

FGM Type	Description
I	Partial or complete removal of the glans clitoridis and/or the prepuce clitoridis ("Sunna")
Ia	Removal of the prepuce clitoridis ("circumcision")
Ib	Removal of glans and prepuce clitoridis ("clitoridectomy")
II	Partial or complete removal of the glans clitoridis and/or the labia minora with or without excision of the labia majora ("excision")
IIa	Removal of the labia minora only
IIb	Partial or complete removal of the glans clitoridis and the labia minora with or without removal of the prepuce clitoridis
IIc	Partial or complete removal of the glans clitoridis, the labia minora, and the labia majora with or without removal of the prepuce clitoridis
III	Removal and apposition of the labia minora or labia majora with or without excision of the prepuce and the glans clitoridis, thereby narrowing the vaginal opening by forming a covering scar plate ("infibulation", "pharaonic circumcision")
IIIa	Apposition of the wound surfaces after removal of the labia minora
IIIb	Apposition of the wound surfaces after removal of the labia majora
IV	Not classifiable according to types I–III or all other types of injuries to the female genitals for non-medical reasons (e.g., piercing, cutting, cauterizing, burning, etc.)

Note: In "clitoridectomy", only the tip of the clitoris and possibly a part of the clitoral body (corpus clitoridis) is removed. The clitoral body/part of the clitoral body, the clitoral legs (crura clitoridis), and the erectile bodies (bulbi vestibuli) remain intact

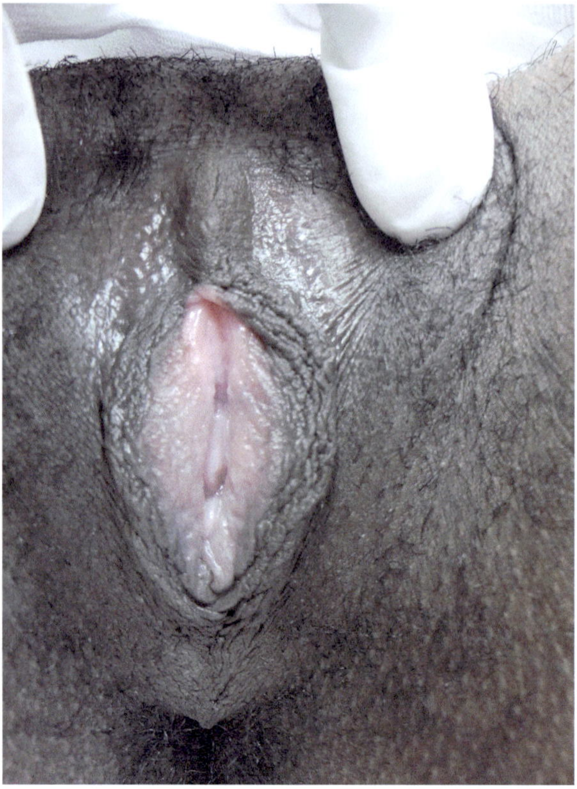

Fig. 21.2 FGM Type Ib: Excision of the clitoral tip (Glans clitoridis) and the prepuce

21.5 Health Consequences

Immediate consequences are distinguished from long-term consequences, as well as the physical and psychological effects of FGM. In addition to direct effects such as injury to neighboring organs, bleeding, and infection, there is a high mortality rate of up to 25% due to hemorrhagic shock or sepsis (WHO 2018).

The long-term consequences often cause lifelong suffering and significant impairment of quality of life.

Recurrent urinary tract infections, dysmenorrhea, dyspareunia, and chronic pain are among the most important chronic complications of FGM. In type III, the obstruction can lead to prolonged urination time, but also to accumulation of menstrual blood and recurrent urogenital infections. Inclusion cysts or neuroma formation are less common.

Obstetrically relevant is the obstruction of the birth canal due to the scar in FGM type III. In countries with inadequate obstetric care, birth complications, which are associated with increased fetomaternal morbidity and mortality, are

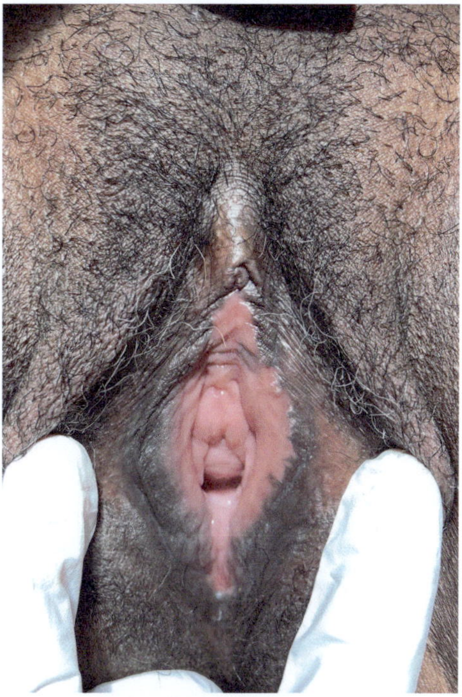

Fig. 21.3 FGM Type IIb: Bilateral Excision of the Labia minora and partial resection of the Glans clitoridis and the prepuce

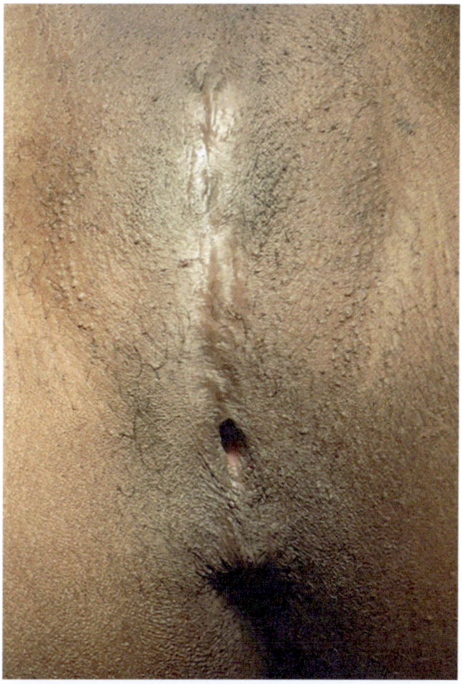

Fig. 21.4 FGM Type IIIb: Radical amputation of the external genitalia and subsequent closure (Excision of the Labia majora and minora and probably also the clitoral tip, which can be preserved under the scar in Type III). Remaining opening of approx. 5 mm

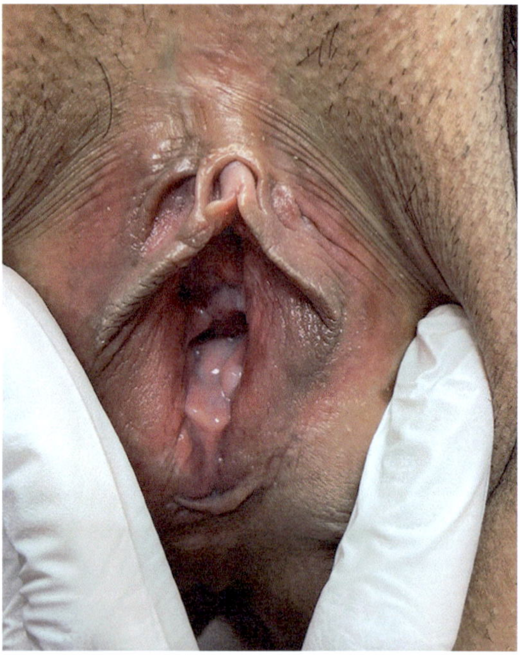

Fig. 21.5 FGM Type IV (from En-Nosse et al. 2022): Lateral scarred notch on the right and point-shaped scarred pit on the left, as well as partially resected prepuce with intact Glans clitoridis. Incision and cauterization in a Kurdish patient

therefore more common (En-Nosse et al. 2022). Fistula formations can occur due to prolonged or obstructed labour or the aforementioned Gishiri method (Ampofo et al. 1990). According to a WHO study, genital mutilations are estimated to lead to one to two perinatal deaths per 100 births, the risk increases in the case of extensive techniques (Banke et al. 2006).

The psychological effects such as trauma sequelae, post-traumatic stress disorders (PTSD), disorders of self-image, higher incidence of anxiety disorders,depression and sexual disorders must also be taken into account (Wacker and Zerm 2020)

The health consequences are summarized in Table 21.2.

21.6 Therapy Options for FGM

In general, the so-called Defibulation ("opening operation") for type III needs to be distinguished from the reconstruction of the external genitalia, which can become relevant for all FGM forms.

The goal of Defibulation is to remedy the obstructive complaints and restore normal body functions such as regular urination and menstruation, sexual intercourse, and vaginal birth. The reconstruction aims to restore the anatomy and function of the vulva, especially the sensitivity in the area of the clitoris.

Table 21.2 Consequences of FGM. (En-Nosse et al. 2022)

Direct Consequences	Extreme pain during the procedure Psychological trauma Infections/Sepsis due to unsterile tools (including HIV, Hepatitis, Tetanus) and lack of hygiene during wound healing High blood loss up to hemorrhagic shock Injury to neighboring structures (e.g., urethra, anus) Hematomas or fractures due to restraining the affected person Death
Long-term Consequences	Psychological consequences with PTSD, anxiety disorder, depression, and self-image disorder Obstetric complications, such as higher-grade birth injuries, prolonged labour, postpartum hemorrhage urogenital fistula formations Dyspareunia/Apareunia, lack of clitoral sensitivity Dysmenorrhea, prolonged menstrual duration, hematocolpos Urination problems due to infibulationsuch as prolonged urination time, dysuria, recurrent urinary tract infections, urinary retention or a deviating urinary stream, urolithiasishydronephrosis, renal insufficiency Chronic vulvovaginal pain keloids, neuromas Recurrent urogenital infections Retention cysts

The defibulation is a fundamentally simple surgical procedure that should be part of the surgical training of every gynecologist and obstetrician (En-Nosse et al. 2022). It improves, based on evidence, the fetomaternal obstetric outcome in women with FGM (WHO 2018; Raouf et al. 2011). A type III FGM is never a reason for a cesarean section! Unfortunately, cesarean sections are still performed too often due to FGM. This is usually due to the lack of knowledge of the health Professionals.

The defibulation can be performed under local, regional, or general anesthesia.

International guidelines prefer the operation to be performed under local anesthesia (RCOG 2015; WHO 2018).

A detailed explanation to the patient is very important for compliance and for avoiding re-traumatization during the procedure. The patient should be explained that the procedure will result in anatomical and physiological changes that can affect her own cultural, psychological, or emotional body image.

21.6.1 Management of FGM during Pregnancy and Childbirth

The ideal time for the defibulation (opening of the scar in type III) is before the onset of pregnancy. However, women often become pregnant with FGM type III, even when penetration is not possible.

Table 21.3 Timing of defibulation. (Advantages +, Disadvantages –)

Before a pregnancy	2nd trimester	During childbirth
++ Ideal	+ well planable + time for wound healing and adjustment to the new situation + monitoring in pregnancy and during childbirth (e.g., cervical length, Bishop score) + probably less urogenital infections in pregnancy + less frequent desire for re-infibulation	+ avoidance of the surgical procedure during pregnancy
	– low risk for the pregnancy or subjective association with pregnancy-related complications	– no assessment of the cervix in pregnancy – performed by respective service personnel and not necessarily by experts

There is no consensus among international medical societies about the optimal timing of defibulation during pregnancy (Esu et al. 2017). Defibulation is often performed during childbirth. However, there are advantages to performing it in the 2nd trimester of pregnancy, which is why this timing is often chosen in Germany and Switzerland. There is evidence that de-infibulation before childbirth avoids the desire for postpartum re-infibulation (reclosure), possibly because the changes caused by defibulation are not associated with childbirth (Abdulcadir et al. 2016a, b; Abdulcadir et al. 2018).

Since there are no evidence-based data on the optimal timing of defibulation, the patient's and her partner's wishes, as well as the expertise of the attending staff, should be included in the decision-making process. This should also be discussed with the patient early on so that an informed decision can be made. Arguments for defibulation before and during childbirth are summarized in Table 21.3.

De-infibulation should be avoided in the first trimester so that a possible spontaneous miscarriage is not associated with the operation.

The individual surgical steps for the practical implementation of the defibulation are explained below:

Practical Implementation of Defibulation (En-Nosse et al. 2022)

1. Lithotomy position, disinfection of the surgical area externally, possibly irrigation disinfection of the scar posterior wall with a bladder syringe; sterile draping.
2. In case of local anesthesia: fan-shaped infiltration of the scar.
3. Marking the median line for the incision.

4. Probing the scar plate using blunt clamp/Overholt/finger: checking for adhesions (e.g., towards the meatus urethrae) behind the scar, lifting the scar ventrally.
5. Gradual opening of the scar along the median line with scissors or scalpel until the meatus urethrae becomes visible (Fig. 21.6).
6. Placement of a single-use or permanent catheter to secure the meatus urethrae.
7. Further median opening up to approx. 1–1.5 cm cranial of the meatus urethrae. CAUTION: Do not cut too deep, risk of injuring the preserved or partially removed clitoris! In any case, the degree of opening should be determined in advance with the patient.
8. Treatment of the bilateral lateral wound surfaces with absorbable continuous intracutaneous suture (e.g., Monosyn 3.0 or 4.0) or single button sutures, e.g., with Vicryl 3.0 or Vicryl 4.0 (Fig. 21.7).
9. Depending on the situation, the bladder catheter can be removed or left in place.
10. Application of fatty ointment, fat gauze or estrogen-containing ointment to prevent adhesions.

Adequate pain therapy in the first postoperative days is obligatory. Usually, level I of the WHO analgesicladder is sufficient. By applying fatty ointment, burning pain in the wound area during urination can be reduced and re-adhesion, especially in the cranial wound area, can be avoided (Abdulcadir et al. 2018)

21.6.2 Reconstruction

The topic of clitoral and external genital reconstruction should not be forgotten in the care of FGM-affected women. This is not an option for every woman, but she should be informed about this possibility by the treating physician. Many affected women are not even aware that this option exists. However, some women specifically ask about the procedure and report a high level of psychological distress due to the mutilation and often a feeling of "incompleteness". Reports suggest that the operation can reduce psychological suffering, but it is controversially discussed whether this can also be achieved through appropriate psychotherapeutic and sexual medical care (Mohamed et al. 2020).

The data on the positive physical outcome of clitoral reconstruction is sparse, which significantly complicates informed counseling. Foldès et al. conducted the largest study to date with 2958 subjects who received clitoral reconstruction. At the 1-year follow-up, only about a third of the operated women appeared, of which 60.7% reported an improvement in clitoral sensitivity, but even 22.6% reported a deterioration in orgasmic ability (Foldès et al. 2012).

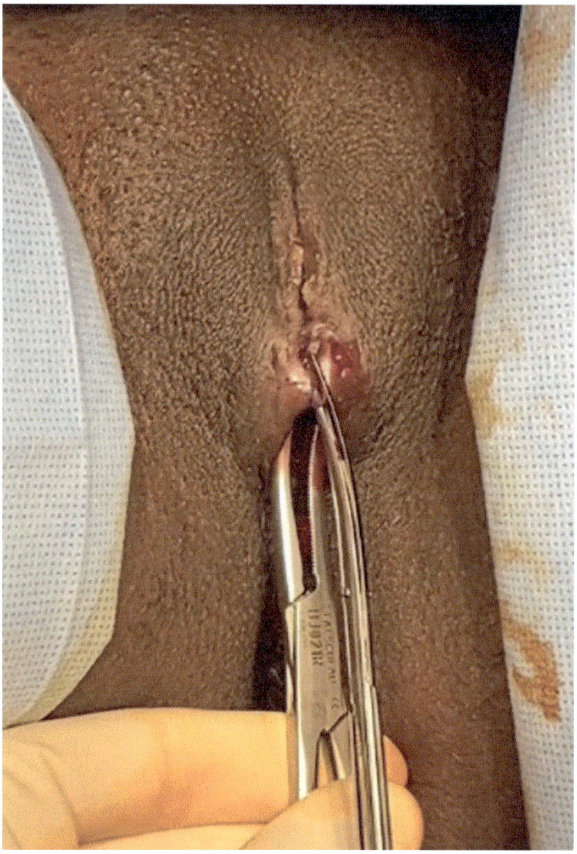

Fig. 21.6 FGM-Type IIIa, Defibulation (from En-Nosse et al. 2022). Excision of the labia minora on both sides and the clitoris, as well as closure. Gradual opening of the scar along the median line

Berg et al. conducted a systematic review of the data collected so far on clitoral reconstruction after FGM and showed a very heterogeneous data situation with insufficient comparability of individual studies and concluded that women who wish for a reconstruction should be informed about the lack of data and also the potentially negative consequences of a reconstruction (Berg et al. 2017). In addition, there are various techniques and only a few centers worldwide that perform this procedure with high expertise. The "Foldès technique" is based on a "re-exposition" of the retracted cutclitoral stump, mobilization by dissecting the Lig. Suspensorium clitoridis and refixation of the cliroral stump. This surgical technique is most commonly used worldwide and waspartially modified by other authors (Berg et al. 2017; Von Fritschen et al. 2020).

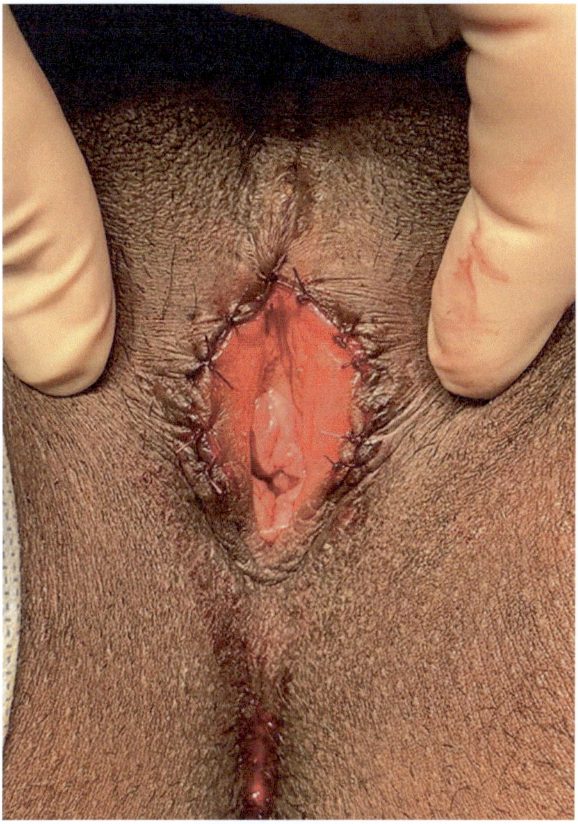

Fig. 21.7 FGM-Type IIIa, Defibulation (from En-Nosse et al. 2022). Wound closure with Vicryl 3.0 single button sutures

Another surgical technique is based on the principles of nerve microsurgery and the re-innervation of the clitoral stump by re-implantation of the Nervi clitoridis ("NMCS-Procedure", "Neurotizing and molding of the clitoral stump") (O'Dey 2019). O'Dey developed this technique after extensive studies on anatomical body donors (cadavers) and initially for the reconstruction of the genitalia after vulvectomy in vulvar carcinoma. In addition, based on the knowledge gained about angiosomes in the area of the external vulva, he developed a pedicled flap (aOAP-Flap), which allows for the reconstruction of the inner labia when there is a significant tissue loss for example, after FGM-Type IIIb (O'Dey 2019).

Long-term follow-up data are still pending, but the innovative method by O'Dey has already been integrated into German guidelines, recent data show a significant improvement in clitoral sensation and overall satisfaction after reconstruction with O'dey technique. (S2k guideline Reconstructive and Aesthetic Operations of the Female Genitalia 2022).

Further prospective and comparative studies are needed to investigate the benefits of reconstruction more precisely. In principle, women who wish for a reconstruction should be treated in a center that has sufficient experience with the procedure.

21.7 Legal Framework and Prevention

Numerous conventions and resolutions of the United Nations (UN), the European Union (EU), and Germany classify FGM as a severe violation of human rights (Plan International 2018).

FGM is considered gender-based violence. In Germany, FGM is considered serious bodily harm under § 226 StGB. In many countries, FGM type III is traditionally re-closed after birth. This is also not permissible in Germany under § 226 StGB for medical personnel and should be communicated to the patient in advance.

Internationally, many prevalence countries have already banned the practice of FGM and there are numerous campaigns by governments and non-governmental organizations against FGM. However, in Asian and Latin American countries, FGM is still not illegal, e.g., in Indonesia (End FGM European Network 2020).

In 2012, the United Nations General Assembly adopted a resolution to abolish FGM and in 2015, the 193 countries unanimously agreed on a new global goal within the Sustainable Development Goals to abolish FGM by 2030 (Sustainable Development Goal, SDG 5) (End FGM European Network 2020).

For long-term successful prevention work regarding FGM, it is essential to always involve the affected communities (Lessan e. V. 2022). In this country, interpreters or cultural mediators specialized in FGM should be involved to overcome cultural and language barriers. Also, more focus should be placed on the training of multipliers.

In Germany, the so-called "Federal Protection Letter" was recently published, which is intended to support families when traveling to their home country against the socio-familial pressure to protect their daughters from an FGM (Federal Government 2022).

Answers to the Initial Questions

1. D. Worldwide
2. C. Schizophrenia
3. D. 4

References

Abdallah Z, Dehne C, Wacker J (1996) Stellungnahme zum Problem der Beschneidung der Frau Frauenarzt 37:1460–1464
Abdulcadir J, Catania L, Hindin M et al (2016a) Female genital mutilation: a visual reference and learning tool for health care professionals. Obstet Gynecol 128(5):958–963. https://doi.org/10.1097/AOG.0000000000001686
Abdulcadir J, McLaren S, Boulvain M et al (2016b) Health education and clinical care of immigrant women with female genital mutilation/cutting who request postpartum reinfibulation. Int J Gynaecol Obstet 135:69–72. https://doi.org/10.1016/j.ijgo.2016.03.027
Abdulcadir J, Marras S, Catania L et al (2018) Defibulation: a visual reference and learning tool. The J Sex Med 15(4):601–611. https://doi.org/10.1016/j.jsxm.2018.01.010
Ampofo EK, Omotora BA, Otu T, Uchebo G (1990) Risk factors of vesico-vaginal fistulae in Maiduguri, Nigeria: a case control study. Trop Doct 20:138–139
Assad MB (1980) Female circumcision in Egypt: current research and social implications. In WHO/EMRO technical Publications 229
Banke et al (2006) Female genital mutilation and obstetric outcome: WHO collaborative prospective study in six African countries. WHO study group on female genital mutilation and obstetric outcome. The Lancet. https://doi.org/10.1016/S0140-6736(06)68805-3
Berg R, Taraldsen S, Said M et al (2017) The effectiveness of surgical interventions for women with FGM/C: a systematic review. BJOG 125(3):278–287. https://doi.org/10.1111/1471-0528.14839
Bundesregierung 2022 Schutzbrief gegen weibliche Genitalverstümmelung. https://www.bmfsfj.de/resource/blob/179278/5f99211073d955cc2202b1fb50f8de91/schutzbrief-gegen-weibliche-genitalverstuemmelung-deutsch-data.pdf. Zugegriffen: 16. Jan. 2022
Dehne KL, Wacker J, Nadembega J, Ira R (1997) Female genital mutilation in the north of Burkina Faso. Curare 20:221–242
End FGM European Network. Female Genital Mutilation/Cutting: a call for a global response (2020). https://www.endfgm.eu/editor/files/2020/03/Gloabl-Report-FGM_PR.pdf. Zugegriffen: 27. Apr. 2022
En-Nosse M, Runge I, von Saldern C, Mürdter E, Schmidt NC (2022) Female Genital Mutilation in Deutschland – erkennen und behandeln in der gynäkologischen Praxis und Klinik. VNR: 2760512022161722964. https://doi.org/10.1055/a-1631-3677, Frauenheilkunde up2date 2022; 16(4):305–326. ISSN 1439-3719 © 2022 Thieme
Esu E, Udo A, Okusanya B et al (2017) Antepartumorintrapartum deinfibulation for childbirth in women with type III female genital mutilation: a systematic review and meta-analysis. Int J Gynaecol Obstet 136(Suppl. 1):21–29. https://doi.org/10.1002/ijgo.12055
Europäisches Netzwerk zur Prävention von weiblicher Genitalverstümmelung. Wie sprechen wir über das Thema weibliche Genitalverstümmelung (2016). https://www.endfgm.eu/content/documents/EFG-004-16-position-paper_DE_FINAL_TDF_.pdf. Zugegriffen: 18. Dez. 2021
Female Genital Mutilation and its Management (2015) RCOG Greentop Guideline No. 53, 10.07.2015, Royal College of Obstetricians and Gynaecologists
Foldès P, Cuzin B, Andro A (2012) Reconstructive surgery after FGM: a cohort study. The Lancet 380(9873):134–141. https://doi.org/10.1016/S0140-6736(12)60400-0
Lessan e. V. (2022). https://lessan.eu/multiplikatoren-schutzbrief. Zugegriffen: 28. Apr. 2022
Mohamed F, Wild V, Earp B et al (2020) Cliroral reconstruction after FGM/C: a review of surgical techniques and ethical debate. The J Sex Med 17(3):531–542. https://doi.org/10.1016/j.jsxm.2019.12.004
Momoh C, Ladhani S, Lochrie DP, Rymer J (2001) Female genital mutilation: analysis of the first twelve months of a Southern London specialist clinic. BJOG 108:186–191

O'Dey D (2019) Vulvar reconstruction Following Female Genital Mutilation/Cutting (FGM/C) and other acquired deformities. Springer Nature Switzerland AG 2019, Springer

Plan International (2018) Weibliche Genitalverstümmelung im Flüchtlingskontext. Herausforderungen und Handlungsempfehlungen. 2018. https://lessan.eu/wp-content/uploads/2019/06/FGM-C-im-Flüchtlingskontext-Publikation-final-.pdf. Zugegriffen: 28. Apr. 2022

Raouf SA, Ball T, Hughes A, Holder R, Papaioannou S (2011) Obstetric and neonatal outcomes for women with reversed and non- reversed type III female genital mutilation. Int J Gynecol Obstet 113(2):141–143

Royal College of Obstetricians and Gynecologists. Green Top Guideline 2015. https://www.rcog.org.uk/media/au0jn5of/gtg-53-fgm.pdf. Zugegriffen: 25. März 2023

S2k Leitlinie Rekonstruktive und asthetische Operationen des weiblichen Genitale (2022), AWMF 009/019, Version 1.1, August 2022. https://register.awmf.org/de/leitlinien/detail/009-019. Zugegriffen: 25. März 2023

Terre des Femmes (2022) Dunkelzifferstatistik zu weiblicher Genitalverstümmelung in Deutschland (2022). https://www.frauenrechte.de/images/aktuelles/2022/FGM/2022_Dunkelzifferschätzung_final.pdf. Zugegriffen: 25. März 2023

Terre des Femmes. Geschlechtsspezifische Gewalt in Herkunftsländern (2021). https://www.frauenrechte.de/informationen/dokumentationsstelle/geschlechtsspezifische-gewalt-in-herkunftslaendern/category/2-laenderberichte-zu-geschlechtsspezifischer-gewalt. Zugegriffen: 18. Dez. 2021

The Womans Stats Project. Female Genital Mutilation scaled 2020. https://www.womanstats.org/maps.html. Zugegriffen: 25. März 2023

UNICEF (2021) Percentage of girls and women aged 15–49 years who have undergone FGM (by place of residence and household wealth quintile). 2021. https://data.unicef.org/topic/child-protection/female-genital-mutilation/. Zugegriffen: 20. Jan. 2022

UNICEF (2022) Indonesia. https://data.unicef.org. Zugegriffen: 22. Aug. 2022

Von Fritschen U, Strunz C, Scherer R (Hrsg) (2020) FGM – Medizinische Beratung und Therapie genitalverstümmelter Mädchen und Frauen. De Gruyter. https://doi.org/10.1515/9783110481006

Wacker J, Zerm C (2020) Über die Bedeutung von FGM bei schwangeren Migrantinnen Geburth Frauenheilk 80:31–34

Wacker J, Zida A, Briegel J, Hüser A, Feldmeier H, Richter J (2013) „Bourouwel" – traditioneller Glaube oder medizinische Erklärung für ein grausames Ritual. Geburtsh Frauenheilk 73:299–303

World Health Organisation (2018) Care of girls and women living with Female Genital Mutilation – a clinical handbook (2018). https://www.who.int/reproductivehealth/publications/health-care-girls-women-living-with-FGM/en/. Zugegriffen: 18. Dez. 2021

Health in Migration: Influencing Factors in Women before, during and after childbirth

22

Tobias Vorburg, Melanie Marwitz and Nicole C. Schmidt

Contents

T. Vorburg
Fachbereich „Früherkennung besonderer Schutzbedarfe und psychischer Erkrankungen“, Refugio München, München, Germany
e-mail: tobias.vorburg@refugio-muenchen.de

M. Marwitz
HebaVaria g.e.V., München, Germany
e-mail: Melanie.marwitz@t-online.de

N. C. Schmidt (✉)
Fakultät für Soziale Arbeit/ Faculty of Social Work, University of Applied Science/ Katholische Stiftungshochschule München (KSH), Munich, Germany
e-mail: Nicole.Schmidt@ksh-m.de

N. C. Schmidt
Gynaecology Division, Department of Paediatrics, Gynaecology and Obstetrics, University Hospitals of Geneva, Geneva, Switzerland

J. Wacker et al. (eds.), *Global Women's Health*,
https://doi.org/10.1007/978-3-662-69700-9_22

Introductory Questions

1. What percentage of the world's population were international migrants in 2020, according to the International Organization for Migration (IOM)?
   A. Approximately 1–2%
   B. Approximately 4–5%
   C. Approximately 7–8%
   D. More than 10%
2. What is the main reason for international migration worldwide?
   A. Refugee migration
   B. Labor migration
   C. Family reunification
3. Approximately what percentage of migrants living in Germany in 2021 had a so-called migration background?
   A. Approximately 15%
   B. Approximately 20%
   C. Approximately 25%
   D. Approximately 30%

This chapter deals with international migration. The first part presents figures on migration worldwide, followed by a focus on female international migration to Germany. The last part sheds light on factors influencing the health of migrant women "around birth". The completion of the chapter coincided with the start of the Russia-Ukraine conflict (March 2022). At this point, there was hardly any reliable data available on the target group of Ukrainian refugees. However, the authors of this chapter assume that Ukrainian refugees also face many of the challenges described. Further differences of this target group will only be able to be recorded and described in detail in the course of 2022.

22.1 International Migration Worldwide

Concept of migration: Depending on the context (legal, administrative, or statistical), definitions of the terms migration, migrant woman, or migrant can vary. These different definitions often do not include the same temporal and spatial dimensions, and also differentiate in terms of the reason for migration. Temporally, various sources often distinguish long-term (>12 months) from short-term migration. In the spatial context, it is important to distinguish international from internal migration. While internal migration refers to migration within a state, international migration refers to the spatial relocation of a person's center of life across internationally recognized state borders (DESTATIS 2021a, b). Although the majority of people migrating worldwide do not cross international borders , this chapter focuses on international migration.

In 2020, according to the International Organization for Migration (IOM), 3.6% of the world's population were international migrants. The number had almost doubled compared to 1990 (from 150 million to 281 million), although the percentage of the world's population changed relatively little (from 2.9 to 3.6%) (McAuliffe and Triandafyllidou 2021). Of the international migrants, 48% were women and almost three-quarters were of working age (i.e., between 20 and 64 years). The main target regions of migration were Europe and Asia, with the main European target countries being Germany, the Russian Federation, England, France, Spain, and Italy (Mcauliffe and Triandafyllidou 2021).

The main reasons for international migration were usually work motivation and the securing of personal and/or family livelihoods. Thus, more than 40% of all international migrants worldwide were born in Asia, especially in India, China, but also in Southeast Asian countries such as Bangladesh, Pakistan, or Afghanistan. Other causes of migration were educational reasons as well as political, social, and environmental challenges or conflicts. In this context, migrants usually live with a residence permit in the country or are in the process of recognition. This situation differs from that of irregular migrants who live without a residence permit in a country whose nationality they do not possess.

22.2 International Migration in Germany

In 2020, 21.9 million people with a so-called migration background lived in Germany. According to the definition commonly used in Germany, a person has "a migration background if they themselves or at least one parent was not born with German nationality" (DESTATIS 2021a, b). Thus, about a quarter of the population in Germany had a migration background. About a third were born in Germany; two-thirds had migrated to Germany during their lifetime. More than a third of people with a migration background came from countries of the European Union (EU) and almost 30% from European countries outside the EU (such as Turkey) and the Russian Federation (DESTATIS 2021a, b).

Although migration is often discussed in the context of people with a refugee background, by the end of 2020, around1.86 million people were actually seeking protection. Thus, only about 9% of people with a migration background living in Germany (and about 2% of the total population in Germany) were registered as protection seekers. Most had a recognized protection status and more than 60% came from Syria, Afghanistan or Iraq. About a third of the protection seekers were female (DESTATIS 2021b).

This critical look at the numbers is important to clarify that people with a migration background are a very heterogeneous group. On the one hand, they may be exposed to specific health risks, but on the other hand, they may also have special health-relevant resources, such as in terms of dietary habits or rejection of substance use (Lemmens et al. 2017). Also, often younger, healthy people migrate, who may have a lower mortality rate compared to the population of the destination country (so-called "Healthy Migrant Effect") (among others, David and Razum 2019). However, it should also be noted that with increasing length of stay, the health risk due to lifestyle-related acculturation and experiences can increase (RKI 2020).

22.3 Factors Influencing the Health of Migrant Women in Germany before, during and after childbirth—A Multiprofessional Perspective

Most professionals in the field of women's health can draw on experiences on the topic of migration before, during and after childbirth. The following presents thoughts, experiences, and perspectives of the authors, who come from the fields of midwifery, social work, and medicine.

Structurally, according to the International Organization for Migration (IOM), four main areas can be identified that can positively or negatively influence the health of migrants (IOM 2019). These are influences on a) the individual health of migrants ("Migrant Health") or b) the health of the general population through migration ("Public Health"). The other two areas are effects on health through c) the national health policy of a country or d) the political response between states.

In this chapter, the focus is on the individual health of migrant women before, during and after childbirth, with overlaps particularly noticeable in the area of national health policy. The individual health of migrant women during this period is not only influenced in the "destination country", but also by the effects of migration on the individual throughout their life course (before, during, after migration or upon return) (Spallek et al. 2011). Influences in the home country (such as infectious diseases like tuberculosis, but also a fruit or vegetable-rich diet) can have positive or negative effects on health in the destination country. Similarly, the experience during migration (such as gender-specific experiences of violence in the context of forced displacement—and/or irregular migration) can influence mental or somatic health. In the destination country, individual stressors and resources, as well as differences in disease behavior, play an additional role, which should also be considered across generations (Spallek et al. 2011). The Berlin Perinatal Study was able to show in terms of these individual factors that differences in the disease or health behavior of migrant women can also have a positive effect on pregnancy compared to the population of the destination country. Among other things, it was found that migrant women with a low degree of acculturation behaved healthier in terms of cigarette consumption during pregnancy than non-migrant women (David and Razum 2019).

Looking at stress or coping resources, studies and reports also suggest that especially women in migration often face a lack of family support during pregnancy, childbirth, and the postpartum period. This can increase the risk of mental health problems. Particularly burdened are women with a refugee experience, who have a higher risk of perinatal or postpartum depression (Tobin et al. 2019; zu Sayn-Wittgenstein et al. 2019).

> ▶ **Important** A generalization of the health relationship of migrant women before, during and after childbirth should be avoided, as the health of this heterogeneous group is influenced by a complex interplay of protective and damaging factors.

In addition to these individual factors, the health of migrant women in Germany is also influenced—as described by the IOM—by areas of the health system as well as by integration and health policy. Even though Germany has an excellent health system, migrant women during pregnancy and childbirth in Germany may face differences in health care compared to the population of the destination country. Differences in health care can be shown, according to Mielck and Hemmert, among other things by differences in health insurance (or supplementary insurance), residence status, but also by differences in doctor-patient communication (Mielck and Hemmert 2016). Even though the literature is not conclusive, women in the asylum process or in irregular migration are very likely to have a higher risk for unfavorable maternal outcome parameters. Among other things, studies reported a higher maternal morbidity among asylum seekers (Gieles et al. 2019), a lower use of antenatal care during pregnancy in women without a regular migration status (David and Razum 2019; Eslier et al. 2020), a higher risk for preterm births or a low birth weight (Salmasi and Pieroni 2015). Differences in the health system are cited as one cause (Bollini et al. 2009; El-Gamal and Hanefeld 2020). In Germany, this includes, for example, restricted access to health services for asylum seekers according to § 4 and § 6 Asylum Seekers Benefits Act. Furthermore, there are further differences with regard to the health system, such as lower knowledge about existing health structures or a lower health literacy in migrants (Quenzel et al. 2016). In addition, differences in access, but also in utilization due to experiences or risks of discrimination are described (Bartig et al. 2021).

Especially women in the context of experiences of forced migration represent a particularly vulnerable group. This will be explained in the following using two case examples.

22.4 Challenges of Pregnant Women After Forced Migration

To understand the challenges of pregnant women after and to intervene if necessary, a lifeworld-oriented view and a culturally sensitive approach are required. This is exemplified below using two case examples from the author's practice. This includes both the situation of women during and after successful completion of the asylum process.

Case Example 1

Ms. M. (28 years old) fled from the Democratic Republic of Congo to escape a looming forced marriage. She was held captive and sexually abused multiple times. Even during her escape , Ms. M. repeatedly became a victim of sexualized violence and was exposed to existential threats (dependence on human traffickers, forced prostitution, homelessness, etc.). In Germany, she was found to be 10 weeks pregnant a immediately after her arrival; she was also found to be HIV-positive.. According to Ms. M.'s statements, both were consequences of one of the rapes she suffered. Ms. M. is considering an abortion and consults the social service of the initial reception facility. Due to her foreign law status, Ms. M. is not legally insured. Therefore, connecting to regular care is a particular challenge, as cost coverage by the social welfare office must first be clarified and presented. As a result, Ms. M. is repeatedly forced to provide information about the origin of her pregnancy. As her mental state has deteriorated in the meantime, she is connected to a psychosocial counseling center. Ms. M. tells the social worker that she now feels like a perpetrator herself. ◀

In Germany, there are so far hardly any reliable figures on unwanted pregnancies as a result of sexualized violence in women who are in or have completed the asylum process (Khan-Zvornicanin 2018; Ernst et al. 2017). Nevertheless, it must be assumed that women and girls are particularly exposed to gender-specific violence in their home country and during migration. This is also evident in the case example presented and professionals should assume a high number of unreported cases. Therefore, it is important to pay appropriate attention to this group of vulnerable women.

A Pregnancy associated with sexualized violence represents an extreme form of stress for the affected woman and all other parties involved in the case (Ernst et al. 2017). Therefore, gynecological care cannot be considered in isolation, as the treatment of post-traumatic symptoms also appears necessary and is of crucial importance for the further course of gynecological treatment. Ernst et al. describe in their review of the care situation for pregnant refugee women affected by violence a conflict situation in which the women find themselves to be trapped in. The fact of "non-identification with the mother role" and the opposing thought of "not wanting to kill" the child drives the women into a psychological extreme situation. This aspect also becomes visible through the described case vignette. Professionals should be aware of this. If the woman affected by violence decides to continue the pregnancy, the physical changes occurring during pregnancy (such as increase in abdominal and chest circumference) as well as gynecological vaginal examination methods represent triggers that can provoke flashbacks and re-traumatization (ibid.). In addition, the special status under foreign law complicates access to medically necessary services, discriminates against this target group and, as illustrated in the case example, can lead to additional trauma (Lammers 2015).

Therefore, a trauma-sensitive approach within gynecology and obstetrics, which is carried out in cooperation with psychosocial institutions, should be understood and established as the gold standard for successful care. With regard to the still non-existent low-threshold access options, professional associations and providers of free welfare services should show support in the sense of patient-oriented work and advocate for structural changes within the care landscape of refugee women.

▶ **Important** For professionals working with women with a refugee background, it is important to cooprtate within an interdisciplinary network,. This network of care should include specialists from the medical, psychological, social and legal fields, as well as representatives from communities as well as language and culture mediators.

Case Study 2

Ms. T. (30 years old) from Eritrea has been living in Germany since 2015. Her asylum application was accepted by the Federal Office for Migration and Refugees and a residence permit was issued. Since then, Ms. T. has been receiving benefits from the local job center. She reports that learning German is difficult for her, as she had no opportunity to attend school in her home country. A few months ago, Ms. T. gave birth and now comes to the counseling center with several letters. The job center has repeatedly demanded her to apply for child benefits as a primary service from the family fund under threat of sanctions. She feels overwhelmed with the content of the letters and does not understand why she now has to apply and what this has to do with the birth of her child. She is also mostly alone with her child, her partner works and social contacts are limited. Ms. T. describes feelings of overwhelm and helplessness. In her home country, she would have received the support of her family as a young mother. Here she feels alone, which makes her sad. When shopping at the local supermarket, she perceives derogatory looks from others. Ms. T. explains this to herself by saying that the Germans would think that she is exploiting the state, does not want to work and only has children. She feels increasingly burdened and depressed. ◄

The case example described above shows that stressors do not suddenly disappear after forced migration and recognition of protection, and social integration does not happen on its own (Schick 2019). Refugee women are particularly vulnerable during or after pregnancy, as comprehensive system knowledge is rarely given. In addition, the local host society is not free from stereotypes and racism. Above all, bureaucratic hurdles and the existing intersectionality (woman, migrant, dark-skinned, headscarf-wearing etc.)[1] with associated feelings of discrimination pose challenges for this target group.

In the case study, the client does not understand that due to statutory obligations to cooperate, an application for benefits from primary benefit providers—here the application for child benefit from the family fund—is a duty when receiving social benefits according to the German Social Code II ("Sozialgesetzbuch", SGB II, §12a) and can be reduced or even completely denied if neglected (§ 66 Abs.1 SGB I). According to the client, the existence in Eritrea is secured by the family and not by state institutions. Therefore, it seems understandable that the local system feels abstract and incomprehensible. Furthermore, the client mentions in the counseling setting that she lived in extended family-like structure in her home country, post-migration she now lives in a nuclear family.

[1] The term intersectionality refers to social categories, such as gender, ethnic background, national affiliation, not being considered in isolation, but the resulting social disadvantage being analyzed in their interaction with each other.

The system change experienced here poses a major challenge, especially for mothers, as in many countries of origin, men are responsible for economic security, while women ensure the healthy development of children through care and support. However, the stabilizing effect of the extended family-like structure is missing in the host-country , and women are left to cope with this task on their own (Abdallah-Steinkopff 2015). The resulting strain can lead to depressive symptoms, as can be seen in the case study. Stereotypes and feelings of discrimination are also described, which may result in social exclusion and isolation. These can also be found in other social structures, for example in access to the labor market. Thus, the results of the Citizen-Science project "Women's Science" (Pallmann and Ziegler 2020) provide an impressive insight into the situation of refugee women. One participant reported that a member of the staff of the employment office told her that she should not even think about studying as a veiled woman.

The described problems (bureaucracy, changed living environment, stereotypes and racisms) represent aggravating factors for pregnant refugee women or refugee women with toddlers in terms of social integration, even after positively completed asylum procedures.

> **Important** So far, little attention has been paid in research to women after successfully completing asylum procedures . Professionals should be aware of the challenges of this target group. It is also necessary to empirically capture the difficulties more precisely in order to be able to respond to them in an interdisciplinary and needs-based manner.

The presented case studies illustrate that it is crucial to consider the situation of each pregnant woman, woman in labor or woman after childbirth individually in order to understand different stress factors and coping resources. Figure 22.1

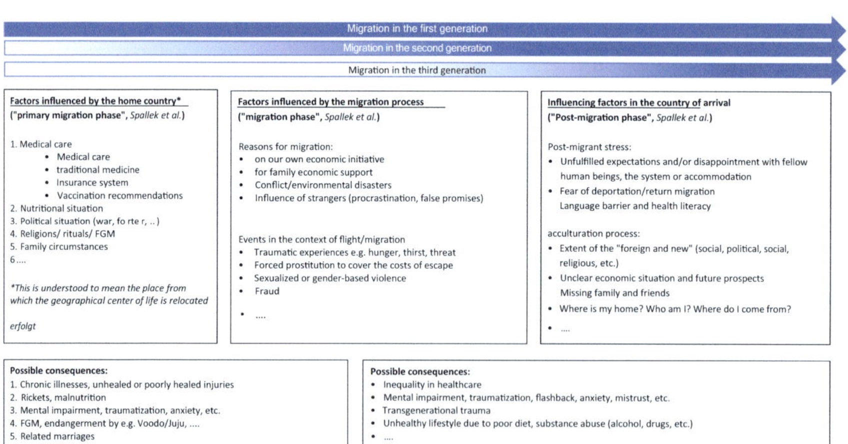

Fig. 22.1 Extended patient history to capture factors impacting on the health of migrant women. Modified according to the life course model by Spallek et al. (2011) to support midwifery care.

exemplarily presents for midwifery care which questions may additionally arise for professionals in the context of migration before, during and after childbirth. Based on the already mentioned life-cycle epidemiology according to Spallek et al., possible influencing factors in the life course are graphically presented in excerpts (Spallek et al. 2011).

22.5 Communication before, during and after childbirth

In addition to the influencing factors described so far, the importance of communication should be explicitly addressed . International studies report that language barriers lead to negative obstetric outcomes. These include, among other things, a higher risk of cesarean section deliveries, but also transfers of newborns to postnatal wards, etc. (Almeida et al. 2013; Bastola et al. 2020). However, the Berlin Perinatal Study could not confirm an increased cesarean section rate among migrants for the three hospitals in Berlin included in the study (David and Razum 2019). It was found that migrants with limited German language skills "even had a generally lower risk for both types of cesarean sections, especially for elective cesarean sections" (David et al. 2015).

How can these differences be explained? From the authors' experiences, language barriers pose a significant challenge for both pregnant women or women in the postnatal period and health care professionals. Whether existing language barriers are associated with negative effects for migrants currently depends primarily on how institutions and professionals in the health and social sectors deal with them. Since there is currently no nationwide regulated cost coverage or organization of services to overcome language barriers within regular care in Germany, dealing with language barriers depends on solution strategies at the micro level (e.g., the individual), meso level (e.g., the institution), or macro level (e.g., federal state or federal level). Especially at the individual level, so-called ad-hoc interpreters are often used. These are people who translate spontaneously because they speak both the provider's language (e.g., doctor) and the user's (patient or client) language. These interpreters can be family members or other professionals in the institution, but these people are usually not prepared for the task, have no appropriate training, and there are no standards compared to professional language mediation. As a result, the quality of medical treatment can be adversely affected, as can satisfaction with the doctor-patient communication (Wasserman et al. 2014; Boylen et al. 2020). Language barriers can cause uncertainties on both sides. Especially as to patients or clients, these sometimes lead to fears or frustration. Against the background of these problems, institutions (hospitals, social institutions in the health sector) are increasingly resorting to trained interpreters either in person, by phone, or via video-call. Institutions, such as the University Hospital Charité in Berlin, which participated in the aforementioned Berlin Perinatal Study, also offer training series on intercultural and interprofessional competence, where, among other things, dealing with language barriers or working with professional interpreters is addressed. Here, either the institutions themselves bear the costs or they sometimes cooperate with cities or municipalities (meso or macro level), which grant cost coverage upon application. Unfortunately, these support offers to overcome language barriers are not always easy to identify. For this reason, professionals in the health or social sector who work with migrants should inform themselves,

- to what extent an institution provides access to professional language mediators,
- what offers for language mediation exist at the level of the municipality or district (contact persons of the local health or social welfare offices often provide important information here),
- whether there are support offers from local mgrant organizations ,
- which recognized information platforms on the relevant subject area from other recognized organizations or structures (such as the web portal Zanzu[2] of the Federal Center for Health Education/BZgA) are available.

22.6 Summary

- Migrant women before, during and after childbirth" represent a very diverse, heterogeneous group in different life situations.
- Professionals in the health and social sector who work with migrant women should be aware of the different stress factors/post-migration stressors and coping resources and build interdisciplinary networks.
- Influencing factors on health in the critical life phase before, during and after childbirth should be individually analyzed in order to develop participatory solutions.

Answers to the initial questions

1. B. approx. 4–5% (3.6% according to McAuliffe and Triandafyllidou 2021)
2. B. Labor migration
3. C. approx. 25%

[2] Information on the Zanzu web portal of the BZgA: "The web portal zanzu.de provides simple explanations in 13 languages on the topics of body knowledge, pregnancy and birth, contraception, HIV and other sexually transmitted infections. It also explains the rights and laws in Germany. The portal is primarily aimed at multipliers (doctors, counseling centers) who work with various migrant groups. The portal can also be used by adult migrants themselves, who can find quality-assured, science-based and neutral information on a sensitive topic here." (https://shop.bzga.de/zanzu-infoflyer-nr-2-englisch-70930003/. Last accessed: 31.03.2022)

References

Abdallah-Steinkopff B (2015) Kultursensible Elternberatung bei Flüchtlingsfamilien. Zeitschrift für systemische Therapie und Beratung, 3/2015, 33. Jhg.: 109–117, Verlag modernes lernen. https://www.jfs.bs.ch/dam/jcr:74a385d8-380e-403d-b42a-f6a84e7fd832/2016-Artikel-Abdallah.pdf. Zugegriffen: 31. März 2022

Almeida LM, Caldas J, Ayres-de-Campos D, Salcedo-Barrientos D, Dias S (2013) Maternal healthcare in migrants: a systematic review. Matern Child Health J 17(8):1346–1354. Zugegriffen: 31. März 2022

Bartig S, Kalkum D, Le HM, Lewicki A (2021) Diskriminierungsrisiken und Diskriminierungsschutz im Gesundheitswesen – Wissensstand und Forschungsbedarf für die Antidiskriminierungsforschung. Im Auftrag der Antidiskriminierungsstelle des Bundes (ADS). https://www.antidiskriminierungsstelle.de/SharedDocs/downloads/DE/publikationen/Expertisen/diskrimrisiken_diskrimschutz_gesundheitswesen.html. Zugegriffen: 31. März 2022

Bastola K, Koponen P, Gissler M, Kinnunen TI (2020) Differences in caesarean delivery and neonatal outcomes among women of migrant origin in Finland: a population-based study. Paediatr Perinat Epidemiol 34(1):12–20. Zugegriffen: 31. März 2022

Bollini P, Pampallona S, Wanner P, Kupelnick B (2009) Pregnancy outcome of migrant women and integration policy: a systematic review of the international literature. Soc Sci Med 68(3):452–461. Zugegriffen: 31. März 2022

Boylen S, Cherian S, Gill FJ, Leslie GD, Wilson S (2020) Impact of professional interpreters on outcomes for hospitalized children from migrant and refugee families with limited English proficiency: a systematic review. JBI Evid Synth 18(7):1360–1388. Zugegriffen: 31. März 2022

David M, Razum O (2019) Perinataldaten besser als gedacht! Zum Einfluss von Migration und Akkulturation auf die Gesundheit schwangerer Frauen und ihrer Neugeborenen. In: Genkova P, Riecken A (Eds) Handbuch Migration und Erfolg. Springer Reference Psychologie. Springer, Wiesbaden

David M, Borde T, Brenne S, Henrich W, Breckenkamp J, Razum O (2015) Caesarean section frequency among immigrants, second- and third-generation women, and non-immigrants: prospective study in Berlin/Germany. PLoS One 10(5):e0127489. Zugegriffen: 31. März 2022

DESTATIS (2021a) Datenreport 2021. Kap. 1: Bevölkerung und Demografie. https://www.destatis.de/DE/Service/Statistik-Campus/Datenreport/Downloads/datenreport-2021-kap-1.pdf?__blob=publicationFile

DESTATIS (2021b) Pressemeldung Zahl registrierter Schutzsuchender im Jahr 2020 um 1 % gestiegen. Pressemitteilung Nr. 340 vom 14. Juli 2021. https://www.destatis.de/DE/Presse/Pressemitteilungen/2021/07/PD21_340_225.html. Zugegriffen: 28. März 2022

El-Gamal S, Hanefeld J (2020) Access to health-care policies for refugees and asylum-seekers. Int J Migr Health Soc Care 16(1):22–45. Zugegriffen: 31. März 2022

Ernst C, Wattenberg I, Hornberg C (2017) Gynäkologische Versorgungssituation und -bedarfe von gewaltbetroffenen Schwangeren und Müttern mit Fluchtgeschichte. Journal Netzwerk Frauen und Geschlechterforschung (Hrsg.) 40:42–51. Zugegriffen: 31. März 2022

Eslier M, Deneux-Tharaux C, Sauvegrain P, Schmitz T, Luton D, Mandelbrot L, Estellat C, Azria E (2020) Association between Migrant Women‘s Legal Status and Prenatal Care Utilization in the PreCARE Cohort. Int J Environ Res Public Health 17(19):7174. Zugegriffen: 31. März 2022

Gieles NC, Tankink JB, van Midde M, Düker J, van der Lans P, Wessels CM, Bloemenkamp KWM, Bonsel G, van den Akker T, Goosen S, Rijken MJ, Browne JL (2019) Maternal and perinatal outcomes of asylum seekers and undocumented migrants in Europe: a systematic review. Eur J Public Health 29(4):714–723. Zugegriffen: 31. März 2022

International Organization for Migration (IOM) (2019) World Migration Report 2020. IOM. Geneva. https://publications.iom.int/system/files/pdf/WMR_2020.pdf. Zugegriffen: 31. März 2022

Khan-Zvornicanin M. 2018 Forschung zur Schwangerschaft und Flucht. Aktuelle Befunde und Forschungslücken. Fachdialog Forschung zu Schwangerschaft und Flucht. 2018; 26. https://www.profamilia.de/fileadmin/publikationen/Fachpublikationen/Schwangerschaft/Fachdialognetz_Forschung_zu_Schwangerschaft_und_Flucht_2018.pdf. Zugegriffen: 29. März 2022

Lammers H (2015) Gesundheitsversorgung von Flüchtlingen – zur gesetzlich festgelegten Zweiklassenversorgung. Public Health Forum. 23(2):93–94. Zugegriffen: 31. März 2022

Lemmens P, Dupont H, Rossen I (2017) Migrants, asylum seekers and refugees: an overview of the literature relating to drug use and access to services. EMCDDA commissioned paper. https://www.emcdda.europa.eu/system/files/attachments/6341/EuropeanResponsesGuide2017_BackgroundPaper-Migrants-Asylum-seekers-Refugees-Drug-use.pdf. Zugegriffen: 28. März 2022

McAuliffe M, Triandafyllidou A (Hrsg.) (2021) World Migration Report 2022. International Organization for Migration (IOM). https://publications.iom.int/books/world-migration-report-2022. Zugegriffen: 31. März 2022

Mielck A, Hemmert U (Hrsg.) (2016) Soziale Ungleichheit und Gesundheit. Handbuch der Gesundheitswissenschaften. Hurrelmann/Razum. 6. ed, Chap 3, pp 493–515 (Kindle Ausgabe) Beltz Juventa

Pallman I, Ziegler J (Hrsg.) (2020) Womens Science. Situationen, Bedarfe und Visionen geflüchteter Frauen. Abrufbar unter: www.minor-kontor.de/abschlusspublikation-womens-science. Zugegriffen: 27. Febr. 2022

Quenzel G, Vogt D, Schaeffer D (2016) Unterschiede der Gesundheitskompetenz von Jugendlichen mit niedriger Bildung, Älteren und Menschen mit Migrationshintergrund [Differences in health literacy of adolescents with lower educational attainment, older people and migrants]. Gesundheitswesen 78(11):708–710. Zugegriffen: 31. März 2022

Robert Koch Institut (RKI) (2020) Gesundheitliche Lage der Frauen in Deutschland. Gesundheitsberichterstattung des Bundes. https://www.rki.de/DE/Content/Gesundheitsmonitoring/Gesundheitsberichterstattung/GBEDownloadsB/Gesundheitliche_Lage_der_Frauen_2020.html. Zugegriffen: 31. März 2022

Salmasi L, Pieroni L (2015) Immigration policy and birth weight: positive externalities in Italian law. J Health Econ 43:128–139. Zugegriffen: 31. März 2022

Schick M (2019) Posttraumatischer Stress und soziale Integration. In: Maier T, Naser M, Schick M, Schnyder U (Hrsg) Trauma – Flucht- Asyl. Ein interdisziplinäres Handbuch für Beratung, Betreuung und Behandlung. Bern, pp 93–103

Spallek J, Zeeb H, Razum O (2011) What do we have to know from migrants' past exposures to understand their health status? A life course approach. Emerg Themes Epidemiol 8(1):6. Zugegriffen: 31. März 2022

Tobin CL, Di Napoli P, Beck CT (2019) Refugee and immigrant women's experience of postpartum depression: a methasynthesis. J Transcult Nurs 29(1):84100. Zugegriffen: 31. März 2022

Wasserman M, Renfrew MR, Green AR, Lopez L, Tan-McGrory A, Brach C et al (2014) Identifying and preventing medical errors in patients with limited English proficiency: key findings and tools for the field. J Healthc Qual 36:5–16. Zugegriffen: 31. März 2022

zu Sayn-Wittgenstein F, Stelzig S, Pinkert C (2019). Schwangerschaft, Flucht und Gesundheit – Die peripartale Versorgungssituation schutzsuchender Frauen in Deutschland. Fachbeitrag IN Fachdialog Forschung zu Schwangerschaft und Flucht. pp 22–31. https://opus.hs-osnabrueck.de/frontdoor/deliver/index/docId/1499/file/Schwangerschaft_Flucht_und_Gesundheit.pdf

Glossary

J. Wacker et al. (eds.), *Global Women's Health*,
https://doi.org/10.1007/978-3-662-69700-9

English	German	French	Arabisch	Ukrainisch
Pregnancy	Schwangerschaft	Grossesse	حمل	Вагітність (wagitnist')
Pregnant woman	Schwangere	Femme enceinte	حامل	Вагітна (wagitna)
Singleton pregnancy	Einlings-schwangerschaft	Grossesse unique	الحمل المفرد	Однoплідна вагітність (odnoplidna wagitnist')
Multiple Pregnancy	Mehrlings-schwangerschaft	Grossesse multiple	حمل متعدد	Багатоплідна вагітність (bagatoplidna wagitnist')
(first day of) last menstrual (LMP)	Erster Tag der letzten Periode	Premier jour des dernières règles	اليوم الأول من آخر دورة شهرية	Перший день останньої менструації (perschuj den' ostan'oji menstruazii)
Naegele´s rule	Nägele-Regel	Formule de Naegele	صيغة نايجل	Правило Негеле (pravulo Negele)
Hegar´s sign	Hegar-Schwangerschaftszeichen	Signe de Hegar	علامة هيجار	Ознака вагітності Гегара (Oznaka wagitnosti Gegara)
Leopold´s manoeuvres	Leopold Handgriffe	Manoeuvre de Léopold	مناورة ليوبولد	Прийоми Леопольда – Левицького (prujomi Leopolda-Lewizkogo)
Gestational age in weeks	Schwangerschaftswoche	Semaine d'aménorrhée	عمر الحمل بالأسابيع	Тиждень вагітності (tyzhden' vahitnosti)
Expected date of delivery (EDD)	Errechneter Geburtstermin	Date probable de l'accouchement	التاريخ المتوقع لـولادة	Розрахована дата народження (rozrakhovana data narodzhennya)
Quickening	Erste Kindsbewegung, die die Mutter spürt	Premiers mouvements actifs	أول حركة تشعر بها الأم للطفل	Перший рух дитини, який відчуває мама (pershyy ruch dutyny, yakyj vidchuvaye mama)
Height of Fundus (HOF)	Symphysen-Fundus-Abstand (SFA)	Hauteur Uterine (HU)	ارتفاع الرحم	Висота стояння дна матки wusota stojannja) (dna matku
Womb, uterus	Gebärmutter	utérus	الرحم	Матка (matka)
Mouth of the womb, cervix	Gebärmutterhals	Col de l´ utérus	عنق الرحم	Шийка матки (schujka matku)
External os	Muttermund	Orifice cervical	فتحة عنق الرحم	Зовнішнє вічко (zownischn'e wichko)
Pelvis	Becken	Bassin	الحوض	Таз (taz)
Pelvimeter	Beckenzirkel	Pelvimetre	دائرة الحوض	Тазове коло (tazowe kolo)

Midpelvis	Beckenmitte	Milieu du Bassin, Détroit moyen	المضيق الأوسط	Малий таз (malyj taz)
Pelvic outlet	Beckenausgang	Detroit inferieur du Bassin	مضيق الحوض السفلي	Вихід з малого тазу (wuchid z malogo tazy)
Pelvic floor	Beckenboden	Plancher du Bassin	أرضية الحوض	Тазове дно (tazowe dno)
Pelvic examination	Beckenaustastung	Examen du Bassin	فحص الحوض	Обслід тазу (obslid tazy)
Birth	Geburt	Accouchement	ولادة	Пологи (pologu)
Woman about to give Birth	Gebärende, Kreißende	Femme en travail, Parturiente	امرأة على وشك الولادة	Породілля (porodilia)
Home Delivery	Hausgeburt	Accouchement à Domicile	الولادة في المنزل	Домашні пологи (domaschni pologu)
Traditional birth practices	Traditionelle Geburtspraktiken	Accouchement traditionnel	الولادة التقليدية	Традиційні пологові практики (traduzijni pologowi praktuku)
Position of Delivery	gebärhaltung	Position pendant l'accouchement	وضع أثناء الولادة	Положення породіллі (pologennya porodilli)
Supine position	Rückenlage	Position dorsale	وضع الظهري	Положення на спині (pologennya na spuni)
Midwife	Hebamme	Sage-femme	قابلة	Акушерка (akyscherka)
Obstetrician	Geburtshelfer (Arzt)	Obstétricien	طبيب توليد	Акушер генікoлог (akyscher genikolog)
Obstetric unit	Geburtshilfiche Abteilung	Maternité	قسم التوليد	Пологове відділення (pologowe widdilennya)
Cephalic presentation	Schädellage	Présentation céphalique	عرض رأسي	Головне предлежання плоду (golowne predlegyannya plody)
Facilitationg an easy delivery	Geburtserleichterung	Facilitation de l´accouchement	تسهيل الولادة	Полегшення пологів (polegschennya pologiw)
Birth at term	Termingerechte Geburt	Naissance à terme	الولادة عند الأوان	Своєчасні пологи (Swoechasni pologu)
First Phase of Labor	Eröffnungsphase	Phase de dilatation du col	مرحلة توسع عنق الرحم	Фаза відкриття (Faza widkruttya)
Uterine Contrations	Wehen	Contraction utérines (CU)	تقلصات الرحم المخاض وانقباضات الولادة	Перейми (perejmu)
Onset of Labor	Wehenbeginn	Début du travail	بداية المخاض	Початок переймів (pochatok perejmiw)
Induction of Labor	Wheneinleitung	Déclenchement di travail	تحريض المخاض	Індукція пологів (Indukzija pologiw)
Progress of Labor	Geburtsfortschritt	Progression du travail	تقدم المخاض	Прогрес пологів (progress pologiw)
Augmentation of labor	Wehen-Stimulierung	Stimulation des Contractions	تحفيز تقلصات الرحم	Стимуляція переймів (stumylyaziya perejmiw)

Monitoring of the labor progress	Geburts-überwachung	Surveillance du Travail/ de l'accouchement	مراقبة المخاض / الولادة	Моніторинг пологів (monitoring pologiw)
Vaginal Examination	Manuelle vaginale Untersuchung	Toucher vaginal	فحص المهبل	Вагінальне дослідження (waginal'ne doslidjennya)
Rupture of Membranes	Blasensprung	Ruptures des Membranes	تمزق الغشاء	Відхід навколоплідних вод (Widchid navkoloplidnuch wod)
Amniotomy	Amniotomie	Amniotomie	فتح الكيس السلوى	Амніотомія (Amniotomiya)
Full dilatation of the Cervix	Muttermund vollständig	Dilatation complete du col	اتساع كامل لعنق الرحم	Зовнішнє вічко повністю (zownischn'e wichko pownistijy)
Second phase of Labor	Austreibungsphase	Phase d´expulsion	المرحلة الثانية من المخاض	Фаза вигнання (faza wugnyannya)
Determining the Level of the presenting part	Höhenstandsmessung des Kopfes	estimation de la hauteur de la présentation	تقدير ارتفاع العرض	Вимірювання висоти голови (wumiryuvannya wusoty golovy)
Fetal head not yet engaged	Kopf ist über Beckeneingang	La tête n'est pas engagée	الرأس فوق المضيق العلوي	Голівка над входом в малий таз (goliwka nad wchodom v maluj taz)
Head is in midpelvis	Kopf ist in Beckenmitte	La descente est engagée a la partie moyenne	رأس في المضيق الأوسط	Голівка в порожнини малого тазу (goliwka w poroznuni mologo tazy)
Head has reached the pelvic outet	Kopf ist in Beckenausgang	La tête a franchi le Detroit inferieur	عبر لرأس المضيق السفلي	Голівка у виході малого тазу (goliwka y wuchodi malogo)
ischial spine	Spina ischiadicae	Epine sciatique	شَوكَةُ الإسْكِيَّة	Сіднична кістка (Sidnuchna kistka)
To bear down, push	Pressen	Pousser	يدفع	Тужся (tyjsya)
Protection of the perineum	Dammschutz	Protection du périnée	حماية العجان	Захист промежини (Sachust promejunu)
Episiotomy	Episiotomie, Dammschnitt	Episiotomie	بضع الفرج	Розріз промежини (rozris promejunu)
Rapid delivery	Rasche Geburt	Accouchement rapide	ولادة سريعة	Швидкі пологи (schwudki pologu)
Third phase of labor	Nachgeburtsperiode	Post partum immédiat	النفاس الفوري	Післяпологовий період (pislyapologowuj period)
APGAR Score	APGAR Score	Score d´APGAR	نتيجة ا بجر	Оцінка APGAR (ozinka apgar)

Resuscitation of the newborn	Reanimation des Neugeborenen	Réanimation du nouveau-né	إنعاش حديثي الولادة	Реанімація новонародженного (reanimazija nowonarodjenogo)
Eye prophylaxis	Augenprophylaxe	Prophylaxie Ophtalmique	الوقاية العينية	Профілактика очей (profilaktuka ochej)
Placenta	Plazenta, Mutterkuchen	Placenta	المشيمة	Плацента, послід (plazenta, poslid)
Umbilical cord	Nabelschnur	Cordon ombilical	الحبل السري	Пуповина (pypowuna)
Woman whohas recently given birth, Woman in childbed, puerpera	Wöchnerin	Accouchée	نفساء	Роділля, поліжниця (rodillya, poligjnutsya)
Postpartum period, the weeks following childbirth	Wochenbett	Suites de couches	بعد الولادة	Післяпологовий період (pislyapologowuj period)
Lochia	Wochenfluß, Lochien	Lochies	إِفْرَازَاتُ ٱلنِّفَاسِ	Лохії (lochij)
Breast-feeding	Stillen	Allaitement	الرضاعة الطبيعية	Грудне вигодовування
				(grydne vugodowyvannya)
Fetal monitoring	Überwachung des Feten	Surveillance du foetus	مراقبة الجنين	Спостереження за плодом (sposterejennya za plodom)
Monitoring of fetal heart beat	Überwachung der kindlichen Herztöne	Surveillance des bruits du Coeur feataux	مراقبة نبضات قلب الجنين	Моніторинг серцевих тонів немовляти (monitoring serzevuch toniv nemovlyatu)
Fetal tachycardia	Fetale Tachykardie	Tachycardie fetale	عدم انتظام دقات القلب لدى الجنين	Тахікардія плода (takhikardiya ploda)
Fetal bradycardia	Fetale Bradykardie	Bradycardie featale	بطء قلب الجنين	Брадикардія плода (bradykardiya ploda)
Asphyxia	Asphyxie	Asphyxie	الاختناق	Асфіксія (asfiksiya)
Respiratory distress syndrome	Atemnotsyndrom	Détresse respiratoire	الضائقة التنفسية	Респіраторний дистрес-синдром (respiratornyy dystres-syndrom)
Cessation of fetal heart sounds	Keine fetalen Herztöne feststellbar	Absence des bruits du cœur fœtaux	عدم وجود أصوات قلب الجنين	Тони серця плода не виявляються (tony sertsya ploda ne vyyavlyayut'sya)
Intrauterine death	Intrauteriner Fruchttod	Mort in utero	الموت في الرحم	Внутрішньоутробна загибель плода (vnutrishn'outrobna zahybel' ploda)

Stillbirth	Totgeburt	Mort-né	ولادة جنين ميت	Мертвонародженість (mertvonarodzhenist’)
Pathology of pregnancy	Pathologie in der schwangerschaft	Pathologie de la grossesse	أمراض الحمل	Патології при вагітності (patolohiyi pry vahitnosti)
Vomiting	Erbrechen	Vomissement	التقيؤ	Блювота (blyuvota)
Vomiting of pregnancy, Hyperemesis gravidarum	Schwangerschaftsbedingtes Erbrechen	Vomissements gravidiques	قيء الحمل	Блювота, пов'язана з вагітністю (blyuvota, pov'yazana z vahitnistyu)
Bleeding in early pregnancy	Blutung in der Frühschwangerschaft	Hémorragie du premier Trimestre de la grossesse	نزيف الثلث الأول من الحمل	Кровотечі на ранніх термінах вагітності (krovotechi na rannikh terminakh vahitnosti)
Threatening abortion	Drohende Frühgeburt	Menace d’accouchement prématuré	التهديد بالولادة المبكرة	Загроза передчасних пологів (zahroza peredchasnykh polohiv)
Spontaneous abortion	Fehlgeburt	Avortement spontané	اجهاض عفوى	Викидень (vykyden’)
Abortion	Fehlgeburt, Schwangerschaftsabbruch	Avortement/ interruption volontaire de Grossesse (IVG)	الإجهاض / الإنهاء الطوعي للحمل	Викидень, переривання вагітності (vykyden’, pereryvannya vagitnosti)
Curettage	Kürettage	Curetage	كشط / كحت الرحم	Кюретаж (kyuretazh)
Punture of pouch of Douglas for the diagnosis of chronic ectopic pregnancy	Douglaspunktion bei Verdacht auf Extrauterin gravidität	Ponction du Douglas pour suspicion de grossesse extra uterine	ثقب ردبة دوغلاس لاستبعاد الحمل خارج الرحم	Пункція Дугласа при підозрі на позаматкову вагітність (punktsiya Duhlasa pry pidozri na pozamatkovu vagitnist’)
Incompetency of the cervix	Zervixinsuffizienz	Insuffisance cervicale, béance cervico-isthmique	قصور عنق الرحم	Цервікальна недостатність (tservikal’na nedostatnist’)
Bleeding in the late pregnancy	Blutung in der Spätschwangerschaft	Hémorragie du deuxième Trimestre de la grossesse	نزيف الثلث الثاني	Кровотеча на пізніх термінах вагітності (krovotecha na piznikh terminakh vahitnosti)
Abruption of Placenta	Plazentalösung	Délivrance	انفصال المشيمة	Відшарування плаценти (vidsharuvannya platsenty)

Supine Hypotensive syndrome	Vena-cava Kompressionssyndrom	Syndrome de compression de la veine cave	متلازمة ضغط الوريد الأجوف	Компресійний синдром (kompressijnuj syndrom)
Pregnancy-induced Hypertension	Schwangerschaft induzierte Hypertonie	Syndrome Hypertensif de la grossesse	متلازمة ارتفاع ضغط الدم أثناء الحمل	Гіпертонія, спричинена вагітністю (hipertoniya, sprychynena vahitnist'yu)
Preeclampsia	Präeklampsie	Toxémie gravidique, prééclampsie	تسمم الحمل	Прееклампсія (preeklampsiya)
Eclampsia	Eklampsie	Eclampsie	الإرجاج تشنج	Еклампсія (eklampsiya)
Premature Labor	Vorzeitige Wehentätigkeit	Travail prématuré	مخاض مبكر	Передчасні перейми (peredchasni perejmu)
Premature ruptur of membranes	Vorzeitiger Blasensprung	Rupture prématurée des membranes/ de la poche des eaux	تمزق الأغشية المبكر / كيس الماء	Передчасний відхід навколоплідних вод (peredchasniy vidchid navkoloplidnuch wod)
Cord prolaps	Nabelschnurvorfall	Procidence du Cordon	تدلي الحبل السري	Випадання пуповини (vypadannya pupovyny)
Amnionitis	Amnioninfektions-syndrom	Infection amniotique	عدوى السائل الأمنيوسي	Синдром амніотичної інфекції (syndrom amniotychnoyi infektsiyi)
Premature Birth	Frühgeburt	Accouchement prématuré	الولادة المبكرة	Передчасні пологи (peredchasni pology)
Postterm Pregnancy	Übertragung	Dépassement de terme	الحمل بعد الأوان	Переношена вагітність (perenoshena vahitnist')
Pathology of Birth	Pathologie der Geburt	Pathologie de l´accouchement	أمراض الولادة	Патологія пологів (patologiya pologiv)
Pelvic contraction	Enges Becken	Bassin rétréci	تضيق الحوض	Вузький таз (Vuz'kyj taz)
Cephalopelvic disproportion	Kephalopelvines Mißverhältnis	Disproportion foeto-pelvienne	عدم التناسق في الحوض	Непропорційність голови плоду (ntproporzijnist' goluwu plody)
Shoulder dystocia	Schulterdystokie	Dystocie de l´épaule	عسر الولادة الكتف	Дистоція плеча (dystotsiya plecha)
Prolonged Labor	Protrahierte Geburt	Accouchement prolonge	مخاض المطول	Затяжні пологи (zatyazhni polohy)
Obstructed Labor	Geburtsstillstand	Arrêt du travail	الولادة المتعسرة	Зупинка родової діяльності (zypunka rodoviji dijal'nosti)

Labor stimulating drug	Wehenstimulierendes Mittel	Médicaments stimulants les contractions utérines	الأدوية التي تحفز تقلصات الرحم	Препарат для стимуляції переймів (preparat dlya stumylyazii perejmiv)
Fetal malpresentation	Pathologische Kindslage	Présentation vicieuse	سوء تمثيل الجنين	Патологічне положення плода (patologichne pologennya ploda)
Labor inhibiting drug	Wehenhemmendes Mittel	Médicaments tocolytiques	دواء مثبط للولادة	Препарат для послаблення перейміів (preparat dlya poslablennya perejmiv)
Sinciput presentation	Vorderhauptslage	Présentation frontale	عرض أمامي	Потиличне предлежання (potuluchne predlejannya)
Face presentation	Gesichtslage	Présentation de la face	عرض الوجه	Лицеве передлежання плода (luzeve predlegyannya plda)
Breech presentation	Beckenendlage	Présentation du siège	عرض المقعد	Тазове передлежання плода (tazove predlegyannya ploda)
Transverse lie	Querlage	Position transverse	وضع الجنين المستعرض	Поперечне передлежання плода (poperechne predlegyannya ploda)
External version	Äußere Wendung	Version par manœuvre externe	قلب من خلال عملية خارجية	Зовнішній поворот (zovnishniy povorot)
Internal podalic version	Kombinierte Wendung	Version par manœuvres mixtes	قلب بمناورات مختلطة	Наружновнутренний класичний поворот (naruzhno-vnutrennyy klasychnyy povorot)
Brandl´s ring	Brandl-Furche	Anneau de Brandl	خاتم براندل	Розрив матки в борозенці (rozryv matky v borozentsi)
Bracht´s manœuvre	Manualhilfe nach Bracht zur Entwicklung von Armen und Kopf	Manoeuvre de Bracht	مناورة براخت	Виведення голівки за Брахтом (Vuvedennya golivky za Brachtom)
Delivery of aftercoming head using the Mauriceau-Smellie-Veit manoeuvre	Entwickeln des Kopfes nach Veit-Smellie	Dégagement de la tête selon la manœuvre de Veit Smellie	خلوص الرأس وفقًا لمناورة Veit Smellie	Виведення голівки за Вейтом-Смеллі (Vuvedennya golivky za Veytom-Smelli)

Classical Arm extraction	Klassische Armlösung	Dégagement des bras	خلوص الذراع	Класичне виведення руки плода (klassuchne vuvedennya ryku ploda)
Manual extraction	Manuelle-Extraktion	Extraction manuelle	الاستخراج اليدوي	Витяг вручну (vytyah vruchnu)
Clavicular Fracture	Klavikularfraktur	Fracture de la Clavicule	كسر الترقوة	Перелом ключиці (perelom klyuchytsi)
Cephalo-haematoma	Kephalhämatom	Cepahlhematome, Bosse sero-sanglante	ورم دموي رأسي	Кефалгематома (kefalhematoma)
Forceps delivery	Entbindung durch Zange	Accouchement par Forceps	الولادات بالملقط	Пологи за допомогою щипців (pologu za dopomogojy shchyptsiw)
Vacuum Extraction	Entbindung nach vakuum	Accouchement par ventouse	الولادات بواسطة كوب شفط	Пологи за допомогою вакууму (pologu za dopomogojy wakyumy)
Caesarean section	Kaiserschnitt, Sektio	Césarienne	عملية قيصرية	Кесарів розтин (kesariv roztyn)
Pfannenstiel incision	Suprasymphysärer querschnitt	Incision transverse supra pubienne	شق عرضي فوق العانة	Розріз Пфанненштиля (rozriz Pfannenshtylya)
Placenta praevia	Placenta praevia	Placenta prævia	المشيمة المنزاحة	Передлежання плаценти (peredlezhannya platsenty)
Cervical laceration	Zervixriß	Déchirure du col de l´utérus	تمزق عنق الرحم	Розрив шийки матки (rozryv shyyky matky)
Vaginal laceration	Scheidenriß	Déchirure du vagin	تمزق المهبل	Вагінальний розрив (vahinal'nuj rozryv)
Perineal tear	Dammriß	Déchirure du périnée	تمزق في العجان	Розрив промежини (rozryv promezhyny)
Retention of Placenta	Placenta retention	Rétention placentaire	المشيمة المحتبسة	Затримка плаценти (zatrymka platsenty)
Postpartum haemorrhage	Verstärkte Blutung in der Nachgeburtsperiode	Hémorragie du postpartum	نزيف ما بعد الولادة	Підвищена кровотеча в післяпологовому періоді (pidvyshchena krovotecha v pislyapolohovomu periodi)
Hemorrhagic shock	Hämorrhagischer schock	Choc hémorragique	صدمة نزفية	Геморагічний шок (hemorahichnyy shok)
(blood) Transfusion	Bluttransfusion	Transfusion sanguine	نقل الدم	Переливання крові (perelyvannya krovi)

Foley catheter	Blasenkatheter	Sonde vesicale	مسبار المثانة	Сечовий катетер (sechovyy kateter)
Laboratory examination	Laboruntersuchungen	Examen de laboratoire	الفحص المخبري	Лабораторні дослідження (laboratorni doslidzhennya)
Urinary set	Urinuntersuchungen	Examen d´urine, Analyse d´urine	تحليل بول	Аналізи сечі (analizy sechi)
Urinary finding	Urinbefund	Resultat des analyses d´urine	نتائج تحليل البول	Результат аналізу сечі (rezyl'tat analizy sechi)
Blood grouping	Blutgruppenbestimmu ng	Groupage sanguin	فصيلة الدم	Групування крові (hrupuvannya krovi)
Bleeding time	Blutungszeit	Temps de saignement	وقت النزيف	Час кровотечі (chas krovotechi)
Fluid balance in and out	Bilanzierung von Ein- und Ausfuhr	Balance hydrique	توازن الماء	Баланс рідини всередину і назовні (balans ridyny vseredynu i nazovni)

MIX
Papier aus verantwortungsvollen Quellen
Paper from responsible sources
FSC® C105338

If you have any concerns about our products,
you can contact us on
ProductSafety@springernature.com

In case Publisher is established outside the EU,
the EU authorized representative is:
Springer Nature Customer Service Center GmbH
Europaplatz 3, 69115 Heidelberg, Germany

Printed by Libri Plureos GmbH
in Hamburg, Germany